NURSES' QUICK REFERENCE TO

Common Laboratory
& Diagnostic Tests

FIFTH EDITION

NURSES' QUICK REFERENCE TO
Common Laboratory
& Diagnostic Tests

MARSHALL BARNETT DUNNING III, BS, MS, PhD
Professor of Medicine and Physiology
Departments of Medicine and Physiology
Division of Pulmonary/Critical Care Medicine
Medical College of Wisconsin
Milwaukee, Wisconsin

Director, Pulmonary Diagnostic Laboratory
Froedtert Hospital
Milwaukee, Wisconsin

FRANCES TALASKA FISCHBACH, RN, BSN, MSN
Associate Clinical Professor of Nursing
School of Nursing
University of Wisconsin-Milwaukee
Milwaukee, Wisconsin

Associate Professor of Nursing (Retd)
School of Nursing
University of Wisconsin-Milwaukee
Milwaukee, Wisconsin

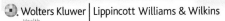

. Wolters Kluwer | Lippincott Williams & Wilkins
Health

Philadelphia • Baltimore • New York • London
Buenos Aires • Hong Kong • Sydney • Tokyo

Acquisitions Editor: Hilarie Surrena
Product Manager: Helen Kogut
Vendor Manager: Cynthia Rudy
Director of Nursing Production: Helen Ewan

Art Director, Design: Joan Wendt
Art Director, Illustration: Brett MacNaughton
Manufacturing Coordinator: Karin Duffield
Production Services: Aptara, Inc.

5th Edition

Copyright © 2011 Wolters Kluwer Health | Lippincott Williams & Wilkins

9 8 7 6 5 4 3 2 1

Printed in China

Library of Congress Cataloging-in-Publication Data

Dunning, Marshall Barnett.
    Nurses' quick reference to common laboratory & diagnostic tests / Marshall Barnett Dunning III, Frances Talaska Fischbach. – 5th ed.
        p. ; cm.
    Order of editors reversed on previous ed.
    Includes bibliographical references and index.
    ISBN 978-0-7817-9616-3 (alk. paper)
    1. Diagnosis, Laboratory—Handbooks, manuals, etc. 2. Nursing—Handbooks, manuals, etc.
I. Fischbach, Frances Talaska. II. Title. III. Title: Nurses' quick reference to common laboratory and diagnostic tests.
    [DNLM: 1. Laboratory Techniques and Procedures—Handbooks. 2. Laboratory Techniques and Procedures—Nurses' Instruction. 3. Diagnostic Tests, Routine—Handbooks. 4. Diagnostic Tests, Routine—Nurses' Instruction. 5. Nursing Diagnosis.   QY 39 D924n 2011]
    RT48.5.N88 2011
    616.07′5—dc22   2009040211

CCS1209

To my dear ones:
Kathleen, Bradley, Deanna, Kevin, and Keri
August, Colin, Trevor, and Henry
MBD

and

To my dear ones:
Jack, Michael, Mary, Paul, and Margaret
Christopher, Matthew, Joseph, and Michael Jonathan
Bennett, Samantha, Dick, Ann, Teri, and Juke
FF

Contributors, Consultants, and Research Assistants

Contributors

Tracy A. Schweitzer, RN, PhD
Clinical Assistant Professor
Course Coordinator & Instructor
Marquette University
Milwaukee, Wisconsin

Consultants and Research Assistants

Patti Cobb, RD, CD
Chief Clinical Dietitian
Food and Nutrition Services
Froedtert Hospital
Milwaukee, Wisconsin

Carol Colasacco, CT (ASCP), CMIAC
Cytotechnologist
Department of Pathology
Fletcher Allen Health Care
Burlington, Vermont

Ann Shafranski Fischbach, RN, BSN
Occupational Health, Case Manager
Johnson Controls
Milwaukee, Wisconsin

Bonnie Grahn, RN, BSN, CIC
Infection Control Coordinator
Froedtert Hospital
Milwaukee, Wisconsin

Gary Hoffman
Manager, Laboratory for Newborn Screening
State of Wisconsin
Madison, Wisconsin

Paul J. Jannetto, PhD, MT (ASCP)
Assistant Professor, Pathology
Director, Clinical Chemistry/Toxicology
Medical College of Wisconsin
Milwaukee, Wisconsin

Karen Kehl, PhD
Associate Professor, Pathology
Department of Pathology
Children's Hospital of Wisconsin
Milwaukee, Wisconsin

Stanley F. Lo, PhD
Associate Professor, Pathology
Department of Pathology
Children's Hospital of Wisconsin
Milwaukee, Wisconsin

Christine Naczek, MT (ASCP)
Manager, Blood Banking and Pre-Transfusion Testing
Department of Pathology
United Regional Medical Services, Inc.
Milwaukee, Wisconsin

Anne Witkowiak Nezworski, RN, BSN
Maternity and Newborn Specialist
Sacred Heart Hospital
Eau Claire, Wisconsin

Joseph Nezworski, BS, RN, BSN
Chief Deputy Medical Examiner
Eau Claire County
Eau Claire, Wisconsin

Hershel Raff, PhD
Professor, Departments of Medicine & Physiology
Medical College of Wisconsin
Director, Endocrine Research Laboratory
St. Luke's Medical Center
Milwaukee, Wisconsin

John Shalkham, MA, SCT (ASCP)
Clinical Assistant Professor—Department of Pathology
Program Director for School of Cytotechnology
State Department of Hygiene
University of Wisconsin
Madison, Wisconsin

Eleanor C. Simms, RNC, BSN
Specialist, Nursing Student Enrichment Program
Coppin State College
Helene Fuld School of Nursing
Baltimore, Maryland

Frank G. Steffel, BS, CNMT
Program Director—Nuclear Medicine Technology
Department of Radiology
Froedtert Memorial Lutheran Hospital
Milwaukee, Wisconsin

Corrinne Strandell, RN, BSN, MSN, PhD
Nursing Research, Home Care and Rehabilitation Specialist
West Allis, Wisconsin

Thudung Tieu, MT (ASCP)
Manager of Quality Assurance & Safety
Dynacare Laboratories
Milwaukee, Wisconsin

Jean M. Trione, RPh
Clinical Specialist
Wausau Hospital
Wausau, Wisconsin

Reviewers

Lippincott Williams & Wilkins, and the authors, Professors Fischbach and Dunning, thank the following instructors for reviewing the revision plan for this edition:

Barbara Celia, RN, MSN, EdD
Clinical Assistant Professor
Drexel University College of Nursing and Health Professions
Philadelphia, Pennsylvania

David Dunham, RN, MS
Assistant Professor of Nursing
Hawaii Pacific University
Kaneohe, Hawaii

Rhonda Lawes, RN, MS
Instructor
University of Oklahoma College of Nursing
Tulsa, Oklahoma

Tami J. Rogers, BSN, MSN, DVM
Professor of Nursing
Valencia Community College
Orlando, Florida

Preface

The purpose of the 5th edition of the *Nurses' Quick Reference to Common Laboratory & Diagnostic Tests* is to provide students, paramedical personnel, clinicians, and nurses with a unique resource that incorporates the nurse's expanded role in providing safe, effective, informed diagnostic care and services. This text provides a foundation for understanding the relatively simple to the most complex and sophisticated diagnostic tests delivered to varied populations in both traditional settings and community environments. It describes the nursing role in depth by directing the application of the nursing process model to all phases of testing—pre-, intra-, and posttest periods. The diagnostic care model focuses on nursing judgments and interventions that are key to achieving desired outcomes and preventing misunderstanding and errors. The description of the nurse's unique role includes basic information for identifying patient needs, intervening, correctly educating patients, and providing timely outcome evaluation.

Throughout the book, emphasis is placed upon communication skills and collaboration between patients and their significant others and among nurses and health care professionals from diverse disciplines. When caregivers see patients in the context of what patients and loved ones are experiencing (ie, situational needs, expectations, previous experiences, and the environment in which they live), only then can they offer meaningful support and care. When patients believe that the caregiver is on their side, they have an increased sense of control. Identifying with patients' point of view leads to a more profound level of communication.

Organization and Unique Features

The book is organized into three chapters and one appendix. Each chapter begins with a functional nursing practice standard. Clinicians adapt their safe practice to changes in society, scientific advances, legal interpretation, and enactment. So, too, do nursing standards emanate from the nursing profession itself and are challenged by these trends.

This book uses terminology that supports the scientific nature of the diagnostic process and collaborative team approach. Nursing diagnoses, interventions, outcome formations, and evaluation are the basis of nursing practice. The suggested nursing diagnoses incorporate approved language of the North American Nursing Diagnosis Association (NANDA), and the interventions are standardized by the

Nursing Intervention Classification (NIC) and nursing outcome by the Nursing Outcome Classification (NOC) taxonomy. Criteria for selecting tests for this book focus on new methods and techniques, those procedures most frequently ordered or mandated, the procedures and tests frequently ordered, performed, or assisted with, as well as the procurement of specimens, their handling, storage, and transport.

Chapter 1 focuses on the nurse's unique role in diagnostic testing and reflects new and innovative methods of meeting patient needs. The first part of the chapter gives an overview of nursing responsibilities, the knowledge and skills needed, and the challenges of nurse-directed testing in various settings and many different environments. The second part of the chapter defines the nursing process care model and demonstrates test examples and how the model may be applied to patient care. The pre-, intra-, and posttest activities and collaborative approaches for the collecting, handling, and transporting of specimens, carrying out and assisting with procedures, administering procedural sedation, managing the environment, and patient monitoring are also described in the second part of Chapter 1.

Chapter 2 focuses on nursing responsibilities and protocol for collecting specimens, handling, storage, and transporting of specimens within specified timelines, observing standard precautions, and educating patients and family members to elicit cooperation and understanding.

Chapter 3 alphabetically lists laboratory tests for specific analytes, hormones, tumor markers, or substances, imaging, invasive, and noninvasive procedures, and special diagnostic studies performed before birth, during a lifetime, and after death.

Part 1 of each test in Chapter 3 lists title, type of procedure, purpose and rationale, indications, normal reference values, clinical implications of abnormal results, procedure steps, specimen needed, and patient involvement. The method of specimen collection and disposal, common or alternative names and abbreviations, and interfering factors that can give false-positive and false-negative results are also discussed.

Part 2 of each test in Chapter 3 defines the nurse's role and lists clinical problems, interventions, and judgments based upon assessment and selective stating of nursing diagnoses (identified in Chapter 1) for all phases of testing: pre-, intra-, and posttest. Clinical alerts, panic or critical lab values, or abnormal procedural findings that demand immediate treatment and follow-up test validation, as well as possible risks involved in testing, adverse outcomes, and contraindications to testing, are part of the vital information.

New to This Edition

Although all tests have been reviewed and revised as applicable, there have been extensive revisions of **coagulation studies, diabetes testing, hormone assays,** and **newborn screening panels,** along with updated references. Elements and concepts new to this edition include the following scientific methodologies and technological advances that provide nurses and clinicians with a greater understanding of the long chain of events from diagnosis through treatment and outcome.

Chapter 1

- Changes in terminology as appropriate (eg, "toxicant" previously referred to as toxin, as used in reference to nerve gas exposure, or "chemical" vs poisoning, as used in the context of terrorism).
- New and unique instrumentation or equipment and analysis methodologies.
- Reference to the U.S. Task Force series of universal diagnostic guidelines.
- Expanded nursing roles.
- More on nurse-directed testing and better training of the diagnostic team (eg, different levels of training to meet the laboratory designation site).
- Follow-up and postcare; importance of notification of results and documentation; follow-up testing.
- More on misinterpretation of tests and importance of "flagging" low or high levels.
- Challenges of privacy, confidentiality, and security.
- Legal and ethical issues and chain of custody as applicable.
- How to contact various governmental regulatory agencies (eg, the Centers for Disease Control and Prevention), as required by pertinent laws, statutes, or regulations

Chapter 2

- Procedures for collection of sexual assault specimens.
- More on breath, hair, nails, and saliva testing.
- Skin and transdermal testing of sweat, drugs of abuse, and therapeutic drug management.
- Specimens for diagnosing possible exposure to chemical or biological terrorism toxicants or agents.

Chapter 3

New tests included in this edition are as follows:

- Aldosterone
- Androstenedione

- Antidiuretic Hormone (ADH)
- High-Sensitivity C-Reactive Protein (hs-CRP)
- D-Dimer
- D-Xylose Absorption
- 25-Hydroxyvitamin D
- Renin Assay
- Salivary Gland Imaging
- West Nile Virus

Appendix

Appendix: Standard Precautions

Responding to the trends and changes in health care, the 5th edition of *Nurses' Quick Reference to Common Laboratory & Diagnostic Tests* is a comprehensive, up-to-date diagnostic reference source that includes information about the nurse's expanded role in diagnostic testing and the many instances of nurse-directed testing with varied populations in varied settings. It incorporates newer technologies, together with the time-honored classic tests that continue to be an important component of diagnostic work. It meets the needs of students and clinicians, educators, researchers, and others whose work and study require this type of resource or reference manual.

Marshall B. Dunning III and Frances T. Fischbach

Acknowledgments

With this 5th edition, Dr. Marshall Dunning leads as first author. As a team, we are committed to the highest educational standards of excellence, the generation of knowledge about providing diagnostic care and services, and describing and "prescribing" behaviors that benefit the health and welfare of patients, as well as being responsive to the health care needs of society as a whole. We continue to adhere to the principles of nursing as a learned and human profession based upon scientific knowledge and guidelines for caring. Principles that reflect ethical behavior, patient rights, and moral choices regarding the value and sanctity of human life are a common thread throughout. Professional nursing aspires to altruism, accountability, honor, integrity, and respect for others. As fellow educators and colleagues, we humbly consider ourselves as respected resources to assist the nursing and student role as the scientist, the nurse as the caregiver, and the nurse as the professional.

Special recognition and thanks are given to all, especially our new contributors: Tracy Schweitzer, Patti Cobb, Paul J. Jannetto, Karen Kehl, Stanley F. Lo, and Hershel Raff; reviewers; researchers; and consultants who helped in the preparation and revisions; and all those unnamed who have provided their expertise in making this edition as up to date and accurate as possible. Recognition and appreciation are also due to the editors and staff, of Lippincott Williams & Wilkins, with special thanks to Helen Kogut and Hilarie Surrena.

While writing a book is truly a challenging but fulfilling undertaking, it both humbles us and makes us thankful to those individuals who have all made it possible. Thanks to all for a job well done!

Marshall B. Dunning III and Frances T. Fischbach

Contents

The Nursing Role in Diagnostic Testing

Nursing Practice Standards

The nurse applies the diagnostic care model to all phases of testing to include the requisite knowledge and skills to provide safe, informed care; acts as a patient advocate; follows professional practice standards; communicates effectively; coordinates and manages the testing environment; supports patients through the process; and uses a collaborative approach to facilitate optimal patient outcomes.

Overview of Nursing Responsibilities

As an integrated part of their practice, professional nurses have long supported patients and their families in meeting the demands and challenges of diagnostic testing. This testing begins before birth and frequently continues even after death. Testing before birth may include amniocentesis, fetal ultrasound, and genetic testing. Testing after death may include autopsy, organ transplant, death reporting, and evidentiary or forensic testing. Nursing responsibilities and interventions extend to all three phases of this testing process: the pretest, intratest, and posttest periods. Each phase requires that its own set of guidelines be followed. Nurses need a sound knowledge and practice base to provide safe, effective care and to bring their unique caring qualities to the diagnostic testing event. The nursing process is a necessary, integral, and ongoing care planning and providing component because the nursing process is the *nursing* frame of reference and foundation for all nursing practice. The sequence of assessment, nursing diagnosis, planning, intervention, and implementation of the plan, together with evaluation, are all necessary sequential steps. Application of the nursing process to diagnostic testing facilitates and establishes a framework and comprehensive plan to provide safe, competent care.

Assessment focuses on procuring a detailed database about the patient to facilitate testing and to correlate test findings with physical findings and other patient status indicators to ensure accurate outcomes. In the assessment phase, the nurse understands the reason and need for the diagnostic test(s) being performed. *Diagnosis* is a clinical judgment that identifies the patient response to an actual or potential health problem during diagnostic evaluation. Its uniqueness lies in the fact that it is nurse-identified and nurse-treated. The diagnostic planning phase has several crucial factors to consider, as the effect of one test may have several implications on/for another. *Planning* flows from the nursing diagnosis. This stage focuses on safety and the physiologic, psychosocial, emotional, and spiritual needs of the patient and family; the nurse develops strategies to meet these needs during diagnostic evaluation.

Collaboration with other clinicians in the care planning is vital. The nurse should include modalities to help patients cope with the actual diagnostic procedure and test outcomes, as well as accommodate patients with special needs, such as hearing or sight impairment, ostomy care, or diabetic care. The comatose, the confused, the child, and the frail, elderly patient also require special consideration.

Nurses and other health care clinicians treat collaborative patient problems simultaneously. During diagnostic tests, the nurse identifies both nursing diagnoses and collaborative problems that require appropriate and independent nursing interventions.

The setting in which testing takes place, age and developmental stage, disabilities, information needs, coping style, and cultural diversity must be considered. Because test preparation and actual testing are often done at home or in a non–acute care setting, care planning is vital for achieving the most desirable outcomes. As society becomes more culturally blended, the need to appreciate, understand, and engage within the realm of cultural diversity is imperative. Interacting with patients and directing them through diagnostic testing can present certain challenges if one is not somewhat familiar with and sensitive to the patient's health care belief system. Something as basic as clear communication in the face of language differences may make it necessary to arrange for a relative or translator to be present at different stages of the testing process. It is important to note that biocultural factors can affect derived diagnostic values. Sensitivity to all of these foregoing issues will frequently influence the patient's response to and adherence with the actual procedure.

Implementation addresses the actual work and process of executing the plans for the pretest, intratest, and posttest phases. It includes specific, measurable nursing interventions and patient activities.

Implementation of specific, independent nursing actions is based on the diagnostic test(s) findings. Emphasis is placed upon proper specimen collection and handling, performance of procedures, administration of drugs and solutions following established guidelines, education, counseling, proper patient preparation, provision of comfort and support, assurance of safety, infection control, and prevention of complications.

Evaluation provides data about interpretation and an understanding of x-rays (or x-ray films) and other test results, whether tests were completed (partially or not at all), effectiveness of care, and patient compliance and reaction to testing. Follow-up testing and treatment modalities are frequently decided in this stage. Comparing actual and expected outcomes, along with initiation of posttest activities, comprises the major evaluation components of the diagnostic phase. Outcomes are neutral concepts or measures that describe patient responses that are influenced by nursing interventions. Goal statements may be general or specific but should be measurable. Reporting and recording the findings, implementing plans, and evaluating outcomes complete the process.

The practice of nursing is based on following certain standards and policies. These standards also influence and govern nursing responsibilities and practice during diagnostic evaluation. *Evidence-based practice* (EBP) refers to those activities that promote the best outcomes. The American Nurses Association (ANA) code, ANA Congress of Nursing Practice, The Joint Commission, Occupational Safety and Health Administration (OSHA) standards, and Centers for Disease Control and Prevention (CDC) precautions, together with agency, institutional, and specialty organization policies and procedures, are categories of standards that nurses are held to (TABLE 1.1). Regulation and accreditation agencies require nursing practice to be evidence-based.

✎ Challenges of the Testing Environment

Diagnostic testing, whether simple or sophisticated, occurs in many different environments. Certain tests can be done in the field, so to speak, where the service is brought to the patient's environment (eg, home, shopping mall, pharmacy, church, mobile unit). Other more sophisticated tests need to be done in a physician's office, clinic, or hospital. If equipment is extremely complex, such as magnetic resonance imaging (MRI), or in ultrasound studies, procedures are commonly performed in freestanding diagnostic centers. The most complex tests, such as endoscopic retrograde cholangiopancreatography (ERCP), cardiac catheterization, or bronchoscopy, usually require hospital services.

(text continues on page 7)

TABLE 1.1 STANDARDS FOR DIAGNOSTIC EVALUATION

SOURCE OF STANDARDS FOR DIAGNOSTIC SERVICE	STANDARDS FOR DIAGNOSTIC TESTING	EXAMPLES OF APPLIED STANDARDS FOR DIAGNOSTIC TESTING
Professional practice parameters of American Nurses Association (ANA), American Medical Association (AMA), American Society of Clinical Pathologists (ASCP), American College of Radiology, Centers for Disease Control and Prevention (CDC), and The Joint Commission health care practice requirements	Use a model as a framework for choosing the proper test or procedure and in the interpretation of test results. Use laboratory and diagnostic procedures for screening, differential diagnoses, follow-up, and case management.	Test strategies include single test or combinations/panel of tests. Panels can be performed in parallel, series, or both.
The guidelines of the major agencies, such as American Heart Association, American Cancer Society, and American Diabetes Association	Order the correct test and appropriately collect and transport specimens. Properly perform tests in an accredited laboratory or diagnostic facility. Accurately report test results. Communicate and interpret test findings. Treat or monitor the disease and the course of therapy. Provide diagnosis as well as prognosis.	Patients receive diagnostic services based on a documented assessment of the need for diagnostic evaluation. Patients have the right to necessary information, benefits, or rights to enable them to make choices and decisions that reflect their need or wish for diagnostic care.

Individual agency and institution policies and procedures and quality-control criteria for specimen collection, procedure statement for monitoring the patient after an invasive procedure, and policy for universal witnessed consent situations. Statements on quality improvement standards. Use standards of professional practice and standards of patient care. Use policy for obtaining informed consent/witnessed consent. Use policies for unusual situations.	Observe standard precautions (formerly known as universal precautions). Use latex allergy protocols and required methodology of specimen collection. Use standards and statements for monitoring patients who receive conscious sedation and analgesia. Vital signs are monitored and recorded at specific times before and after the procedure. Patients are monitored for bleeding and respiratory or neurovascular changes. Record data regarding outcomes when defined care criteria are implemented and practiced. Protocols to obtain appropriate consents are employed and deviations from basic consent policies are documented and reported to the proper individual.	The clinician wears protective eyewear and gloves when handling all body fluids and employs proper hand-washing before and after handling specimens and between patient contacts. Labeled biohazard bags are used for specimen transport. Vital signs are monitored and recorded at specific times before and after the procedure. Patients are monitored for bleeding and respiratory or neurovascular changes. Record data regarding outcomes when defined care criteria are implemented and practiced. Protocols to obtain appropriate consents are employed and deviations from basic consent policies are documented and reported to the proper individual.
State and federal government communicable disease reporting regulations; Centers for Disease Control and Prevention (CDC), U.S. Department of Health and Human Services, Agency for Health Care Policy and Research (AHCPR), U.S. Food and Drug Administration (FDA), and Clinical Laboratory Improvement Act (CLIA)	Clinical laboratory personnel and other health care providers follow regulations to control the spread of communicable diseases by reporting certain disease conditions, outbreaks, and unusual manifestations, morbidity, and mortality data. Findings from research studies provide health care policy makers with evidence-based guidelines for appropriate selection of tests and procedures.	The clinician reports laboratory evidence of certain disease classes (eg, sexually transmitted diseases, diphtheria, symptomatic HIV infection; see list of reportable diseases). Personnel with hepatitis A may not handle food or care for patients, young children, or the elderly for a specific period of time. Federal government regulates shipment of diagnostic specimens. MR and CT scans are used to evaluate persistent low back pain according to AHCPR guidelines.

(table continues on page 6)

TABLE 1.1 (continued)

SOURCE OF STANDARDS FOR DIAGNOSTIC SERVICE	STANDARDS FOR DIAGNOSTIC TESTING	EXAMPLES OF APPLIED STANDARDS FOR DIAGNOSTIC TESTING
U.S. Department of Transportation (U.S. DOT)	Alcohol testing is done in special situations (eg, following a motor vehicle accident, homicide, or suicide, or on an unconscious individual).	Properly trained personnel perform blood, saliva, and breath alcohol testing and use required kits as referenced by federal law.
Occupational Safety and Health Administration (OSHA)	Workplace testing for drug and alcohol abuse, health and wellness screenings, hearing and lung function testing, and TB screening.	The clinician is properly trained, under mandated guidelines, to administer employee medical surveillance and respirator qualification and fit testing.
International Organization for Standardization (ISO) The ISO 15189 standard is specific to medical laboratories, providing both management and technical requirements.	Clinical laboratory requirements for personnel, medical equipment, pre- and postexamination procedures, quality assurance, and reporting of test results. Management requirements include such areas as document control, resolution of complaints, corrective and preventive actions, internal audits, and continual improvement.	ISO accreditation involves a comprehensive review of management, clinical personnel competency, and technical requirements to ensure quality and ongoing improvement. Accreditation of a clinical laboratory by ISO is recognized as a "stamp of quality."

The Joint Commission, formerly, Joint Commission on Accreditation of Healthcare Organizations; HIV, human immunodeficiency virus; MR, magnetic resonance; CT, computed tomography.

With changing methods of health care delivery in today's society, the nurse's unique role in diagnostic evaluation must, of necessity, reflect new and innovative methods of meeting needs, providing quality care, and containing costs. Responsibilities for diagnostic care in various settings and the home, workplace, health care facility, and community at large are summarized in TABLES 1.2 and 1.3.

Home Care Environment

The trend toward shorter hospitalizations for acute illnesses has created a need for continued care in the home setting. The nurse uses astute clinical decision-making skills and recognizes when to initiate physician contact to confirm the need for specific laboratory and diagnostic tests to avoid illness complications, as well as unnecessary exposure, transfer, and hospital admission costs. Specimen collection and testing vary according to home health care agency policies, home location, nursing skills, physician's preference, nature of the illness, and the degree to which immediate intervention is necessary. Often, especially in some community and rural areas, the nurse must be skilled in drawing venous blood, in collecting specimens from invasive lines (or catheters), in obtaining cultures, and in properly labeling, documenting, handling, and transporting of specimens. Sometimes, teaching the patient and significant others how to correctly collect and preserve specimens may be an important part of the entire process. The home care nurse must also be knowledgeable of the patient's cultural and alternative therapeutic practices to facilitate appropriate diagnostic testing procedures and evaluations. In urban or suburban areas, the health care agency frequently contracts with other providers for specimen collection, analysis, and issuing of reported findings. As the care coordinator, the nurse must obtain test results in a timely manner and communicate these findings to the proper clinicians as soon as possible. Test results frequently validate new diagnoses, confirm the need to change medication or dosage, or alert the need for an appointment with the clinician to further evaluate the situation.

The home health care nurse may need to perform selective procedures, procure specimens, or monitor health problems as shown in the following examples:

Diabetes control: Blood glucose testing by fingerstick or venous draw, fasting blood glucose testing using glucometers, or urine glucose testing by test strips.

TABLE 1.2 EXAMPLES OF NURSING ROLES

SETTING	NURSING ROLE
Hospitals/medical centers	Provide emergency room and specialty patient care, collect specimens, take x-rays, conduct nuclear scanning, perform ultrasounds, and conduct pretransfusion, pretransplant complex, and invasive testing
Freestanding clinic	Collect specimens for sexually transmitted diseases
Physician office	Conduct *H. pylori* blood tests for infection; obtain electrocardiograms (ECGs)
Occupational environment	Conduct pre-employment screening for TB, perform case finding for alcohol or drug abuse, perform health and wellness screenings, monitor exposure to hazardous materials (lead, chromium), and perform pulmonary function and blood testing
Insurance examiner	Administer tests in client's home or office, such as a resting ECG, spirometry, urine, blood draw for cholesterol
Forensic (ED and surgery)	Save evidence of crimes and deal with ethical and legal issues
Hospital-based clinic	Administer procedural sedation and analgesia in asthma, cystic fibrosis, pulmonary hypertension, cardiac, and transplant clinics
Long-term care environment	Test urine for diagnosis and treatment of lower urinary tract infections, test blood for glucose levels, collect sputum cultures for various respiratory infections, and perform TB skin testing
Homeless shelter	Conduct HIV testing and vaginal and rectal exams for sexually transmitted diseases; collect sputum cultures to screen for TB; collect and test blood and urine specimens for blood glucose levels
Community and public health	Educate patient, test for HIV and AIDS (blood and saliva), conduct TB (skin and blood) testing, perform stool tests for occult blood as an indication of cancer or food-borne pathogens

SETTING	NURSING ROLE
Home setting	Obtain blood samples to monitor coagulation and diabetes
Health fair	Perform health and wellness screening for diabetes, blood glucose, abnormal cholesterol, risk factors for atherosclerotic heart disease (AHD)
Advanced practice nurse (APN)	Manage the patient testing process, including ordering, performing, and interpreting blood tests, electrocardiograms, x-rays, and computed tomography (CT) scans; perform examinations for rape or sexual abuse, lumbar punctures, and ultrasounds; collect specimens for rape and sexual abuse
Sexual assault nurse examiner (SANE)	Interview, examine, and collect specimens from sexual assault victims; use special kits to obtain vaginal and rectal specimens; take hair samples and photographs of bruises and bite marks
Point-of-care testing (POC)	Order complete blood count (CBC) and differential count for the diagnosis of anemia and infection; conduct PAP smears; perform ECGs; test blood glucose levels; conduct spirometry testing
Blood/plasma center	Ensure donor suitability; collect blood or plasma; maintain product integrity

Cardiac disorders: Blood draw for prothrombin time, for international normalized ratio (INR), and to monitor anticoagulation therapy; cardiac enzymes for symptomatic changes (eg, chest pain); serum lipids (considered risk factors for cardiac disease); peptides to distinguish between cardiac and respiratory causes of dyspnea; serum electrolytes to evaluate diuretic and potassium therapy; digitalis blood levels to detect toxicity.

Hydration/dehydration, nutritional problems: Blood draw for serum electrolytes and other blood chemistry or metabolic panels, particularly albumin for nutritional loss and potassium and sodium for dehydration. Blood draw for monitoring chemotherapy with special attention to red blood cell (RBC), white blood cell (WBC), and differential count.

Infection control: Monitor patients with infectious diseases and resistant organisms with complete blood count (CBC), WBC, and

TABLE 1.3 EXAMPLES OF NURSE-DIRECTED TESTING

TEST	NURSING RESPONSIBILITY
Blood draws for testing (arterial, venous, or capillary)	Monitor blood glucose levels, cardiac enzymes, electrolytes, drug presence (licit or illicit), cell counts (red and white blood cells), alcohol intake, oxygenation levels, acid-base status, presence of bacterial pathogens, hormone levels, tumor markers, antibodies, etc.
Guaiac stool testing	Check for fecal blood, color, consistency, and presence of pathogenic organisms
Tuberculin skin testing	Interpret results; obtain blood and/or sputum for TB testing
HIV/AIDS testing	Obtain blood or saliva and obtain informed consent
Rectal exams	Obtain stool for occult blood, positive guaiac smears as possible sign of rectal or colon cancer
Finger- or heelsticks	Screen newborns and infants for genetic disorders
Pap smears	Perform vaginal swab for diagnosis of precancers and cancers of genital tract; check for the presence of microorganisms
Throat swabs	Swab throat for the diagnosis of *Streptococcus* infections
Urine dipsticks	Determine blood glucose level, alcohol levels, and the presence of bladder infection
Lung function testing	Use spirometer for peak airflow assessment in asthma
Breath alcohol testing	Use specialized devices to detect above-normal levels of alcohol
Audiometric examination	Follow guidelines for hearing deficits
Vision testing	Conduct simple to complex vision tests; follow guidelines for retinal and macular degeneration disorders
Pulse oximetry	Apply special device to monitor arterial oxygenation levels (during rest, walking, exercise)
ECG	Apply leads to identify normal cardiac rhythms, arrhythmias, and myocardial ischemia; evaluate pacemaker function
IV	Draw blood and collect specimens from invasive lines for evaluation

differential count and urine and wound cultures to identify causative agent and to monitor antibiotic effectiveness and immune function.

Neonates and infants: Use photo light and serum to monitor jaundice and bilirubin levels. If home birth, obtain newborn blood sample as indicated by state guidelines and report birth information to local health department.

Renal problems: Blood chemistry tests such as blood urea nitrogen (BUN), creatinine, sodium, potassium; CBC (for anemia) to monitor renal function and effectiveness of home dialysis. Urinalysis and random and timed urine specimens to evaluate kidney status (protein, electrolytes, and urine waste products).

Respiratory disorders: Apnea monitor and pulse oximetry to check respiratory rate and oxygen saturation levels; CBC, with attention to RBC, hematocrit (HCT), and hemoglobin (Hb) to assess blood oxygen carrying–capacity and blood viscosity; sputum cultures to assess and evaluate respiratory infections; arterial blood gases and end-tidal carbon dioxide to assess oxygenation, acid-base status, and ventilation.

✐ Occupational Care Environment

The occupational and environmental health care nurse's responsibilities include screening, case finding to reduce or prevent known workplace hazards, problem evaluation, management of ergonomics, evaluation of interventions, ongoing monitoring of identified health problems, and collaboration with employers and supervisors about job injury sites. The nurse's main role lies in pre-employment baseline screening and testing and periodic monitoring of exposure to potentially hazardous workplace substances. OSHA and employer standards direct the focus of care. Pre-employment drug screens as well as baseline and ongoing tests for the presence of exposure to industrial toxins (eg, chemical and heavy metals) are required. Pre-employment tests will vary according to the type of exposure encountered (eg, lead, chromium), nature of business, or health, service, or occupational role. Screening for tuberculosis (TB) skin or blood testing may also be done. Blood, saliva, and urine specimens; breathalyzer tests; pulmonary function breathing tests; and vision and hearing exams are routinely ordered, and the nurse should be well versed in procuring specimens and administering these tests. Skills in drawing venous blood and knowing how to correctly label and transport specimens are also needed.

Appropriate health counseling and monitoring include proper notification of the employee, employer, and primary physician about test results; performance of follow-up testing; and initiation of measures to prevent and treat exposures to toxic and hazardous materials. Nurses are accountable for monitoring the chain of custody and obtaining properly signed and witnessed consent forms for drug or alcohol testing, for worker's compensation in industrial accidents, for initiation and monitoring of appropriate testing, and for recommendations for changes in work surface, slip hazards, and a worker's job situation, among others.

The occupational and environmental health care nurses' other main role resides in creating healthy and productive workplaces. Health promotion is essential to a healthy and safe work environment. This nurse provides health screenings (eg, blood glucose and cholesterol levels), assessments, education (eg, how to manage diabetes, smoking cessation), and wellness programs that support and promote employee health.

Long-Term Care Environments

With increasing numbers of younger people with complex problems, greater numbers of older adults (those who live into their 90s and 100s), and sick and frail elderly in long-term care settings, nurses play a dynamic role in promoting optimal health status for residents of these facilities while also dealing with ethical and legal issues.

Changes and challenges in long-term care include the following:

- There are more patients with multiple systemic and degenerative problems for which there are no cures.
- Increasing numbers of residents with "full code" (ie, to be resuscitated) status lead to greater volumes and varieties of tests, which raises costs of care.
- Increased awareness of residents' rights (eg, right to refuse tests) and signed advance directive documents allow more decision making by residents and families.
- More pretest, posttest, and follow-up care procedures occur in nursing homes because residents are frequently transferred to hospitals or clinics only for the more complex procedures, such as computed tomography (CT), endoscopy, and angiography. Intratest care includes performing or assisting with procedures such as performing fingersticks for blood glucose monitoring, assisting with x-ray films after falls and compromised respiratory

occurrences (eg, pneumonia), and obtaining portable electrocardio-grams (ECGs) for the onset of chest pain in a patient with a history of cardiac disease and no recent ECG records.

- More confused, combative, or uncooperative behaviors are being cared for in long-term care facilities, and many of these behaviors are related to changes associated with longevity and the aging process; chronic or degenerative diseases; dementia, lack of knowledge, motivation, and concern; and relocation syndrome (ie, moving from one environment to another). Frequently, an attitude of "not wanting to be bothered," fear of findings and treatment, or outright refusal to have tests done make testing difficult. The nurse must understand the meaning of the patient's behaviors, provide the patient with an age-friendly environment to foster safety and comfort, and incorporate appropriate communication strategies and nursing interventions for these special populations.

TABLE 1.4 contains the most common nurse-identified problems found in long-term care settings and their related diagnostic tests.

◢ Public Health Environment

Urban and Rural Communities

The role of the nurse in the community setting is rapidly changing to include serving persons in certain geographical areas and settings. Specializations include the parish nurse, school nurse, clinic nurse, prison nurse, forensic nurse, nurse consultant, nurse case manager, and tele-health nurse. The community-based nurse's role is continu-ally expanding because of societal demands and needs. This trend focuses on providing care to all ages, especially the middle-aged to elderly population, although in nurse-managed clinics for the home-less, many young people are served. Responsibilities include case finding (eg, genetic sickle cell disease), case management, screening for sexually transmitted diseases and TB and wellness screenings (cholesterol levels), vision testing, and referrals for diseases such as diabetes (eg, fasting blood glucose and urine tests), colorectal cancer (eg, rectal exams and stool tests), anemia (eg, blood tests for hemo-globin and hematocrit), or breast cancer (eg, mammograms). Case finding or screening frequently occurs at health fairs or outreach cen-ters, schools, homeless shelters, community health centers, mobile health vans, church settings, and senior citizen residential facilities.

Responsibilities vary but often include providing test information and obtaining saliva, urine, blood, and stool specimens; they may

TABLE 1.4 COMMON NURSE-IDENTIFIED PROBLEMS AND RELATED
DIAGNOSTIC TESTS

NURSE-IDENTIFIED PROBLEMS	DIAGNOSTIC TESTS
Ineffective cardiac output related to altered tissue perfusion	ECG, pulse oximetry, protein, electrolytes, digoxin levels, CBC, chemistry/metabolic panels, heparin/Coumadin anticoagulation levels, nuclear imaging
Risk for altered respiratory function (eg, infection) related to immobility, compromised immune system, impaired gas exchange, aspiration, or ineffective breathing patterns	CBC, differential count, radiology, arterial blood gases (ABGs), pulse oximetry, sputum culture, pulmonary function, endoscopies
Neurosensory alterations related to seizures, cerebrovascular accidents (CVAs), infections, injuries, or ineffective medication control	CAT scans, MRIs, EEGs, anticonvulsant drug levels, therapeutic drug monitoring for psychotropic drugs to review and reduce dosage, CBC, chemistry/metabolic panels, lumbar puncture
Risk for urinary tract infections, retention, altered elimination patterns, or catheter or appliance use	CBC, differential count, urine culture and sensitivity
Altered bowel elimination related to incontinence, constipation, diarrhea, impaction, or obstruction (caused by cancer, adhesions, diverticulitis, food-borne illness, or other intestinal problems)	Abdominal ultrasound, gastrointestinal (GI) x-rays, stool specimen, CBC, chemistry/metabolic panels, nuclear scans
Acute pain related to falls, injuries, infections, or acute head, chest, or abdominal problems	X-rays, CBC, chemistry/metabolic panels, nuclear scans
Management of therapeutic regimen related to requirements of rehabilitation program for acute and chronic conditions	X-rays, hematology tests, and chemistry/metabolic panels
Altered thought processes related to confusion, social isolation, hyperthermia, impaired gas exchange, or organ failure (eg, brain, kidney, heart, liver)	Chemistry/metabolic panel, CBC, ABGs, x-rays, and scans

NURSE-IDENTIFIED PROBLEMS	DIAGNOSTIC TESTS
Risk for injury related to falls, impaired mobility, muscular weakness, paralysis, sensory/perceptual alterations, and confusion	X-rays, nuclear and duplex scans, Holter monitoring, chemistry metabolic/panel, CBC, ABGs, and stress testing
Altered nutritional intake related to a lack of appetite, poor eating habits, pretest fasting, chewing difficulties (eg, edentulous, poor dentition), impaired swallowing, depression or confusion, food-borne illness, infection	Prealbumin, albumin/globulin (A/G) ratio, swallow tests, GI x-rays, stool sample, chemistry/metabolic panel, CBC, and nuclear scans
Fluid volume deficit related to inability to swallow, incontinence, urinary fluids, vomiting, diarrhea, or other GI disorders	Blood tests to evaluate electrolytes, hemoglobin, and hematocrit; stool sample, chemistry/metabolic panel; GI x-rays; GI scans, endoscopy
Altered tissue perfusion (all types) related to anemia, inadequate nutritional intake, occult bleeding, food-borne illness, numerous blood draws, digestive disorders, malabsorption of nutrients	CBC, chemistry/metabolic panel, iron tests, x-rays, stool sample, occult blood tests, GI x-rays, and swallowing procedures
Impaired skin integrity related to venipunctures, with greater risk for infection, infectious processes, draining wounds, immobility, altered peripheral tissue perfusion, or decubitus ulcers	Wound cultures, chemistry panel, potassium, CBC, and differential count

extend to performing procedures (eg, Pap smears), transporting and preparing specimens for analysis, or performing actual test analysis. The patient or guardian must give his or her consent before the test is performed.

Homeless Environment

Many homeless people who come to nursing clinics are young people or mature men with alcohol or drug addiction. The population is difficult to contact or locate, so many of the laboratory tests done at the nursing clinic are blood fingersticks (eg, for detection of diabetes, hematocrit to confirm anemia), which give immediate readings. This screening enables prompt attention to be given to abnormal results.

Dipstick tests of urine for glucose, acetone, and microhemoglobin are done during the first visit, as well as TB skin tests, blood tests for TB, fingersticks, and intravenous (IV) blood draws for certain individuals. A throat swab sample can be tested for *Streptococcus* infection by mixing a reagent with a swab and getting an immediate reading. A guaiac test for blood in stool can also be done immediately. For men older than 50 years, rectal examinations are done to detect blood in stool and to check for prostatic cancer or hypertrophy. Pap smears and rectal examinations are done for female patients.

Indications for IV blood draws include a history of drug abuse or multiple sex partners, HIV (AIDS), hepatitis B and hepatitis C infections, *Chlamydia* infection, basic metabolic panels, CBC, and cholesterol determination.

✐ Special Examiner Roles ─────────────────

Nurse Insurance Examiners

In the setting of an insurance application or claim, nursing responsibilities will vary according to the testing location (usually the patient's home or office). The data collection focus is on obtaining a required medical history; conducting a physical exam (eg, blood pressure, pulse, height, weight, chest, and abdominal measurements done manually); initiating specific interventions, such as obtaining specimens (eg, saliva, dried blood spot by venipuncture [do not draw blood if blood pressure is less than 80/50 mmHg] or fingerstick); using a spirometer for breath testing (eg, timed vital capacity); analyzing a urine sample (eg, dipstick interpretation and reading of glucose and protein); or performing a resting ECG. The required procedures depend on the requests and policies of insurance underwriters. There are several special challenges:

- Dealing with ethical and legal issues, such as using tamperproof tape, following chain-of-custody requirements, obtaining properly signed and witnessed consent forms (eg, for HIV testing and urine drug testing), and maintaining confidentiality of records.
- Assembling and using required kits and equipment (eg, use of scale with 300-lb capacity, tape measure, urine dipstick, container with label showing timing and color chart instructions, and portable spirometer to measure lung volume).
- Assessing risk for fainting or convulsions during or after a blood draw and risk for cotton allergy triggered during saliva testing.
- Following special policies for minors.

- Being cautious with urine preservative tablets (eg, risk for mild injury if person ingests the tablet); if needed, contacting the poison control center, family physician, or emergency department.
- Correctly using dipstick tests and interpreting and reporting results.
- Correctly using bar codes as part of a complete and proper specimen identification.
- Correctly using kits for blood and saliva testing and ensuring proper handling and shipping of specimens.
- Properly positioning patients for blood draws (sitting), ECGs (on a flat surface near an electrical outlet), and breath testing (sitting or standing).
- Intervening appropriately when special situations occur (eg, interpreter is required, patient cannot read or write, patient refuses to sign forms, patient is unable to void, nurse is unable to obtain required blood specimens, and simultaneous specimen collection is required for multiple companies).

Advanced Practice Nurses (APNs)

In many states, roles in patient management for advanced practice nurses (APNs) are expanding, including ordering and interpreting diagnostic studies. The spectrum of responsibilities for diagnostic testing may vary from patient notification and follow-up counseling about physician-ordered studies to independent ordering, performance, and interpretation of diagnostic studies.

Studies previously reserved for specialized physician practices are becoming a routine part of APN practice, including obtaining diagnostic specimens for culture, DNA amplification, and biopsies for pathology; performing rapid assays, including newer bedside tests for serum chemistries and drugs of abuse; conducting common tests for *Streptococcus* species and pregnancy; and performing simple microscopy.

As part of the patient workup, the APN may perform some of the diagnostic studies needed to make a medical diagnosis. APNs retain ultimate accountability for their orders, the procedures they perform, and the decisions made on the basis of data collected, regardless of the circumstances with respect to physician supervision, physician consultation, state regulations, or practice protocols.

Sexual Assault Nurse Examiners (SANEs)

Sexual assault nurse examiners (SANEs) are clinicians who have had advanced training in forensic or criminal examination of sexual assault victims. SANE programs have helped standardize evidence collection in a compassionate environment and create a victim-sensitive system of response to sexual assault. *Sexual assault or abuse* is defined as sexual contact of one person with another without appropriate legal consent, as outlined in state and local laws.

Interviews and examinations should be conducted promptly in a compassionate environment by a trained examiner with special attention to the medical and psychological needs of the victim as well as the collection of evidence for medical-legal purposes. Communication with involved law enforcement officials is critical, as well as obtaining informed consent, preserving the chain of custody, and providing detailed documentation, including photographs.

The nurse obtains informed consent from the victim before conducting any examination or collecting any evidence. Victims may refuse evidence collection and request only medical treatment. The victim should be discouraged from eating, drinking, smoking, washing, or urinating prior to the examination.

All specimens collected must be packaged with the kit provided, following labeled instructions. Specimens for DNA evidence to identify the perpetrator may include victim's clothing, fingernail scrapings, dried secretions, pubic hair, external genital swabbing, vaginal secretion specimens, specimens and photographs obtained during colposcopy, and urine sample.

Report of victim findings and examiner's exhibits must be carefully reported and documented using a diagram of the human body to point to abrasions, bite marks, areas of bleeding, and so forth.

✐ Basics of Diagnostic Care ─────────────────

In this high-tech era, health care delivery involves many different disciplines and specialties, and clinicians must have a working knowledge of many areas of expertise, including diagnostic evaluation and diagnostic services. Safe, informed diagnostic care includes basic knowledge and skills regarding the following: test background information, normal reference values, test purpose, indications for testing, actual procedures, specimen collection and handling, clinical implications of abnormal test outcomes, interfering factors, patient pretest care and preparation, patient intratest care, patient posttest care, clinical alerts for special cautions, interpretation of test results, and correlation of results with the patient's signs and symptoms.

Laboratory and diagnostic tests are assessment tools to gain additional information about the patient. By and of themselves, they are not therapeutic. However, when joined with a thorough history and physical examination, these tests may confirm or rule out a diagnosis or may provide valuable information about a patient's status and response to therapy that may not be apparent from the history and physical exam alone. Generally, a tiered approach to selecting tests is used that includes the following:

- Basic screening (frequently used with wellness groups and case finding).
- Establishment of initial diagnosis.
- Differential diagnosis.
- Evaluation of current medical case management and outcomes.
- Evaluation of disease severity.
- Monitoring of course of illness and response to treatment.
- Group and panel testing.
- Regularly scheduled screening tests as part of ongoing care.
- Testing related to specific events, certain signs and symptoms, or other exceptional situations (eg, sexual assault, drug screening, pheochromocytoma, or postmortem tests).

Normal Values and Findings

Knowledge of test terminology, test purpose, process, and normal or reference ranges and outcomes is vital. Theoretically, the term "normal" can refer to the ideal health state, to average reference values, or to types of statistical distribution. Normal or expected values are those that fall within 2 SDs from the mean value for the normal population. The reported reference range for a test can vary according to the laboratory, the method used, the population tested, the conditions of collection, and specimen preservation. Each laboratory must specify its own normal ranges.

The term "normal findings" for procedure test outcomes refers to expected anatomical and physiologic parameters, for example, normal organ size (no enlargement), function (eg, gastric fluid clear or opalescent, no obstruction of blood flow), clear x-ray visualization, ultrasound and Doppler echoes revealing no pathologic processes, and nuclear scan uptake expected and symmetric. There can also be a distinction between "diagnostic" versus "therapeutic" normal values. *Diagnostic normal* typically refers to the range of measurements (generally the 95% confidence interval) over which disease is absent and anything outside the range is considered to be abnormal. *Therapeutic normal* describes the range of measurements over which treatment may not be indicated or beneficial. The greater the degree of test abnormality, the more likely the outcome will be more serious.

Critical (panic) values are abnormal or unexpected values that fall significantly outside the "normal" range and may imply a life-threatening situation for the patient. The nurse must immediately notify the appropriate clinician with the critical value so that there will be no significant delays in (potential) treatment. Critical (panic) value lists, policies, and procedures are institutional specific. All diagnostic tests (eg, imaging, blood tests, and ECGs) can have "critical values" associated to them. Accreditation by The Joint Commission requires critical value reporting to the physician in a timely manner along with proper documentation. Federal law also requires critical value reporting as part of the Centers for Medicare & Medicaid Services (CMS) guidelines.

There may be circumstances in which a diagnostic test does not provide a clear result. As such, reporting of the result(s) may fall into one of three categories: (1) uninterpretable, that is, test did not meet specific procedural protocols or standards; (2) indeterminate, that is, test results are equivocal; and (3) intermediate, that is, test falls between a positive result and a negative result.

✐ Interfering Factors

Many factors may affect values and influence the determination (range) and normal findings. These factors may produce values that are normal under the prevailing conditions but are outside the limits determined under other circumstances. Age, sex, race, culture, environment, posture, diurnal and other cyclic variations, foods, beverages, caffeine or nicotine intake, patient movement, retained barium and intestinal gas, fasting, postprandial state, drugs, and exercise may all affect the values derived. (Most normal values for blood tests are determined by measurement of "fasting" specimens.)

The influence of drugs upon test outcomes must always be considered. Drugs that most often affect test outcomes include anticoagulants, antibiotics, anticonvulsants, homeopathic and alternative drugs, and hormones.

The influence of posture is important when plasma volume is measured because it is 12% to 15% greater in a person who has been supine for several hours. When the position changes from supine to standing, values increase for hemoglobin, RBCs, hematocrit, calcium, potassium, phosphorous, aspartate aminotransferase (AST), phosphatases, total protein, albumin, cholesterol, and triglycerides. When position changes from upright to supine, values decrease for hematocrit, calcium, total protein, and cholesterol. There is a 1% decrease when going from the standing to sitting position for breathing tests, and hemoconcentration occurs following a stress test. A tourniquet applied for more than 1 minute produces an increase in values for protein (5%), iron (6.7%), AST (9.3%), and cholesterol (5%) and a decrease in values for potassium (6%) and creatinine (2.3%).

SI Values

Scientific publications and many professional organizations (eg, World Health Organization) are changing the reporting of clinical laboratory data from conventional units to Système International d' Unitēs (SI units). Currently, much clinical laboratory data are reported in conventional units, with SI units placed in parentheses. This conversion is to establish a common language for laboratory measurements.

The SI system uses seven dimensionally independent units of measurement to provide a logical and consistent measurement. For example, SI concentrations are written as amount per volume (moles or millimoles per liter) rather than as mass per volume (grams, milligrams, or milliequivalents per deciliter, 100 milliliters, or liters). Sometimes, numerical values differ between systems. However, they may be the same. For example, chloride is the same—95 to 105 mEq/L (conventional) and 95 to 105 mmol/L (SI).

Margins of Error

The nurse recognizes the existence of margins of error. If a patient has a metabolic panel or battery of chemistry tests, the possibility exists that some tests will be abnormal owing purely to chance. This can occur because a significant margin of error arises from the arbitrary setting of limits. Moreover, if a laboratory test is considered normal up to the 95th percentile, the result can indicate an abnormality in 5 of 100 tests, even though a patient is not ill. A second test performed on the same sample will probably yield the following: 0.95×0.95 or 90.25%. This means that for 9.75 of 100 tests, the result will show an abnormality, even though the person has no underlying health disorder. Each successive testing will produce a higher percentage of abnormal results. If a patient has a group of tests performed on one blood sample, some of the test results may be abnormal due to chance.

Test Reliability

The clinical value and reliability of a test are related to its *diagnostic accuracy*. Measures of diagnostic test accuracy include sensitivity, specificity, and incidence of disease in the population tested. Sensitivity and specificity do not change with different populations of ill and healthy patients. The predictive value of the same test can be very different when applied to people of differing ages, sex, and geographic locations. *Specificity* refers to the ability of a test to correctly identify those individuals who do *not* have the disease. The formula for computing specificity follows:

$$\% \text{ of specificity} = \frac{\text{persons without disease who test negative}}{\text{Total number of persons without disease}} \times 100$$

Sensitivity refers to the ability of a test to correctly identify those individuals who truly have the disease. The formula for computing sensitivity is as follows:

$$\% \text{ of sensitivity} = \frac{\text{persons with disease who test positive}}{\text{Total number of persons tested with disease}} \times 100$$

Incidence of disease refers to prevalence of disease in a population or community. The predictive value of the same test can be very different when applied to people of differing ages (eg, newborns), sex, and geographic locations.

Predictive values refer to the ability of screening test results to correctly identify the disease state. *Positive predictive values* correctly identify individuals who *have* the disease, whereas *negative predictive values* identify individuals who *do not have* the disease. Positive predictive value equals the percentage of positive tests that are true positives (ie, individuals who do have disease). *Negative predictive values* refer to the percentage of negative tests that are true negatives (ie, individuals who do not have disease).

Application of Diagnostic Model to Pretest, Intratest, and Posttest Phases

The *pretest focus* is upon selecting the appropriate test, obtaining proper consent, assessing risk, preparing and educating the patient, providing emotional and physical support, and communicating effectively. These interventions are key to achieving desired outcomes and preventing misunderstanding and errors (FIG. 1.1).

The *intratest focus* is on managing the testing environment, collecting and handling specimens, providing supplies and equipment, using special kits, providing comfort and reassurance, preparing or administering drugs and solutions, performing or assisting during procedures, and positioning and monitoring the patient during procedures. Invasive procedures place patients at greater risk for complications and require increased vigilance and observation. Moderate sedation/analgesia (also known as conscious sedation), local and systemic anesthesia, and IV drugs administered to counteract other test medications are a frequent part of the scenario. Monitoring fluid intake and loss, body temperature, and respiratory and cardiovascular systems and treating problems in these domains require critical thinking and quick responses. A collaborative team approach to achieve patient-centered care is necessary.

The *posttest focus* is upon follow-up activities: explaining medical, pharmacologic, or surgical treatment; observing and monitoring to prevent serious complications; and implementing appropriate referrals and repeat or additional testing. Test outcome evaluation, test interpretation, counseling, documentation, reporting, and record keeping are also major components of this phase.

Pretest Care: Elements of Safe, Effective, Informed Care

Assessment Parameters

Consider the following factors:

- Age and developmental stage, pertinent health history data (eg, family history, allergies; medication history; alternative health interventions, prior surgical experiences, vision, hearing, speech,

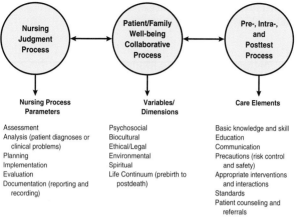

Nursing Process Parameters	Variables/ Dimensions	Care Elements
Assessment Analysis (patient diagnoses or clinical problems) Planning Implementation Evaluation Documentation (reporting and recording)	Psychosocial Biocultural Ethical/Legal Environmental Spiritual Life Continuum (prebirth to postdeath)	Basic knowledge and skill Education Communication Precautions (risk control and safety) Appropriate interventions and interactions Standards Patient counseling and referrals

**Specific Nursing Process Parameters Applied to
Pre-, Intra-, and Posttest Phases of Care**

PRETEST	INTRATEST	POSTTEST
• Assess test indications, interferences, and contraindications. • Know test terminology, and translate into language patient understands. • Identify risk-prone patients. • Develop appropriate diagnosis. • Prepare and educate patient/family. • Obtain appropriate consent. • Use standards and precautions. • Apply requisite knowledge. • Document, report, and monitor proper records. • Consider ethical and legal aspects.	• Observe standard/universal precautions and institutional policies. • Perform and assist with procedures. • Collect and transport specimens. • Provide support and reassurance • Permit family presence during procedures. • Prevent/treat complications. • Communicate and collaborate. • Monitor appropriately. • Document and report • Prepare or administer drugs and solutions	• Interpret results, evaluate outcomes if abnormal, assess compliance. • Know how to treat critical values. • Provide support for unexpected outcomes. • Monitor/teach to watch for complications. • Implement infection control plan. • Order follow-up tests at appropriate intervals, and explain posttest treatment. • Evaluate the effectiveness of managed care. • Summarize diagnostic process with documentation and reporting to patient, clinician, and others as mandated by government bodies.

This model provides specific guidelines and standardized language based on North American Nursing Diagnosis Association (NANDA) and the Nursing Intervention Classification (NIC) taxonomies.

FIGURE 1.1 A diagnostic care model for safe, effective, informed patient care.

and mobility deficits), and social history and habits (eg, drugs, smoking, alcohol, sexually transmitted diseases).
• Ability to follow instructions and cooperate in procedural protocols (eg, anxiety, mental confusion, and physical weaknesses or limitations, such as casts, immobilization, and diseases); coping

strategies, phobias, and other limitations such as cultural differences or language barriers; nutritional status (eg, special nutritive requirements—tube feeding, gastrostomy tube, IV lines, central indwelling lines); and need for information (eg, level of understanding; knowledge about condition, tests, and procedures; possible nondisclosure about tobacco, IV drug, or alcohol use; hepatitis risk status; and sexually transmitted diseases).

Factors That Influence Testing

Drugs are an important factor. The following factors may influence test outcomes:

- Prescribed medications
- Over-the-counter drugs
- Vitamins
- Minerals
- Iron preparations
- Use of herbs
- Pretest diet
- Fluid intake
- Undisclosed drug, smoking, or alcohol use
- Exposure to toxic agents

The additional factors that may confound test results are as follows:

- Stress
- Elevated anxiety levels
- Fear
- Confusion
- Improper specimen collection
- Strenuous exercise
- Age
- Gender
- Weight and body build
- Communication errors (improper labeling and/or specimen identification)
- Nondisease factors (pregnancy)
- Physical impairment
- Past illness
- Present health status
- Altered mental state
- Alternative health therapies
- Injuries
- Testing environment (many test sites have shifted into community settings)

Testing Contraindications

Assess for contraindications to testing, such as pre-existing conditions (eg, severe heart disease, pregnancy); an inability to comprehend or to follow directions, or to physically cooperate with testing; disorientation; allergies to contrast agents (eg, iodine), drugs, or latex; influence of previous testing procedures; and presence of bleeding disorders and infections.

Risk Factors

Assess for risk factors by performing a safety assessment; eliciting a history of falls, cerebrovascular accidents, fainting, neuromuscular conditions, loss of balance, and the need for ambulatory assistive devices; and identifying risk-prone patients. The following elements potentiate risk, although they do not mean incidents or complications will occur:

- Age older than 70
- Balance problems
- Paresthesias
- Weakness
- Pain
- Impaired meaning
- Illogical thinking and judgment
- Use of diuretics
- Sedatives
- Gastric motility
- History of falls
- Unsteady gait
- Fatigability
- Hearing impairment
- Visual problems
- Seizures
- Aggressive behaviors
- Analgesic use
- Drug use

Patients at risk for adverse outcomes include the following:

- *High-risk indicators:* a history of cancer, latex allergy, radiation therapy, organ transplants, HIV-related or other serious illnesses, seizure disorders, neuromuscular conditions.
- *Increased risks for infection or injury:* invasive procedures involving venous or arterial access devices, specific positioning requirements, urinary devices and catheters, endoscopes, enemas, catheters, nasogastric and other suctioning devices, conscious sedation, and analgesia. Infection and injury can occur as a result of any invasive procedure in spite of adherence to rigid protocols and careful technique.
- *Additional risk factors:* possible dehydration; altered nutrition that does not meet body requirements, caused by prolonged fasting for extensive testing; and inadequate vitamin, fluid, and mineral intake.

All of these assessment parameters are used as the basis for nurse's formulation of appropriate patient diagnoses.

Nursing Diagnoses

The most common nursing diagnoses and nurse-identified clinical problems are (1) deficient knowledge (most important), (2) risks (very important), and (3) fear and anxiety (important). Examples of these diagnoses are grouped together, followed by a listing of other appropriate diagnoses in numbers 4 to 13:

1. Deficient Knowledge
   - related to need for patient education.
   - related to lack of or a misinterpretation of a diagnostic test, purpose, and process (eg, for diabetes testing, timing of specimen collection and how it relates to disease control).
   - related to lack of understanding about test outcome abnormalities or deviations and need for lifestyle change and treatment.
2. Risks
   - related to nursing judgment about invasive procedures, adverse outcomes, complications, and patient indicators of high risk.
   - related to risk for injuries during invasive procedures (eg, IVs, arterial access); special preparation (eg, prolonged bowel preparation for a patient who is elderly, frail, and chronically ill); complex procedures (eg, cardiac catheterization); administration of radiopharmaceuticals or contrast agents; perforation; or other events.
   - related to injury pertaining to limited physical mobility and need for assistance and positioning required for many procedures.
   - related to injury about positioning requirements during some procedures.
   - related to ineffective breathing patterns associated with conscious sedation and claustrophobia fears during MRI.
   - related to latex allergy reaction as a result of the use of latex products during diagnostic procedures.
   - related to injury caused by adverse or allergic reactions to drugs and solutions used in testing.
   - related to injury from radiation exposure to multiple, repeat x-rays and fluoroscopy.
   - related to fluid volume excess from the absorption of large amounts of endoscopic irrigant fluid into the circulatory system.
   - related to impaired tissue integrity caused by extravasation or local infiltration of IV medication into surrounding tissue during a scan procedure.
   - related to decreased cardiac output as a result of the administration and systemic absorption of local anesthetic.

- related to infection from arterial, venous, or other invasive lines (eg, insult to skin integrity); endoscopic procedures; or arteriograms.

3. Fear and Anxiety
   - related to patient need for support, comfort, and counseling regarding outcomes and need for further testing and treatment.
   - related to possible need for further treatment and possible pain during the process.
   - related to memories of past invasive procedures.
   - related to separation from parents, family, or significant others during procedures.
   - related to anticipated discomfort or pain during the procedure.
   - related to medical personnel who participate in complex procedures and an unfamiliar environment.

4. Altered Family Dynamics
   - related to sense of comfort or pain.
   - related to lengthy and complicated diagnostic test regimens or life-threatening diseases.
   - related to nutrition meeting less than body requirements resulting from fasting and fluid test restrictions.
   - related to an altered sense of comfort or pain resulting from pre-existing disease, tissue trauma, biopsy, diagnostic procedure, or positioning.
   - related to anticipatory grieving over unexpected test results that may indicate serious disease.

5. Body Image
   - related to patient's need for sensitive interventions.
   - related to disturbance of body exposure during procedure, potential invasion of privacy, and embarrassment.

6. Denial
   - related to difficulty managing decisional conflict.
   - related to inability to accept negative outcome of testing.
   - related to difficulty in managing therapeutic regimen or environment caused by the lack of adequate support services.

7. Decisional Conflict
   - related to the need for individual consent.
   - related to choices among several treatment options based upon test result interpretation.

8. Discomfort
   - related to the need for relief measures.
   - related to procedures that require the patient to lie still (ie, no movement for specified lengthy periods).
   - related to physical immobility during orthoscopy.

9. Ineffective Individual Coping
   * related to the need for special consideration.
   * related to an inability to accept diagnosis of a serious disease.
10. Impaired Communication
    * related to the need for special nursing measures.
    * related to a language barrier and/or lack of an interpreter; an inability to read or understand test instructions.
    * related to denial or nonacceptance of test results or a need for lifestyle changes.
11. Ineffective Health Maintenance (Compliance, altered) to Test Protocols
    * related to nurse's judgment about reasons for inability to comply.
    * related to anxiety, confusion, weakness, denial, refusal, or inability to follow specific instructions (eg, fasting, no oral intake [NPO], and antidiabetic medications); preparation (eg, timed tests); and failure to keep appointments.
12. Potential Ineffective Health Maintenance (Compliance, altered)
    * related to nurse's judgment regarding abnormal vital signs.
    * related to sedation and impaired breathing pattern and analgesia affecting gas exchange or potential central nervous system (CNS) depression.
    * related to disbelief of abnormal test results and that follow-up treatment is needed in the absence of overt disease signs and symptoms.
13. Powerlessness
    * related to the need for regaining sense of control.
    * related to the lack of control over unfamiliar procedures, strange environment, cultural differences, or unknown diagnosis.

Planning Parameters
Include Pretest, Intratest, and Posttest Nursing Orders in the Care Plan

Consider the patient's age, language, cultural diversity, compliance, understanding, and care setting. Consider legal and ethical implications, including the patient's right to information, explanation, and instructions concerning risks, as well as the benefits of tests and properly signed and witnessed consent forms. The nurse and other clinicians have certain duties that reflect basic ethical considerations: to maintain privacy and confidentiality of information; to honor the patient's right to consent to, question, or refuse diagnostic tests; to report certain infectious diseases to governmental agencies; and to respect the dignity of the individual. The clinician who orders the test

has a responsibility to inform the patient about test results, to interpret test results, and to discuss further testing and follow-up care.
Other caregivers can provide additional information and clarification. Caregivers have the right to know the diagnoses of the patients
they care for so that they can minimize their own risks.

A properly executed consent form includes dates and witnesses,
as required. The patient's signature must be correct. A parent or
guardian signs for a minor. For patients who are not competent to
sign consent forms, an advance directive (ie, durable power of attor-
ney for health care) or living will can protect their personal health
care (including diagnostic care) and decision-making autonomy.
When incompetent patients have no advance directives, many states
have a Surrogate Act that permits a surrogate decision maker to make
treatment decisions depending on medical diagnoses (including consent forms) on behalf of patients who lack the capacity to make these
decisions. The act usually identifies the order of priority for potential
surrogates (ie, patient's guardian, spouse, children, parents, siblings,
grandparents, close friend, and estate guardian). This responsibility
is crucial for the most vulnerable patient (eg, the elderly, mentally ill,
and homeless) to protect the autonomy of these persons.

Schedule Tests and Procedures

A plan that allows the patient to maintain dignity and some control
over scheduling and participation in the process is the ideal. Fasting
screening tests are scheduled first. Procedures using contrast agents
are scheduled before nuclear scans and after blood testing work. Less
invasive tests are done before more invasive procedures (eg, ECG
before cardiac catheterization).

Serial procedures are scheduled over a period of days (eg, nuclear
scan, tumor imaging, tests for infections). Some tests reflect diurnal
activity and must be scheduled at the proper time (eg, early morning).
Collaborate with diagnostic laboratories about scheduling certain
procedures because a limited number of tests may be done in a certain day (eg, myelogram, cardiac catheterization). Some procedures
are done immediately in emergency situations and delay regularly
scheduled procedures. Planning also includes privacy for the patient,
safety, prevention of complications, and management of risks.

Intervention Parameters

Prepare Patient and Family

Provide information about the testing site, give directions for locating
the facility, and allow time to enter the facility and find the specific testing laboratory. Provide a safe environment for the patient at all times.

Because of apprehension or fears related to testing and the technical environments in which it takes place, nurses must be sensitive to patients' perceptions, concerns, fears, and anxieties and to the special needs of persons with physical limitations or disabilities, ostomies, and diabetes, children, the elderly, and the culturally diverse.

Facilitate Family Presence During Procedures

Involving family members in the diagnostic care process has helped families by including them as active participants. Their presence may provide the opportunity to calm the patient, offer additional comfort to the patient, and reduce anxiety and fear. However, some families may find the option of observing procedures to be distressing or uncomfortable; other patients may not want family members present. Nurses acting as patient advocates recognize the importance of supporting the patient's need for reassurance and the family's need and right to be present during diagnostic procedures.

Provide Culturally Competent Care

Do not stereotype or judge patients according to a personal frame of reference. Cultural behavior is learned, not inborn, and develops out of a necessity for survival and acceptance in the cultural group. Poverty is a problem of all cultures. Many characteristic responses that are described as cultural limitations are actually the consequence of poverty (eg, seeking medical care late). Solving these problems may be a question of locating adequate financial sources rather than overcoming cultural influences.

Many cultures have diverse beliefs about diagnostic testing that requires blood sampling. For example, alarm about having a blood specimen drawn or concerns regarding the disposal of body fluids or tissue may require health care workers to demonstrate the utmost patience, sensitivity, and tact when communicating information about blood tests.

Consider biocultural variables when interpreting test results. Examples of physiologic differences that occur as a result of biocultural processes and their interpretation follow:

Orthopedic x-rays: African Americans have longer arms and legs and shorter trunks than Caucasians. African-American women have wider shoulders and narrower hips but have more abdominal adipose tissue than Caucasian women. Caucasian men exhibit more abdominal adipose tissue than African-American men. Native Americans and Asians have larger trunks and shorter limbs than African Americans and Caucasians. Asians tend to have wider hips and narrower shoulders.

Bone density measurements: The greatest bone density occurs in African-American men, African-American women, and Caucasian men. Caucasian women have the least-dense bones. Persons of Chinese, Japanese, and Eskimo ethnicity (men and women) have bone densities that are less than those of Caucasian Americans. Bone density decreases with age.

Cholesterol levels: At birth, African Americans and Caucasians have similar cholesterol levels, but during childhood, African Americans develop higher cholesterol levels. African-American adults, however, have lower cholesterol levels than Caucasian adults.

Hemoglobin and hematocrit levels: The normal hemoglobin level for African Americans is 1 g lower than for other groups. Given similar socioeconomic conditions, Asian Americans and Mexican Americans have higher hemoglobin and hematocrit levels than Caucasians.

Individualize Patient Education

Place special emphasis on patient education. Children, adolescents, and older, frail adults should be approached in a manner different from that of the average adult. Growth, developmental stages, and cognitive levels must be considered. Children, adolescents, or adults may have heard "horror stories" from peers. Preconceived perceptions frequently influence reactions to the total testing experience.

All patients require honest, simple, easily understood explanations; nurturance; active participation; and respect for identity and body image. Listening well is paramount to effective communication. Give accurate and precise instructions according to the patient's level of understanding and condition. Avoid medical jargon. Ascertain communication barriers (eg, impairments of cognition, language, hearing, or vision). Provide sensory and objective information about the test. Talk about the process, sensations that might be felt, equipment used, noises, anticipated length of procedure, personnel present, and physical environment. Develop "listening eyes and ears." Reinforce information about the diagnostic process, time frames, and the patient's role in testing and use resource people when necessary.

Legal and Ethical Implications

Consider the following legal and ethical implications:

- "Chain of custody" is a legal term descriptive of a procedure to ensure specimen integrity from collection to transport to receipt to analysis and specimen storage. A special form is used to provide a written record.

- The right to informed consent before certain tests and procedures pertains to patient autonomy, the ethical right of self-determination, the legal right to be free of procedures to which one does not consent, and to determine what will be done to one's own person. Risks, benefits, and alternatives are explained and written consent is obtained well in advance of the procedure.

- The patient must demonstrate appropriate cognitive and reasoning faculties to sign a legally valid consent. Conversely, a patient may not legally give consent while under the immediate influence of sedation, anesthetic agents, or certain classes of analgesics and tranquilizers. If the patient cannot validly and legally sign a consent form, an appropriately qualified individual may give consent for the patient.

- Guidelines and wishes set forth in advance directives or "living will"–type documents must be honored, especially in life-threatening situations. Such directives may prevent more sophisticated invasive procedures from being performed. Some states have legislated that patients can procure do-not-resuscitate (DNR) orders and medical DNR bracelets that indicate their wishes. A copy of a patient's advance directives in the health care record can be helpful in unpredictable situations.

- A collaborative team approach is essential for responsible, lawful, and ethical, patient-focused care. The clinician who orders the test has a responsibility to inform the patient about risks and test results and to discuss alternatives for follow-up care. Other caregivers, including the nurse, can provide additional information and clarification and can support the patient and the family in achieving the best possible outcomes.

- The duty to maintain confidentiality, to provide freedom of choice, and to report infectious diseases may result in ethical dilemmas. Recently, the Health Insurance Portability and Accountability Act (HIPAA) set forth regulations regarding patient confidentiality. HIPAA addresses protected health information (PHI) as any information, whether oral, written, electronic, magnetic, or recorded in any form, that is received or created by a health care provider; relates to the patient's past, present, or future health care treatment; identifies the patient (eg, name, Social Security number, medical record number); or can be used to identify a patient. HIPAA also provides rights to the patient (eg, right to request, amend, correct, restrict, or limit his or her PHI).

- Respect for the dignity of the individual reflects basic ethical considerations. Patients and family have a right to consent, to question, to request opinions, and to refuse diagnostic tests. Conversely,

caregivers have the right to know the diagnoses of the patients they care for so that they can minimize the risks to themselves.
• Patients have a right to a correct and proper diagnosis and prognosis.

🖊 Intratest Care: Elements of Safe, Effective, Informed Care

Collect Samples for Testing and Assist With or Conduct Certain Diagnostic Procedures

The most commonly collected specimens are blood, urine, stool, saliva, and sputum. Chapter 2 provides the specific techniques of specimen collection and handling. Types of assisted procedures include endoscopy, lumbar puncture, and cardiac catheterization. Diagnostic procedures the nurse often performs independently include Pap smears, centrifugation of blood samples, ECGs, breathing tests, and pulse oximetry. (See Chapter 3, Procedures.)

Institute Infection Control

Use special measures and sterile techniques as appropriate. It is important to identify patients at risk for infection, to prevent skin and tissue infections, to use aseptic technique as needed, and to institute strict respiratory and contact isolation as necessary. The nurse must ensure proper collection, transport, and receipt of specimens and use properly cleaned instruments. The Appendix offers more information on standard or universal precautions for safe practice and infection control and isolation. These precautions direct all persons exposed to body fluids and tissues to protect themselves and assume that every direct contact is potentially infectious from any person—living or dead (eg, blood, tissue, and other body fluids, specimens, and cultures are designated as potentially infectious).

Use Required Kits, Equipment, and Supplies

• Use special kits and containers for obtaining many specimens: for heelsticks and fingersticks, blood alcohol saliva, or oral fluid and urine specimens. Do not use a package if you notice a defect (eg, moisture, pinholes, tears). Do not use kit or specimen supplies more than once (eg, finger- or urine strips). If the glucometer does not produce a response or urine dipstick does not change colors, gather new materials and begin the test over.
• Use tape with caution, especially when skin integrity can be easily compromised in the frail, elderly patient.

- Provide proper urine containers for specimens obtained at home.
- Require, in some instances, the operation of special equipment, such as video monitors for endoscopic procedures.
- Use barrier drapes as directed. For example, arthroscopy drapes are positioned with the fluid control pouch at the knee or during catheterizations when collecting urine samples.
- Use and maintain aseptic technique during certain procedures (eg, cystoscopy, bone marrow biopsy).

Position for Procedures

Proper positioning involves placing the patient in the best possible position for the procedure and aligning the body correctly for optimal respiratory and circulatory function. These include the jackknife, prone, lithotomy, sitting, supine, and Trendelenburg positions. Using positioning devices, arranging padding, and repositioning the patient are important measures to prevent skin pressure and skin breakdown. The potential adverse effects of various positions, especially during lengthy procedures, include skin breakdown, venous compression, sciatic nerve injury, muscle injury, and low back strain, among others. Necessary positioning skills include ensuring that the patient's airway, IV lines, and monitoring devices are not compromised and identifying those at potential risk for injury (eg, elderly, thin, frail, or unconscious patients) before positioning. If wounds, skin breakdown, abrasions, or bruises are present, accurately document their presence and location before the procedure.

Administer Drugs and Solutions

All drugs and solutions administered during diagnostic procedures are given according to accepted practices. Drugs are given by mouth, rectally, intranasally, by intubation, by injection (IV, IM, or subcutaneously), and by local or topical skin applications. IV fluids and endoscopic irrigating fluids are also commonly administered.

Recognize the potential for adverse reactions. Before the procedure begins, confirm previous drug reactions with the patient. Risks for injury are related to hypersensitivity, allergic or toxic reactions, drug-drug reactions, impaired drug tolerance caused by liver or kidney disease, extravasation of IV fluids, and absorption of irrigating fluids into the systemic circulation. Required skills include managing airways and breathing patterns; monitoring fluid intake and loss; monitoring body, skin, and core temperature; and observing the effects of sedation and analgesia (eg, vital signs, skin inspection for rashes, edema). The primary drugs used for moderate procedural sedation and analgesia include the benzodiazepines and opiates. The most commonly used drugs include diazepam (Valium), midazolam (Versed), lorazepam (Ativan), meperidine (Demerol), fentanyl (Sublimaze), morphine, and ketamine (Ketalar). Diphenhydramine HCl (Benedryl) can be used for sedation or allergic reactions. Some of these drugs work as CNS depressants and therefore may be contraindicated in certain conditions.

Manage the Environment

The main goal of environmental control is safe practice to ensure that the patient is free from injury related to environmental hazards and is free from discomfort. Be attentive to temperature and air quality; the patient's temperature; exposure to radiation, latex, and noxious odors; room signage; infection control; and sanitation and cleanliness.

Remember to:

- Take latex and rubber allergy precautions.
- Eliminate or modify sensory stimuli (eg, noise, odors, sounds).
- Post a PATIENT AWAKE sign if the patient is awake during a procedure.
- Be sensitive to conversation among team members in the presence of the patient. At best, it can be annoying to the patient; at worst, it may be misinterpreted and have far-reaching negative effects and consequences.
- Assess, treat, and document a patient's pain and discomfort, nausea, and vomiting. Use a pain scale, when appropriate, as an indication of how well the patient is responding to pain management treatment. Follow safe practice precautions.

Posttest Care: Elements of Safe, Effective, Informed Care

The focus of the posttest phase is on patient aftercare and follow-up activities, observations, documentation, and monitoring necessary to prevent or minimize complications. Recently, there have been tremendous strides made in the area of *translational medicine*, sometimes referred to as "bench to bedside." Translational medicine has its basis in disciplines such as "proteomics," "oncogenomics," and "pharmacogenomics," as well as other cutting-edge diagnostic technologies. *Proteomics* is the analysis and identification of proteins in biological samples. These disease-associated proteins can be used as biomarkers and have the potential to change the way we approach patient treatment and care. *Oncogenomic* molecular profiling, or gene sequencing as it relates to cancers, and *pharmacogenomics*, the genetics of drug interactions, all have the potential to be used in the area of "personalized" medicine. Evaluation of outcomes and effectiveness of care, follow-up counseling, discharge planning, and appropriate posttest referrals are the major components of this phase. It has been shown that verbal and nonverbal behaviors by the clinician can have either a positive impact or a negative impact on patient compliance with recommendations and treatment plans. Positive verbal behaviors include empathy, reassurance, courtesy, and clarification. Positive nonverbal behaviors include head nodding, direct focus on the patient, and body orientation. Behaviors that should be avoided include being dominant or inattentive.

Evaluate Diagnostic Care

The nurse will:

- Incorporate EBP into his or her clinical assessment.
- Measure progress toward established goals or anticipated outcomes and identify unexpected or abnormal test outcomes. Nursing-sensitive outcomes are neutral concepts, indicators that describe patient outcomes influenced by nursing interventions that relate to the nursing diagnosis. For example, for the diagnosis of anxiety and apprehension about remaining in the MR scanner for the total required time, based on the patient's prior indication of claustrophobia, patient status outcomes for anxiety would be anxiety controlled or coping successfully to measure coping outcomes. The specific indicators are that the patient uses effective strategies, such as breathing techniques. Nursing interventions are as follows: use anxiety control measures and teach breathing techniques. A goal (outcome) may be that the patient can tolerate the diagnostic procedure to its completion. A goal statement may be general or may include specific indicators. Outcomes must be subjectively or objectively measurable. They can be adjusted or modified to reflect what is realistic regarding an outcome (eg, MRI will be repeated in an open scanner at another facility).
- Compare the current and previous test results. Employ the proper sequence of data gathering from records. Review the most recent data first to determine the current status of patient and then work backward to evaluate trends or changes from previous data.
- Modify nursing interventions accordingly when unexpected or abnormal outcomes or critical values occur (eg, positive culture results, abnormal test results for newborns, high or low potassium levels).

- Report to and collaborate with other clinicians and employers when the plan of care needs to be modified or when changes in medical care management may be necessary as a result of test outcomes.
- Document as mandated by licensure regulations and institutional policies.
- Evaluate outcomes using the following steps:
  1. Encourage the patient to take as much control of the situation as possible.
  2. Recognize that the different stages of behavioral responses to negative results may last several weeks or longer.
  3. Monitor changes in patient affect, mood behaviors, and motivation. Do not assume that persons who initially have a negative perception of their health (eg, denial of diabetes) will not be able to integrate better health behaviors into daily life once they accept the diagnosis.
  4. Use the following strategies to lessen the impact of a life-threatening prognosis:
     - Offer appropriate comfort measures.
     - Allow the patient to work through feelings of anxiety and depression. At the appropriate time, reassure the patient that these feelings and emotions are normal initially. Be more of a therapeutic listener than a talker.
     - Assist the patient and family in making necessary lifestyle and self-concept adjustments through education, support groups, and other means. Emphasize that risk factors associated with certain diseases can be reduced through lifestyle changes. Be realistic.

Examples of expected and unexpected test outcomes follow:

EXPECTED OUTCOMES	UNEXPECTED OUTCOMES
Anticipated outcomes will be achieved.	Some anticipated outcomes may not be achieved. Reasons may be related to specific patient behaviors that interfere with care interventions (eg, a patient does not appear for testing appointment, did not fast or withhold medications as directed before testing, did not return for TB skin test reading).

The patient and the family should be able to describe the testing process and purpose, and the patient should be able to properly perform expected activities. Information contributes to empowerment.

If test outcomes are abnormal, the patient will make appropriate lifestyle changes and adopt healthy behaviors.

The patient does not develop complications; he or she remains free from injury.

Should complications occur, they will be optimally resolved.

Anxiety and fears will be alleviated and will not interfere with the testing process. The patient is helped to balance fears with recognition of potential for developing coping skills.

With support and education, the patient is able to cope with test outcomes revealing a chronic or life-threatening disease. Hope is inspired and generated, and the patient feels "cared for."

Inability to fully participate in the teaching/learning process as evidenced by verbal and nonverbal cues. Inability to properly perform expected activities. Misinterpretation and misinformation of diagnostic process results in panic, avoidance behaviors, and refusal to have tests done.

Nonadherence with test preparation guidelines and posttest recommended lifestyle changes. Hides test results or minimizes or exaggerates the meaning of test outcomes.

The patient exhibits untoward signs and symptoms (eg, allergic response, shock, bleeding, nausea, vomiting, or retention of barium).

Complications are not fully resolved; the health state is compromised; there is a need for more extensive testing and care.

Because of anxiety, fear, and uncertainty, the patient is unable to collect specimens properly or accurately comply with procedure steps. The nurse is unable to calm and reassure the patient. Invasive tests may be canceled if the patient is too anxious or fearful.

The patient exhibits a lack of appropriate problem-solving behaviors, uncertainty and/or denial about test outcomes, an inability to cope with test outcomes, extreme depression, and abnormal patterns of responses; refuses to take control of the situation or to cooperate with prescribed regimens. Anxiety, grief, and/or guilt and the social stigma of illness persist. The patient uses alcohol or drugs. Caregivers are seen as uncaring.

Refer and Treat

Referrals for further testing and beginning treatment are a part of the collaborative process. For example, the nurse practitioner refers patients with abnormal Pap smears to the specialist for a colposcopy or biopsy. When abnormal blood glucose testing indicates diabetes, the clinician contacts specialists for further evaluation and medical management, including the dietician for nutritional assessment. The clinician refers the parent to the dietician for dietary therapy for genetic disorders, such as phenylketonuria (PKU), in the newborn.

Initiate Posttesting Modalities

- Ensure patient safety by monitoring for complications and other risks. The most common complications after invasive procedures are bleeding, infection, respiratory difficulties, perforation of organs, and adverse effects of conscious sedation and local anesthesia. Watch for signs and symptoms related to these such as redness, swelling, signs of skin irritation, pain or tenderness, dyspnea, abnormal breath sounds, cyanosis, decreased or increased pulse rate, abnormal blood pressure, signs of laryngospasm, agitation or combative behavior, pallor, and complaints of dizziness. If adverse reactions or events occur, contact the physician immediately and initiate treatment as soon as possible.
- Take special safety measures and precautions when contrast agents such as iodine are given, when barium has been used, when latex rubber products are used, or when moderate procedural sedation and analgesia have been administered.
- Follow established agency protocols for discharge to home after testing is completed. For complex procedures that are invasive or require sedation, be certain that a responsible individual escorts the patient home. Provide specific instructions regarding infection control, barium elimination, iodine sensitivity, resumption of pretest activities, and diet.
- Intervene promptly when critical (panic) laboratory values are too high or too low. The health care professional reviews records for any sudden change in values that may also signal alarm (eg, new diagnoses of leukemia, sickle cell anemia, aplastic crisis). Critical laboratory values represent serious medical conditions that may be life threatening unless immediate actions are taken. Notification and collaboration with the clinician and other members of the health care team must take place when critical values are identified so that prompt treatment can begin (eg, a blood glucose level <70 or >300 mg/dL [<4 or >17 mmol/L]; an increased bleeding time [>15 minutes]; a hemoglobin <7.0 or >20 g/dL

[<70 or >200 g/L]; a brown to black-gray urine upon standing, with an increasing pH value; or elevated digoxin >2.00 mg/mL [>2.6 mmol/L]).

Provide Discharge Planning and Follow-up Counseling

• Frequently, patients are discharged with unresolved medical problems and unscheduled follow-up tests and postdischarge appointments with their physician. It is important to schedule these appointments with and/or for the patient upon discharge, as it has been shown that this can decrease these appointment times by up to 23%.*

• Counsel the patient regarding test outcomes and their implications for further testing, treatment, and possible lifestyle changes. Provide time for the patient to ask questions and voice concerns regarding the entire testing process.

• Test outcome interpretation involves reassessment of interfering factors and patient adherence if test outcomes significantly deviate from normal and previous results.

• Recognize that no test is perfect; however, the greater the degree of abnormality indicated by the test result, the more likely that this outcome deviation is significant or represents a real disorder.

• Notify the patient about test results after consultation with the clinician. Treatment may be delayed if test results are misplaced or not communicated in a timely manner.

• Help patients interpret the results of community-based testing.

• Identify differences in the patient's view of the situation, the clinician's viewpoint about tests and disease, and the health care team's perceptions.

• Be sensitive to the implications of genetic or metabolic disorders. Realize that genetic counseling should be provided by a specially trained person. Informing the patient or family regarding the genetic defect requires special training in genetic science, family coping skills, and an understanding of legal and ethical issues. Confidentiality and privacy of information are vital.

• Be familiar with crisis intervention skills for patients who experience difficulty dealing with the posttest phase, abnormal test results, or confirmation of disease or illness.

*Adapted from Greenwald, J. L., Denham, C. R., & Jack, B. W. (2007). The hospital discharge: A review of a high risk care transition with highlights of a reengineered discharge process. *Journal of Patient Safety, 3*(2), 97–106.

- Encourage the patient to take as much control of the situation as possible.
- Recognize that the different stages of behavioral responses to negative or abnormal results may last several weeks or longer (see the following text).

Immediate Response	Secondary Response
Acute emotional turmoil, shock, disbelief about diagnosis, denial, bargaining, acceptance	Insomnia, anorexia, difficulty concentrating, depression, difficulty in performing work-related responsibilities and tasks
Anxiety will usually last several days until the person assimilates the information.	Depression may last several weeks as the person begins to incorporate the information and to participate realistically in a treatment plan and lifestyle adaptation.

- Monitor changes in patient motivation. Do not assume that a person who initially has a negative perception of his or her health (eg, denial of the seriousness of diabetes) will not be able to integrate better health behaviors into daily life.
- Isolation or quarantine may be used under certain circumstances in an effort to protect the public. *Isolation* refers to the separation of the infected individual who is ill from those individuals who are healthy, whereas *quarantine* is the separation and restriction of movement of the individual who may have been exposed to an infectious agent but is not ill. (*Note:* State regulations regarding mandatory quarantine vary widely, and in some cases can result in a criminal misdemeanor if violated by the individual.)

Documentation and Reporting Parameters

The patient's health care record is the only way to validate the need for diagnostic care, the quality and type of care given, and the patient's response to the care and to ensure that current standards of medical and nursing care and diagnostic testing are being met. The medical record may also be the basis for reimbursement for diagnostic tests by government (Medicare) or private insurance programs. Accuracy, completeness, objectivity, and legibility are of utmost importance in the documentation process.

Documentation for laboratory and diagnostic testing includes recording all pretest, intratest, and posttest care:

- Indicate the time, day, month, and year of entries. This information can assume great importance in the office or clinic setting. Enter appropriate assessment data and note the patient's concerns and questions that help define the nursing diagnoses and focus for care planning. Document specific teaching and preparation of the patient before the procedure. Avoid generalizations.
- When an interpreter is present, document his or her name and relationship to the patient. Record that patient consent to give confidential test information through an interpreter was obtained before actually revealing the information. Record any deviations from basic witnessed consent policies (eg, illiteracy, non–English-speaking client, sedation immediately before the request for a consent signature, consent by telephone) and include nurse measures employed to obtain appropriate consent for the procedure.
- Record that the preparation, side effects, expected results, and interfering factors have been explained. Document the information given and the patient's response to that information. Keep a record of all printed and written instructions. Record medications, treatments, food and fluids, intake status, beginning and end of specimen collection, and procedure times, outcomes, and patient condition during all phases of diagnostic care. If the patient does not appear for testing, document this fact and include any follow-up discussion with the patient. Completely and clearly describe side effects, symptoms, adverse reactions, or complications along with follow-up care and instructions for posttest care and monitoring.
- Record a patient's refusal to undergo diagnostic tests. Note the reasons, using the patient's own words if possible. Document significant nonadherent behaviors such as refusal or inability to fast, restrict or increase fluid or food intake, incomplete timed specimens, inadequate or improperly self-collected specimens, and missed or canceled test appointments. Place copies of letters sent to the patient in his or her chart.
- Notify patients regarding test outcomes in a timely fashion and document that the patient or family has been notified regarding test results. Document follow-up patient education and counseling.
- Report results to designated professionals. Report critical values immediately and document to whom results were reported, orders received, and urgent treatments initiated. Also, report *vital values*, laboratory results that although outside of the reference range may not be life threatening but could have an adverse affect on the patient.

- Report all communicable diseases to appropriate agencies.
- Report and document situations that are mandatory by state statute (eg, suspected elder abuse and child abuse, as evidenced by x-rays).

Reportable Diseases and Conditions

The nurse reports a single case of a disease of known or unknown origin that may be a danger to the public health. Unusual manifestations of a communicable disease are also reportable to the local health department. An outbreak of a disease of known or unknown origin that may be a danger to the public health is reported immediately by telephone or electronic means (Display 1.1).

As an example, the Annotated Code of Maryland, Health-General Article § 18-205, requires the director of a medical laboratory to submit a report to the health officer for the county where the laboratory is located within 48 hours after an examination of a specimen shows any evidence of being a communicable disease or condition. The report should include the date, type, and result of the test; the name, age, sex, and residence address of the patient from whom the specimen was taken; and the name and address of the physician who requested the test. For reports of HIV infection, the report should include the unique patient identifying number; age, sex, and ZIP code of the residence address of the patient; and the name and address of the physician.

Conclusion and Importance of Communication

Nurses engage with people not so unlike themselves in many ways. These individuals present with their perceptions of what the diagnostic process and their illnesses mean to them and their loved ones. When nurses see patients in the context of what the patient and loved ones are experiencing (eg, their situational needs, expectations, previous experiences, and the environment in which they live), only then can they offer meaningful support and care. When patients feel that the nurse is on their side, they will have an increased sense of control.

Negative communication by caregivers is often experienced by patients as an uncaring attitude and results in a sense of discouragement. As caregivers and patient advocates, nurses must go beyond a superficial level and try to "take on the mind" of another. They must be willing to show sympathy and empathy. Identifying with the patient's point of view leads to a more profound level of communication. The

DISPLAY 1.1 Diseases and Conditions Reportable by Health Care Providers

AIDS and symptomatic HIV infection*
Amebiasis
Anaplasmosis
Animal bites[†]
Anthrax[†]
Arboviral (checklist)
Babesiosis
Botulism[†]
Brucellosis[†]
Campylobacter infection
Chancroid
Chlamydia infection
Cholera[†]
Coccidioidomycosis
Creutzfeldt-Jakob disease
Cryptosporidiosis
Cyclosporiasis
Dengue fever[†]
Diphtheria[†]
E. coli 0157:H7 infection[†]
Ehrlichiosis
Encephalitis
Epsilon toxin of *Clostridium perfringens*
Giardiasis
Glanders
Gonococcal infection
Haemophilus influenzae, invasive disease
Hantavirus infection[†]
Harmful algal bloom related illness

Hemolytic uremic syndrome, postdiarrheal
Hepatitis, viral (A, B, C, and other types undetermined)*
HIV infection*
Influenza-associated pediatric mortality
Influenza, novel influenza A virus infection[†]
Isosporiasis
Kawasaki syndrome
Legionellosis[†]
Leprosy
Leptospirosis
Lyme disease
Malaria
Measles (rubeola)[†]
Meningitis (infectious)
Meningococcal, invasive disease[†]
Mumps (infectious parotitis)
Mycobacteriosis, other than tuberculosis and leprosy
Pertussis[†]
Pertussis vaccine adverse reactions
Plague[†]
Pneumonia in a health care worker resulting in hospitalization
Poliomyelitis[†]
Psittacosis
Q-fever[†]
Rabies[†]

Ricin toxin[†]
Rocky Mountain spotted fever
Rubella (German measles) and congenital rubella syndrome[†]
Salmonellosis (nontypical)
Septicemia in newborns
Severe acute respiratory syndrome (SARS)[†]
Shiga-like toxin producing enteric bacterial infections
Shigellosis
Smallpox and other orthopoxvirus infections[†]
Staphylococcal enterotoxin B[†]
Streptococcal invasive disease Group A and Group B
Streptococcus pneumoniae invasive disease
Syphilis
Tetanus
Trichinosis
Tuberculosis and suspected tuberculosis[†]
Tularemia[†]
Typhoid fever (case, carrier, or both, of *Salmonella typhi*)[†]

(display continues on page 46)

DISPLAY 1.1 (continued)		
Varicella (chickenpox), fatal cases only	Vibriosis, noncholera types Viral hemorrhagic fevers (all types)[†]	Yellow fever[†] Yersiniosis

From State of Maryland Department of Health and Mental Hygiene. Epidemiology and Disease Control Program (reviewed: December 2008).

*Diseases and conditions reportable by those personnel listed in State of Maryland Department of Health and Mental Hygiene, Epidemiology and Disease Control Program, and in occurrence to the programs' policies and procedures.

[†]Reportable immediately by telephone.

diagnostic care nursing model is an effective method for providing safe, effective, informed care throughout all phases of the diagnostic process, including the sensitive communications necessary for a therapeutic relationship to occur.

The cardinal rule for communicating with and educating patients and families is to recognize at all times that the patient operates within distinct physiologic, psychological, emotional, and spiritual parameters that unite to make this person a unique, holistic, human being. The use of the nursing process enables the nurse to better discern those characteristics that define each patient's desires, concerns, and care needs during diagnostic evaluation.

2

Nursing Standards and Protocols for Specimen Collection

The Nurse's Role

Nursing Practice Standard

The nurse should follow proper procedures and guidelines for collecting, handling, and transporting specimens, at the same time being cognizant of standard precautions and sterile techniques. Nursing interventions include collecting proper specimen amounts, using appropriate containers and media, processing specimens correctly, and storing and transporting specimens within specified time lines. Explaining procedures to the patient or family in appropriate terminology, taking into account cultural background, developmental level, and socioeconomic factors, normally elicits cooperation and understanding of the collection process and procedures within the pretest, intratest, and posttest periods.

Overview of Nursing Responsibilities

The nurse's role varies according to the specimen type, test purpose, patient age and gender, health status, and clinical setting. Specific protocols for nursing are governed by the setting in which the testing is done. Appropriate skills and practical methods for educating patients and coordinating teamwork are necessary for smooth functioning. Specimens collected can include blood, urine, stool, sputum, oral fluids, tissue, hair, and nails. Adherence to principles, protocols, and standards related to specimen collection prevents invalid test results, specimen rejection, and patient injury and mitigates health hazards because of excessive blood draws, infection, and psychological stress.

Recently, with the introduction and use of *interpretive reports*, especially in the primary care area, instances of misinterpretation (health care provider has received correct laboratory values but does not take correct action) of results have been reduced. Interpretive reports often provide an explanation or reason for an abnormal result, along with suggestions for additional testing and the need for immediate treatment or follow-up. These types of reports are often used in conjunction with toxicology, endocrinology, and hematology test results. The use of interpretive reports has been shown to improve patient care and outcome.

Nursing Interventions
Interfering Factors

- Actions that may interfere with accurate test results include incorrect specimen amounts and collection, improper handling and labeling, wrong preservative or lack of preservative, delayed delivery, improper storage (eg, improper temperature or container) or transport of the specimen, clotting of whole-blood specimens or hemolysis of blood, incomplete specimen collection, and incorrect or incomplete patient preparation.
- Other factors that can alter test results include pretest diet; pregnancy; time of day; age and gender; drug and alcohol ingestion history; plasma volume; past and present illness or current health status; incomplete patient knowledge, understanding, or compliance; body position or activity at the time of specimen collection; physical or emotional stress; noncompliance (not following pretest instructions); and fasting or nonfasting status.

Preparation of the Patient

- Proper preparation of the patient is crucial for obtaining accurate test results. Fasting, special diets, activity restrictions, withholding of selected medications, or other special preparations are some pretest phase components. When in doubt about withholding medication, confer with the laboratory staff and the patient's physician.
- Isolation precautions must be observed when necessary. Mandatory standard precautions must prevail at all times.

Legal Implications Related to Specimen Collection

- The patient's right to information includes knowing the purpose, risks, and outcome of the test. A properly signed and witnessed consent form may be required. Drug abuse testing involves unique protocols. For instance, legal *chain of custody* may be required to protect the specimen for drug testing. This means that each time the specimen is transferred, the person receiving it becomes the documented holder of the specimen and therefore becomes responsible for the specimen's integrity. It may be necessary to verify the patient's identity by photograph for validation before collecting the specimen and at every other stage of the process.

Ethical Implications
- Confidentiality must be maintained. This becomes especially relevant when obtaining specimens for HIV testing or genomic studies (gene sequencing). Reporting certain infectious diseases to state and federal centers for disease control may be mandatory, even if the patient objects. (See Chapter 1 for ethical considerations and reporting standards for special circumstances.)

Safety Measures
- Patient safety and well-being should be optimized by preventing or detecting complications. Before and after testing, the patient's behavior, complaints, appearance, and degree of compliance should be observed and documented. Nurses also are at risk for infection when procuring, handling, and processing specimens and need to observe standard precautions. Protocols for dealing with spillage need to be clearly stated. Other issues to consider are electrical and fire safety, proper use of supplies, equipment, handling of radioactive materials, and disposition of biohazard materials and sharps.

Infection Control and Standard Precautions
- Standard precautions are always followed according to government Occupational Health and Safety Act (OSHA) standards. Appropriate protective clothing and personal protective equipment (PPE) must be used. (The Appendix provides the guidelines for standard precautions.) Isolation precautions should be followed according to the type of infection identified or suspected per hospital and governmental regulations (eg, the Centers for Disease Control and Prevention [CDC]). The importance of proper hand-washing cannot be overemphasized.

Storage and Transportation of Specimens
- Routines for specimen collection, processing, handling, temperature storage, and transportation may vary depending on agency protocols and clinical settings. The primary objectives in the storage and transport of diagnostic specimens are to maintain the integrity of the sample and to minimize hazards to the specimen handlers. Specimens should be collected and transported as quickly as possible (within 2 hours is recommended). The nurse must follow instructions carefully.

Immediate Specimen Transport
- After the specimen is collected, it should be placed in a biohazard bag and transported to the laboratory immediately for prompt processing and analysis to prevent specimen deterioration. If the blood sample cannot be transported to the laboratory in a reasonable

time, the blood can be centrifuged to prevent deterioration of the specimen, or refrigerated or placed on ice. Consult with laboratory personnel for proper storage and temperature.

- Unacceptable specimens lead to increased costs and wasted time for everyone concerned, including the third-party payer. Exposure to sunlight, warming, cooling, and air or other substances can all alter specimen integrity. "STAT" tests should always be hand-carried to the laboratory, processed immediately, and documented as such in the health care record.

Transport From Nonacute Care Settings to the Laboratory

- As the trend shifts toward specimen collection in the community, nursing home, clinics, physician offices, and private home care environments, the nurse working in these areas needs to be aware of the procedures and protocols for specimen collection, handling, transport, and, in some cases, actual specimen measurement, that is, point-of-care testing (POCT). The movement toward POCT is an effort to expand and improve the quality of care, health outcomes, and cost-effectiveness.
- The specimen should be placed in a biohazard bag. Include clearly written instructions and specific directions to the laboratory.
- Specimens are also often mailed or transported to specialty laboratories in other areas. To avoid delays in analysis and in reporting the results, follow specific instructions and label correctly.
- Exact time frames must be observed.

Transport to Special Laboratories

- When shipping specimens to specialty laboratories, place the specimen in a securely closed, leak-proof, nonbreakable container such as a test tube, vial, or other appropriate receptacle (ie, primary container). Enclose this primary container within a second, durable, leak-proof container (ie, secondary container). Together, these primary and secondary containers should then be enclosed in a sturdy, strong, outer shipping container.
- Appropriately label biologic and tissue agents or biomedical material. If the package becomes damaged or leaks in transit, the carrier is required by federal regulations to isolate the package and to notify the Biohazards Control Office of the CDC in Atlanta, GA. The carrier must also notify the sender. Understandably, this can cause a significant delay in medical diagnosis and treatment.
- Regulations regarding the mode of shipping or packaging, whether domestic or international, change frequently. Check with the laboratory for the most recent guidelines.

CLINICAL ALERT

- Code of federal regulations governing the shipment of biologic agents, S72.2: *Transportation of diagnostic specimens, biologic or etiologic products, and other materials; minimum packaging requirements:* "No person may knowingly transport or cause to be transported in interstate traffic, directly or indirectly, any material, including but not limited to, diagnostic specimens and biologic products that such person reasonably believes may contain an etiologic agent unless such material is packaged to withstand leakage of contents, shocks, pressure changes, and other conditions incident to ordinary handling in transport."

Examples of special laboratory requirements for transporting, packaging, and mailing of specific specimens follow:

SPECIMEN	CAUTIONS FOR PACKAGING AND MAILING
Routine urinalysis of random, mid-stream specimen	Preferred transport container is a plastic, yellow screw-top tube that contains a tablet that preserves any formed element (eg, crystals, casts, cells) and prevents alteration of chemical constituents caused by bacterial overgrowth. Pour urine into the tube, cap the tube securely, and invert to dissolve the tablet.
Urine culture	Use a culture and sensitivity transport kit containing a sterile plastic tube and transfer device for collection. This tube contains a special urine maintenance formula that prevents rapid multiplication of bacteria in the urine. Pour the urine specimen into the tube and seal properly.
Urine for calcium, magnesium, and oxalate	Use acid-washed plastic containers for collection and transport of the specimen. If urine pH is >4, the results may be inaccurate. Do not collect urine in metal-based containers such as metal bedpans or urinals.
Blood for trace metals	Observe contamination control in sample collection. Most blood tubes are contaminated with trace metals; all plastic syringes with black rubber seals contain aluminum, varying amounts of zinc, and all heavy

(continued)

SPECIMEN	CAUTIONS FOR PACKAGING AND MAILING
	metals (eg, lead, mercury, cadmium, nickel, chromium). The trace metal sample should be collected first—once the needle has punctured the rubber stopper, it is contaminated and should *not* be used for trace metal collection. Use ChloraPrep (chlorhexidine gluconate) to clean skin; avoid iodine-containing disinfectants; use only stainless steel phlebotomy needles. Blood for serum testing of trace elements should be collected in a royal blue–top (sodium heparin anticoagulant) trace element blood collection tube. After collecting and centrifuging, place in a 5-mL metal-free, screw-capped polypropylene vial; do not use a pipette to transfer serum to the container. Cap vial tightly, attach specimen label, and send to laboratory cooled or frozen. All specimens that are stored for more than 48 hours should be frozen and sent on dry ice. (Depending on geographic location, keep the specimen cool with *frozen* coolant in April–October and *refrigerated* coolant in November–March.)
Frozen specimen	If a delay of more than 4 days is anticipated before specimen examination, freezing the specimen is preferred. Place the specimen in a plastic vial (not glass). The container should not be more than three-fourth full to allow for expansion when frozen. Store in the freezer or on dry ice until specimen is picked up by a carrier or transported to the lab. Label vial with patient's name, date, and type of specimen.
Refrigerated specimen	Urine, respiratory exudates, and stool or feces must be refrigerated before transport. *Note:* Specimens that cannot be refrigerated before the inoculation of media include spinal fluids and other body fluids, specimens for *Neisseria gonorrhea* isolation, blood, and wound cultures. Place the

specimen in the refrigerator for storage (iced or cooled) before pickup. When packaging, place the specimen container into a zip-lock bag, with the required coolant put into the outer pouch. If dry ice or a refrigerant is used, it must be placed between the secondary container and the outer shipping container. Shock-absorbent material should be placed in a way such that the secondary container does not become loose inside the outer shipping container as the dry ice evaporates. Styrofoam containers are recommended when shipping the specimen on dry ice to prevent CO_2 buildup as the dry ice evaporates.

Blood for photosensitive analysis
Avoid exposure to any type of light (artificial or sunlight) for any length of time. These specimens need to be enclosed in an aluminum foil wrap or a brown plastic or glass container. Specimens for assays of vitamins A and B_6, beta-carotene, porphyrins, vitamin D, and bilirubin are examples of substances that need to be protected from light.

Anaerobic microbes
Aspiration with a needle and syringe, rather than a swab, is the preferred method of specimen collection for anaerobic bacteria. Once collected, the specimen must be protected from ambient oxygen and kept from drying until it can be processed in the laboratory. The transport container for anaerobic specimen includes the following components:

Syringe and needle attached to the syringe for aspiration—dispose of needle in sharps container and replace with a blunt adaptor for transport.

Tube or vials—tube is used primarily for insertion of swab specimens; vials are used for inoculation of liquid specimen.

Swab/plastic jacket system—the plastic tube or jacket is fitted with a swab and
(continued)

Specimen	Cautions for Packaging and Mailing
	contains transport or prereduced medium. The culturette system also includes a vial or chamber separated by a membrane that contains chemicals that generate CO_2 catalysts and desiccants to eliminate any residual O_2 that may enter the system.
	Biohazard bag or plastic pouch system—a transparent plastic bag that contains a CO_2-generating system, palladium catalyst cups, and an anaerobic indicator. The bag is sealed after inoculated plates have been inserted and the CO_2-generating system is activated. The advantage of this system is that the plates can be directly observed for visualization of early colony growth.
Stool specimen	Use a special 1000-mL container, such as Nalgen™, for total sample collection or a 100-mL white polypropylene container for a portion of a large sample (aliquot) for feces collection. Each container should have a similar label affixed before giving to the patient (Fig. 2.1).
Stool, homogenized	For a homogenized (blended) specimen, the required mailed specimen is an 80-mL portion of homogenized feces. Homogenize and weigh according to laboratory protocol. Pour the homogenate into container as soon as possible to avoid settling. On a request form, indicate the specimen's total weight and the amount of water added. Include the period of collection on the request form. Send the homogenized specimen at the preferred transport temperature listed in the agency specimen requirements protocol.
Infectious material	An etiologic agent label must be affixed to all patient specimens transported as body fluids that have been recognized by the CDC as directly linked to the transmission of HIV (AIDS) or hepatitis B virus (HBV). Standard precautions apply to

---

Only fill to this line

Duration: ___ Random ___ 24 hrs

___ 72 hrs ___ 48 hrs

Other _____

Is this the entire collection?

_____ Yes _____ No

Total number of containers sent: _____

Patient Name: _____

When container is given to the patient, provide the following instructions: Test to be done and specimen requirements, diet requirements, collection and storage of specimen, two 1000 ml Nalgene™ containers provided for timed collection and one 100 ml container for a random collection specimen; information on how to obtain additional containers, if necessary, and instructions for **not filling** any container more than 3/4 full (indicated line on label).

At the time that the patient returns the container(s) to the clinic, the health care worker fills in the label with the correct information. If "other" is checked, list on line on label. If more than one container is sent, be sure to indicate total number sent on the line.

FIGURE 2.1 Stool collection container label.

handling these fluids and include special handling requirements for blood, blood products, semen, vaginal secretions, cerebrospinal fluid, synovial fluid, pleural fluid, peritoneal fluid, pericardial fluid, amniotic fluid, and concentrated HIV and HBV. A biohazard label must be affixed to all microbiology specimens, including anaerobic and aerobic bacteria, mycobacteria, *(continued)*

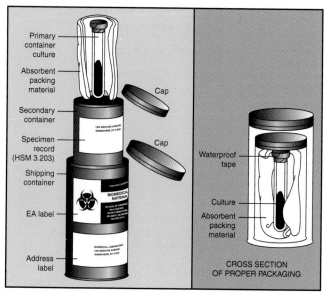

FIGURE 2.2 Proper technique for packaging of biologically hazardous materials. (CDC Laboratory Manual, DHEW publication no. [CDC] 74-8272, Atlanta, GA: Centers for Disease Control and Prevention, 1974.)

SPECIMEN	CAUTIONS FOR PACKAGING AND MAILING
	fungi, and yeast. The specimen must be sent on an agar slant tube in a special transport container (a pure culture, actively growing; FIG. 2.2); do not send on culture plates. The outer shipping container of all etiologic agents transported through interstate traffic must be labeled as illustrated in FIGURE 2.3.
Specimens requiring exceptional handling	Clearly and accurately label each specimen with patient's full name, sex, birth date, identification number, time and date of specimen collection, name of practitioner ordering specimen, and signature of person collecting specimen. The test order form and name of sample contents should be checked for a match and transported in a single package.

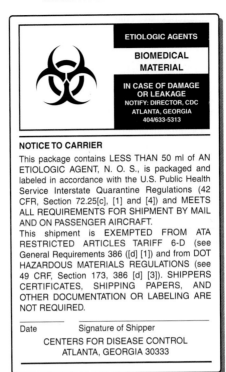

ETIOLOGIC AGENTS

BIOMEDICAL MATERIAL

IN CASE OF DAMAGE OR LEAKAGE
NOTIFY: DIRECTOR, CDC
ATLANTA, GEORGIA
404/633-5313

NOTICE TO CARRIER

This package contains LESS THAN 50 ml of AN ETIOLOGIC AGENT, N. O. S., is packaged and labeled in accordance with the U.S. Public Health Service Interstate Quarantine Regulations (42 CFR, Section 72.25[c], [1] and [4]) and MEETS ALL REQUIREMENTS FOR SHIPMENT BY MAIL AND ON PASSENGER AIRCRAFT.

This shipment is EXEMPTED FROM ATA RESTRICTED ARTICLES TARIFF 6-D (see General Requirements 386 ([d] [1]) and from DOT HAZARDOUS MATERIALS REGULATIONS (see 49 CRF, Section 173, 386 [d] [3]). SHIPPERS CERTIFICATES, SHIPPING PAPERS, AND OTHER DOCUMENTATION OR LABELING ARE NOT REQUIRED.

Date   Signature of Shipper

CENTERS FOR DISEASE CONTROL
ATLANTA, GEORGIA 30333

FIGURE 2.3 Etiologic agents logo and "notice to carrier" that must be affixed to the outside of any package containing potentially hazardous and infectious biologic materials.

Note: In the event of a damaged package, the carrier should immediately isolate the package and contact the CDC. In the event that a package is not received within 5 days of the anticipated delivery date, the sender should contact the CDC.

Nursing Protocols for Blood Specimen Collection

- Blood samples may be procured through skin puncture (ie, capillary blood), venipuncture (ie, venous blood), arterial puncture (ie, arterial blood), or bone marrow aspiration. The type of blood sample needed—whole blood, plasma, or serum—varies with the specific test. Equipment (ie, automated or manual system), blood sample type, collection site, technique, and the patient's age and condition determine the methods of collection.

• Blood collection tubes have color-coded stoppers to indicate which types of additives are present. Additives preserve the specimen, prevent specimen deterioration and coagulation, and block the action of certain cell enzymes. The choice of additives is dictated by the test ordered. In general, most hematology tests use liquid ethylenediaminetetraacetic acid (EDTA) as an anticoagulant. Tubes with anticoagulants should be gently but completely inverted end over end 7 to 10 times after collection. This action ensures complete mixing of anticoagulants with blood to prevent clot formation. Even slightly clotted blood invalidates the test, and the sample must be redrawn. The following guide shows which specimens belong to which color-coded collection tubes:

Collection Tube Color and Additives	Use and Precautions
White (gel and K_2 EDTA)	For HIV and hepatitis C virus (HCV) viral load testing, genotyping, blood bank, plasma testing in molecular diagnostic studies
Green-top tube with heparin (sodium heparin, lithium heparin, ammonium heparin)	For heparinized plasma specimens; arterial blood gases (ABGs), special tests such as ammonia levels, hormones, plasma testing for chemistry panels, and electrolytes; invert tube 7–10 times to prevent clot formation
Gray-top tube with potassium oxalate and sodium fluoride [acidification of the blood with NaF and EDTA (K_2EDTA/NaF) has been shown to inhibit glycolysis]	Serum or plasma glucose levels, lactate, and alcohol measurements. *Note*: The placing of the collection tube in ice slurry can help stabilize the glucose.
Lavender-top tube with K_2 or K_3 EDTA	For whole blood and plasma, hematology, genetic, immunosuppressant, HbA_{1c}, and red blood cell (RBC) folate. The use of EDTA for hematology and complete blood cell counts (CBCs) prevents filled tube from clotting. If tube is less than half filled, the ratio of anticoagulant to blood may be altered enough to give unreliable laboratory test results. Invert tube 7–10 times to prevent clotting.

Light blue–top tube with sodium citrate	For plasma-coagulation studies such as prothrombin times and partial thromboplastin times. The tube must be allowed to fill to its capacity, or an improper blood-to-anticoagulant ratio will invalidate coagulation test results. Invert tube 7–10 times to prevent clotting.
Royal (dark) blue–top tube with Na, EDTA, or sodium heparin	For cadmium and mercury; toxicology and nutritional chemistry; trace element–free tube; invert tube 7–10 times.
Royal (dark) blue–top tube without EDTA or sodium heparin	For aluminum, arsenic, chromium, copper, nickel, and zinc; trace element–free tube (no additives) (use anticoagulant—blood will clot).
Tan-top tube with heparin	For heparinized plasma specimens for pediatric lead levels; lead-free tube; invert tube 7–10 times.
Yellow-top tube with 5.95 mg of sodium polyanethole sulfonate (SPS) [0.35% in 14.4 mg of NaCl (0.86%)]	For collection of blood cultures in microbiology; use aseptic technique for blood draw; invert tube 7–10 times to prevent clot formation.
Gold- or red-marbled tube; serum separator tube (SST)	For serum samples such as chemistry serum analysis, SSTs should be gently inverted (completely, end over end) five times after collection to ensure mixing of clot activator with blood and clotting within 30 minutes. After 30 minutes, centrifuge promptly at relative centrifugal force (rcf) 1000–1200 *g* (virtual gravity) for 15 ± 5 minutes to separate serum from cells. Serum can be stored in gel separator tubes after centrifugation for up to 48 hours. Do not freeze SSTs. If a frozen specimen is needed, separate serum into a labeled plastic transfer vial. SSTs must not be used for therapeutic drug levels. The gel may lower values.
Red-top, plain tube; no additive	For a wide range of chemistry tests, blood bank, therapeutic drug testing, all

(*continued*)

Collection Tube
Color and
Additives   Use and Precautions

antibody tests, collecting a clotted blood
specimen; no preservatives or anticoagulant. After drawing blood, it is necessary
to allow the blood to clot at room temperature for 30–45 minutes. Then, centrifuge
the specimen at rct 1000–1200 g for 15 $\pm$
5 minutes and transfer the serum portion
to a properly labeled plastic transfer vial.
*Prolonged exposure of the serum to the
clot can invalidate some test results.*

Nursing Interventions

The nurse's role in blood collection varies according to the type of
specimen collected, the patient's age and condition, and the clinical
setting. Standard precautions must be observed at *all* stages of the
blood collection process, including disposal activities.

CLINICAL ALERT

- Several factors increase the risk for infection to nurses and patients
  during blood collection. Infection needs four conditions to exist simultaneously: (1) a sufficiently large amount of the infectious agent, (2) a
  sufficiently virulent or deadly form of the agent, (3) an opportune portal
  of entry into the host (eg, open cut, nasal passages, needle stick), and
  (4) a sufficiently lowered level of resistance in the host. The likelihood
  of developing an infection is greatly reduced or eliminated if one or
  more of these conditions is removed.
- Transmission of blood-borne pathogens presents greater risk during
  blood collection than during injection.

In acute care settings, the nurse prepares the patient for blood testing and assists laboratory or medical personnel as necessary. However,
in a rural or community setting, the nurse may procure the specimen,
process or centrifuge the sample, and transport specimens.

Skin Puncture for Capillary Blood

Proper specimen collection depends on correct technique and accurate timing. Capillary blood is preferred for a peripheral blood smear,
and it can be used for other hematologic studies. Adult capillary
blood samples require a skin puncture, usually of the fingertip. For

children, the tip of the finger is also often the choice. Infants younger than 1 year and neonates yield the best samples from the great toe or side of the heel.

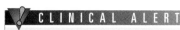

CLINICAL ALERT

• In patients diagnosed with leukemia, agranulocytosis, or lowered immunologic resistance, fingerstick punctures are more likely to cause infection and bleeding than venipunctures. If a capillary sample is necessary, wash the site with soap and water and dry with sterile gauze before and after blood collection.

Pretest Care

Explain the procedure and purpose of blood sampling to the patient or parents. Obtain informed consent if necessary. A warm compress may be applied to the anticipated puncture site area for about 10 minutes before the procedure to dilate the blood vessels for easier access. Assess for the following interfering factors:

• Inadequate available blood supply may occur because of cold, cyanosis, swelling, or edema of the site or because of an improper collection process.
• Blood sample dilution can occur because of improper pressure (ie, squeezing) on the puncture site or neglecting to wipe away the first drop of blood. Such dilution alters blood composition and invalidates test results.
• Residual alcohol applied at the site before puncture affects red cell morphology.
• Epithelial or endothelial cells present in the first drop of blood cause incorrect results.

Intratest Care

• Observe standard precautions; gloves must be worn.
• Assess the puncture site. *Avoid using the lateral aspect of the heel where the plantar artery is located.*
• Clean the puncture site using soap and water. Use a circular motion and then wipe dry with sterile gauze.
• Create blood stasis by pressing on a distal joint to produce engorgement at the tip of the finger.
• Puncture the skin with a disposable sterile lancet (no deeper than 2 mm) quickly and deeply enough for blood droplet formation. Wipe away the first drop of blood. Collect subsequent drops in a microtube or prepare a smear directly from a drop of blood.

- After collection, briefly apply pressure to the site and then cover the site with a small, sterile dressing or adhesive strip.
- Label the specimen properly, and enclose it in a biohazard bag. Send the sample to the laboratory promptly. Document pertinent information.

Dried Blood Spot

In this method, a lancet is used and the resulting droplets of blood are collected by blotting them with filter paper directly. Check the stability of equipment and integrity of supplies when performing a fingerstick. If provided, check the humidity indicator patch on the filter paper card. If the humidity circle is pink, do not use this filter paper card. The humidity indicator must be blue to ensure specimen integrity.

- After wiping the first drop of blood on the gauze pad, fill and saturate each of the circles in numeric order by blotting the blood droplet with the filter paper. Do not touch the patient's skin to the filter paper; only the blood droplet should come in contact with the filter paper. If an adult has a cold hand, run warm water over it for approximately 3 minutes. The best flow occurs when the arm is held downward, with the hand below heart level, making effective use of gravity. If there is a problem with proper blood flow, milk the finger with *gentle* pressure to stimulate blood flow or attempt a second fingerstick; do not attempt more than two. When the saturated blood circles penetrate through to the other side of the filter paper, the circles are fully saturated.

Posttest Care

- The dressing may be removed after a few hours if bleeding has stopped. Occasionally, a small bruise or some discomfort may occur. Notify the laboratory or clinician if bleeding does not stop with pressure on the site within a reasonable period. Evaluate the patient's medication history for an anticoagulant, nonsteroidal anti-inflammatory drug (NSAID), or aspirin-type drug ingestion.

Venipuncture for Venous Blood

Most blood studies require venous blood samples. Venipuncture allows for procurement of larger quantities of blood than capillary collection. Care must be taken to avoid sample hemolysis or hemoconcentration and to prevent hematoma, vein damage, infection, and discomfort. The median cubital vein located in the antecubital fossa is the most commonly used venipuncture site because of easy access, followed by the cephalic vein and the basilica vein. Sometimes, the wrist area, forearm, or dorsum of the hand or foot must be used. Blood values should remain consistent for all of these venipuncture sites.

Pretest Care

- Diagnostic blood tests may require certain dietary restrictions or fasting for 8 to 12 hours before the test.
- Drugs taken by the patient should be documented on all appropriate forms, requisitions, and computer screens because they may affect results.
- Application of warm, moist compresses to the blood draw site for 10 to 20 minutes before venipuncture or lowering the arm well below the heart level before the procedure may help distend veins that are difficult to find. For young children, warming the draw site should be routine to distend small veins.
- Be ready to provide assistance if the patient becomes lightheaded or faints.

 CLINICAL ALERT

- Strenuous activity immediately before a blood sample draw can alter results because body fluids shift from the vascular bed to the tissue spaces and produce circulatory blood hemoconcentration. It may take 20 to 30 minutes of rest and reduced stress to reestablish fluid equilibrium.
- Assess for other interfering factors, including cellulitis, phlebitis, venous obstruction, lymphangitis, or arteriovenous fistulas or shunts. To avoid spurious test results because of an actively infusing solution, do not draw blood above an intravenous (IV) catheter or infusion site. If necessary, choose a site distal to the IV line site if no other site is available. Be alert to the fact that hemoconcentration may be caused by leaving the tourniquet in place for more than 1 minute at a time.

Intratest Care

- Observe standard precautions. Gloves must be worn. If latex allergy is suspected, use latex-free supplies and equipment.
- Position a snug tourniquet above the puncture site to produce venous distention (ie, congestion). A blood pressure cuff inflated to a range between the person's systolic and diastolic pressure can also be used.
- For elderly persons, a tourniquet is not always recommended because of possible rupture of capillaries. Instruct the patient to make a tight fist. Do not pump the fist, because this activity may increase plasma potassium levels by as much as 1 to 2 mmol/L, potentially resulting in a significant diagnostic alteration.
- Disinfect skin area with ChloraPrep and allow to dry.

- To anchor the vein, draw the skin taut over the vein and press the thumb below the puncture site. Hold the distal end of the vein during puncture to decrease the possibility of rolling veins; this is especially important for the frail elderly with friable, tissue paper–like skin.
- Puncture the vein with the needle bevel up according to accepted technique. Usually, for an adult, anything smaller than a 21-gauge needle may make blood withdrawal more difficult and possibly hemolyze the blood. A Vacutainer system syringe or butterfly needle system can be used.
- Hold the collection device with the needle bevel facing up and the needle shaft parallel and angled approximately 15 degrees to the skin. Gently insert the needle into the vein. After the needle enters the vein, the blood fills the attached vacuum tube automatically because of a vacuum within the collection tube. If using a syringe, watch for blood flow back into the needle hub and then gently pull back on the syringe plunger to withdraw blood.
- Transfer the blood from the syringe to the proper vacuum tube by piercing the tube stopper with the needle still attached to the syringe containing the blood sample.
- Release the tourniquet as soon as adequate blood flow is established into the sample container and before removing the needle from the puncture site; otherwise, bruising will occur.
- Remove the needle when the sample has been collected, apply pressure for a few moments, and dress the site with a sterile adhesive strip. The patient should not "bend up" the arm. Instead, keep the arm straight while exerting pressure for 2 to 4 minutes or until active bleeding stops.
- When drawing multiple samples, carefully remove the full Vacutainer tube from the Vacutainer holder while keeping the needle anchored in the patient's vein. Then insert the next Vacutainer tube into the holder and collect another blood sample. The following sequence in which samples must be drawn has been set by the Clinical and Laboratory Standards Institute (CLSI) (formerly the National Committee for Clinical Laboratory Standards) and must be followed:
    1. Yellow-top (SPS) tube (for blood culture)
    2. Gold-top (SST)/red-top nonadditive tube
    3. Light blue–top coagulation tube
    4. Light green–top (plasma separator tube [PST])/green-top additive tube
    5. Lavender-top additive tube

6. Grey-top additive tube
7. Royal blue–top tube with EDTA
8. Royal blue–top tube without EDTA
9. Yellow-top (acid citrate dextrose [ACD]) tube
10. Tan-top tube

- If only a light blue–stoppered coagulation tube is being used for drawing, a small red-top tube should be used first and then discarded to avoid contamination of the blue-top tube with tissue clotting factors.
- After obtaining the blood sample, remove the needle, and discard it in a biohazard container. Do not recap needles because this presents a greater risk for injury and exposure to disease for the phlebotomist.
- Gently invert the collection tubes with a "back-and-forth" motion 7 to 10 times to blend the sample. Do not shake tubes.
- Send the labeled specimen to the laboratory immediately in a bio-hazard bag, and document pertinent information in the health care record.
- Keep red-top tubes upright and undisturbed for at least 30 minutes, but no longer than 1 hour, to allow the blood to clot before centrifu-gation. If red-top tubes cannot be centrifuged within 1 hour, store them upright in the kit and in a chilled cooler, and centrifuge within 8 hours.
- After gloving, centrifuge the red-top tubes at a high speed of at least 2500 to 3400 rpm for at least 15 minutes. Pour the serum from both tubes into the labeled plastic serum transfer tube without disturbing the clot, and seal tightly. Serum must be free of RBCs. Recap the red-top tubes, and for an insurance case, replace in the blood kit.

Posttest Care
- Check the patient and the puncture site. Instruct the patient to lie down and rest if he or she is anxious, experiences vasovagal syn-cope, or develops hematomas or signs of sepsis such as chills, rapid temperature elevation, and a drop in blood pressure. If this happens, notify the attending physician immediately.
- Cold compresses may be applied to the site if the patient complains of discomfort.

Patient Aftercare
- If oozing or bleeding from the puncture site continues for more than a few minutes, elevate the area and apply a pressure dressing. Observe the patient closely. Ask about the use of

anticoagulants, NSAIDs, or aspirin-type products. If venous bleeding is excessive and persists for longer than 10 minutes, notify the physician.

- Occasionally, a patient may become dizzy, faint, or nauseated during venipuncture. If this happens, immediately remove the tourniquet and terminate the procedure. If possible, place the patient in a supine position. If the patient is sitting, lower the head between the legs and have the patient breathe deeply several times. A cool, wet towel may be applied to the forehead and back of the neck. If necessary, an ammonia inhalant may be introduced briefly. If the patient's status remains unchanged, notify the physician immediately.

- Hematomas can usually be prevented by the use of proper technique.

CLINICAL ALERT

Generally, do not draw blood from the same extremity being used for the administration of IV medications or fluids or for blood transfusions. Only as a last resort, if no other site is available, should this be considered as the venipuncture site. In this case, the venipuncture site should be below the IV line site. Avoid areas that are edematous, paralyzed, on the same side as a previous mastectomy, are infected, or exhibit abnormal skin conditions. Sometimes, venipuncture may be the cause of infection, circulatory or lymphatic impairment, or prolonged healing.

After two attempts, a physician or highly trained phlebotomist should be called.

Prolonged tourniquet application causes stasis and hemoconcentration, which alters test results.

Blood samples may be drawn off central lines. The lines must first be flushed with saline prior to the blood draw. A physician's order is normally required. Agency protocols and guidelines must be strictly followed and strict aseptic technique must be maintained.

Arterial Puncture for Arterial Blood

Arterial blood samples are necessary for ABG determinations or when it is not possible to obtain a venous blood sample. "Arterial sticks" are usually performed by a physician or a specially trained nurse or technician because of the potential risks inherent in this procedure. Samples are normally collected directly from the radial, brachial, or femoral artery. If the patient has an arterial line in place (most frequently in the radial artery), samples can be drawn from the line. Be sure to record the amounts of blood withdrawn because significant amounts can be removed if frequent samples are required.

ABG determinations are used to assess the status of oxygenation, ventilation, and acid-base balance. Blood gases are also used to monitor critically ill patients, to establish baseline laboratory values, to detect and treat electrolyte imbalances, to titrate appropriate oxygen therapy, and to qualify a patient for home oxygen use. Arterial puncture sites must satisfy the following requirements:

- Sites must have available collateral blood flow.
- Sites must be easily accessible.
- Sites must be relatively nonsensitive as periarterial tissues.

Pretest Care
- Assess patient for the following contraindications to an arterial stick or indwelling arterial line in a particular area:
  Absence of a palpable radial artery pulse
  A positive Allen's test result, which shows only one artery supplying blood to the hand
  Negative modified Allen's test result, which indicates obstruction in the ulnar artery (ie, compromised collateral circulation)
  Cellulitis or infection at the potential site
  Presence of arteriovenous fistula or shunt
  Severe thrombocytopenia (blood platelet count 20,000/mm^3)
  Prolonged prothrombin time or partial thromboplastin time (>1.5 times the control is a relative contraindication)
- A Doppler probe or finger pulse transducer may be used to assess circulation and perfusion in dark-skinned or uncooperative patients.
- Before drawing an arterial blood sample, record the patient's most recent hemoglobin concentration, mode and flow rate of oxygen, and temperature. If the patient has been recently suctioned or placed on a ventilator or if delivered oxygen concentrations have been changed, wait at least 15 minutes before drawing the sample. This waiting period allows circulating blood levels to return to baseline levels. Hyperthermia and hypothermia also influence oxygen release from hemoglobin at the tissue level.

Intratest Care
- Observe standard precautions and follow agency protocols for the procedure.
- Have the patient assume a sitting or supine position.

- Perform a modified Allen's test by encircling the wrist area and using pressure to obliterate the radial and ulnar pulses. Watch for the hand to blanch and then release pressure only over the ulnar artery. If a positive test result is obtained, flushing of the hand is immediately noticed, indicating that circulation to the hand is adequate. The radial artery can then be used for arterial puncture. If collateral circulation from the ulnar artery is inadequate (ie, negative test result) and flushing of the hand is absent or slow, then another site must be chosen. An abnormal Allen's test result may be caused by a thrombus, an arterial spasm, or a systemic problem such as shock or poor cardiac output.
- Elevate the wrist area by placing a small pillow or rolled towel under the dorsal wrist area. With the patient's palm facing upward, ask the patient to extend the fingers downward, which flexes the wrist and positions the radial artery closer to the surface.
- Palpate for the artery, and maneuver the patient's hand back and forth until a satisfactory pulse is felt.
- Swab the area liberally with an antiseptic agent such as ChloraPrep.
- *Optional:* Inject the area with a small amount (<0.25 mL) of 1% plain Xylocaine (lidocaine), if necessary, to anesthetize site. Assess for allergy first. This allows for a second attempt without undue pain.
- *Note:* Do not use Xylocaine that contains epinephrine; it causes blood vessel constriction and makes the arterial puncture difficult.
- Prepare a 20- or 21-gauge needle on a preheparinized, self-filling syringe, puncture the artery, and collect a 3- to 5-mL sample. The arterial pressure pushes the plunger out as the syringe fills with blood. (Venous blood does not have enough pressure to fill the syringe without drawing back on the plunger.) Air bubbles in the blood sample must be expelled as quickly as possible because residual air alters ABG values. The syringe should then be capped and gently rotated to mix heparin with the blood.
- When the draw is completed, withdraw the needle, and place a 4 × 4-in absorbent bandage over the puncture site. Do not recap needles; if necessary, use the one-handed mechanical, recapping, or scoop technique, or commercially available needles [eg, B-D Safety-Glide™ (Franklin Lakes, NJ) or Sims Portex Pro-Vent® (Keene, NH)]. Maintain firm finger pressure over the site for a minimum of 5 minutes or until there is no active bleeding evident. After the bleeding stops, apply a firm pressure dressing but do not

encircle the entire limb, which can restrict circulation. Leave this dressing in place for at least 24 hours. Instruct the patient to report any signs of bleeding from the site promptly and apply finger pressure if necessary.

- Place the sample on ice slurry, and place it in a biohazard bag for transport to the laboratory. Putting the sample on ice prevents alterations in gas tensions because metabolic processes within the sample otherwise continue after blood is drawn.

> ### CLINICAL ALERT
>
> - Metabolizing blood cells can quickly alter blood gas values (primarily Pa_{O_2}) at normal body temperature ($37°C$). This occurs much slower at $0°C$ (ie, temperature of ice water). An iced sample should remain stable for at least 1 hour. Any sample not placed in ice should be tested within minutes after it is drawn or else discarded. The main effect of cellular metabolism decreases P_{O_2}. Several studies have shown a remarkable fall in Pa_{O_2} if the blood contains more than 100,000 white blood cells/mm^3 (ie, leukocyte larceny), even when the sample is on ice. A white blood cell count of this magnitude (usually in leukemia) should mandate special handling, such as running the sample immediately. Alternatively, check the patient's oxygen saturation by pulse oximetry, which is not affected by extreme leukocytosis.
> - Label the sample with patient's name, identification number, and date and time procured and indicate the type and flow rate of O_2 therapy or whether the patient was on "room air." Do not use blood for ABGs if the sample is more than 1-hour old.
> - In clinical settings such as the perioperative or intensive care environment, ABG studies usually include pH, P_{CO_2}, S_{O_2}, total CO_2 content (T_{CO_2}), O_2 content, P_{O_2}, base excess or deficit, HCO_3, hemoglobin, hematocrit, and the electrolytes chloride, sodium, and potassium.

Posttest Care
- Posttest assessment of the puncture site and extremity includes color, motion, sensation, degree of warmth, capillary refill time, and quality of the pulse.
- Frequently monitor the puncture site and dressing for arterial bleeding for several hours. The patient should not use the extremity for any vigorous activity for at least 24 hours.

> ### CLINICAL ALERT
>
> Some patients may experience lightheadedness, nausea, or vasovagal syncope during the arterial puncture. Treat according to established protocols.
>
> Monitor the patient's vital signs and mental function to determine adequacy of tissue oxygenation and perfusion.
>
> The arterial puncture site must have a pressure dressing applied and frequently assessed for bleeding for several hours. Instruct the patient to report any bleeding from the site and to apply direct pressure to the site if necessary.
>
> For patients requiring frequent arterial monitoring, an indwelling arterial catheter may be inserted. Follow agency protocols for obtaining arterial line blood samples. Procedures vary for neonates and pediatric and adult patients (see Arterial Blood Gases (ABGS), Blood Gases in Chapter 3).
>
> Label all specimens appropriately and document pertinent information in the health care record.

Nursing Protocols for Urine Specimen Collection

Urine specimen testing is a useful indicator for determining a healthy or a diseased state (eg, renal or liver function). It is an integral part of a comprehensive patient examination. Moreover, urine is a readily available and easily collected specimen, and simple laboratory urine tests can reveal much information about the body's functions.

If it is necessary to determine whether a particular fluid is urine, the specimen can be tested for its urea and creatinine content. Both of these substances are more highly concentrated in urine than in any other body fluids.

Because the composition and concentration of urine changes continuously through any given 24-hour period, different types of specimens are ordered. They may include a single, random specimen; second (double)-voided specimen; timed specimen; pediatric specimen; clean-catch midstream specimen; catheter specimen; first morning specimen; fasting specimen; and suspected substance abuse specimen. Random, second-voided, and clean-catch midstream specimens can be collected any time, whereas first morning, fasting, or timed specimens require collection at specific times.

Dipsticks

Although laboratory facilities allow for a wide range of urine tests, some types of tablets, tapes, and dipstick tests are available for urinalysis outside the laboratory setting. They can be used and read directly by patients or clinicians.

Similar in appearance to small pieces of blotter paper on a plastic strip, dipsticks function as miniature laboratories. These chemically impregnated reagent strips can provide quick determinations of pH, protein, glucose, ketones, bilirubin, hemoglobin (blood), nitrite (bacteria), leukocyte esterase, urobilinogen, and specific gravity. Dipsticks are also available to test for phenylketonuria, salicylates, and cystinuria. The dipstick is impregnated with chemicals that react with specific substances in the urine to produce color changes that are matched to predetermined color-coded scales. The color produced when the urine comes in contact with the reagent strip correlates with the concentration of the substance in the urine. Directions for elapsed times between the time the dipstick is in contact with the urine sample and the time the test is read must be observed for the most accurate results. The prescribed elapsed time can vary, depending on which test is being done. More than one type of test may be incorporated on a single stick (eg, pH, protein, and glucose). In this case, the chemical reagents for each test are separated by a water-impermeable barrier made of plastic so that results of each test do not become altered.

If an entire voided amount is to be saved, instruct the patient to use toilet tissue *after* transferring all of the urine from the voiding collection container to the specimen container or bottle. Toilet tissue or other materials placed within the specimen absorb some of the urine available and may also contaminate the specimen. Results of the test could be skewed.

Feces can also contaminate urine specimens. Patients should void and transfer the urine to the collection of specimen receptacle before defecating.

If other discharges, secretions, or a heavy menstrual flow is present, the test may have to be postponed, or an indwelling catheter may need to be inserted to keep the urine specimen free of contamination. In some cases, thorough cleaning of the perineal or urethral area before voiding may be sufficient. If in doubt, communicate with laboratory personnel or the patient's physician.

Using Dipstick Reagent Strips

- Use a fresh urine sample (ie, within 1 hour of voiding or a sample that has been refrigerated).
- Review directions for use of the reagent. Periodically check for changes in procedure, especially if the product is "improved."
- Dip the reagent strip into well-mixed urine, remove it, and compare each reagent area on the dipstick with the corresponding

color-control chart according to the established time frames for reading results. Match colors as closely as possible, and record corresponding results on the health care record.

- If dipsticks are kept in the urine sample too long, the impregnated chemicals in the strip may be dissolved and may produce inaccurate readings and values.
- If the reagent chemicals on the impregnated pad become mixed, the readings will be inaccurate. To avoid this, if not contraindicated, blot off excess urine (by turning the strip on its side onto a piece of paper towel and allowing excess urine to be drawn off—never blot with the reagent strip face down) after withdrawing the dipstick from the urine sample.

CLINICAL ALERT

Precise timing is essential. If not timed correctly, color changes may produce invalid or false results.

The container of unused dipsticks should be kept tightly closed to keep the contents dry, and it should be stored in a cool, dry environment. If the reagents absorb moisture from the air before they are used, they cannot produce accurate results. If a desiccant comes with the reagents, it should be kept in the container.

Follow quality control protocols. Honor expiration dates, even if there is no detectable deterioration of strips. Discard bottles 6 months after opening, regardless of expiration date, unless instructed to dispose of sooner. When opening a new bottle of strips, write the date it was opened on the bottle.

Known positive and negative (abnormal and normal) controls must be run with each new bottle of reagent strips opened and whenever there is a possibility of deterioration.

Nursing Interventions
Pretest Care

- Patient teaching varies according to the type and amounts of urine specimen required and the patient's ability to understand and cooperate with specimen collection. To obtain a specimen that is truly representative of a patient's metabolic state, it is often necessary to regulate certain aspects of specimen collection (eg, time and length of collection period, patient's dietary and medicinal intake, the collection method itself).
- Clear instructions reinforced with written information and pictures or diagrams are key to a successful outcome.

- Provide the patient with the proper urine containers and supplies.
- Assess for interfering factors that may affect test outcomes, including the patient's use of illegal drugs, strenuous activity (ie, causes proteinuria), time of day (ie, urine is concentrated in the early morning), food consumption (ie, glycosuria increases after meals), and the presence of fecal material, toilet paper, vaginal discharge, blood, or semen. These may contaminate and invalidate the specimen. The specimen should be refrigerated or kept in a cool place during the collection period. Urine is an excellent culture medium, and many of its components decompose quickly at room temperature. Failure to follow collection instructions, inadequate fluid intake, certain medications, certain foods, or urine containers contaminated with detergent or sodium chloride may also interfere with accurate test results.
- Assess the patient's usual urinating habits and encourage fluid intake (unless contraindicated).

CLINICAL ALERT

- False-positive or false-negative urine test results may be caused by several factors: failure of the patient or health care worker to follow the proper procedure (ie, most common source of error), specimen contamination, presence of certain organisms, timing of specimen collection, specimen handling, presence of interfering substances (eg, glucose, ascorbic acid, urine cells, bacteria), urine properties (eg, pH, specific gravity, concentrated urine), and physiologic factors (eg, exercise, exposure to cold, prolonged recumbent position, and physical illness).
- In a health care facility, responsibility for the collection of urine specimens should be specifically assigned.

Intratest Care
- Observe standard precautions.
- Ensure that specimens are voided into clean receptacles, transferred into urine specimen containers, and properly sealed.
- Examine urine for amount, odor, color, appearance, blood, mucus, or pus. Document observations.
- Label specimens accurately. Leaking containers are a biohazard to any person handling them and may be rejected.
- Place the specimens in a biohazard bag and send them to the laboratory immediately after collection. Refrigerate the specimen if a delay occurs.
- Transport the specimen according to established protocols.

Random Collection Specimen

- The randomly collected specimen is the most commonly requested specimen.
- These specimens may be collected at any time, but early morning specimens are more concentrated and best for routine urinalysis.
- Provide the patient with the proper container and appropriate instructions before the test. The patient should void directly into the container.

Second-Voided Specimen

- Some diseases or conditions (eg, diabetes testing) require second-voided specimens.
- These specimens provide less concentrated urine but more accurately reflect the urine components.
- Instruct the patient to void and discard the first urine specimen and then drink one glass of water to stimulate urine production. The patients voids 30 minutes later into the proper receptacle.

First Morning and Fasting Collections

- Because it is collected after rest and sleep, the first-voided morning specimen is particularly valuable because it is usually more concentrated and more likely to reveal abnormalities and the presence of formed substances, as well as being relatively free of medication, dietary, and physical activity influences.
- Instruct the patient to void and discard urine at bedtime. For a fasting specimen, restrict food and fluids after midnight.
- Collect the first void in morning. Patients who must void during the night should note the time between the last night voiding and the time of the specimen collection on the specimen label (eg, "urine specimen, 3:20 AM–8:00 AM").

Clean-Catch Midstream Specimen

- The clean-catch method is often used for random collection to reduce the presence of bacterial counts, contaminants, feces, discharges, vaginal secretions, and menstrual blood. The urethral area is thoroughly cleaned with an antiseptic wash before voiding.
- For males, clean or instruct the patient to clean the tip of the penis with antiseptic swabs by wiping in circular motion away from the urethra.
- For females, separate the labia or instruct the patient to do so before cleaning and during collection. Clean each side of the urinary meatus first and then down the center as the last wipe. Always wipe from front to back.

- Instruct the patient to initiate voiding into the toilet, urinal, or bedpan first. The patient stops voiding briefly and then voids into a *sterile* collection container, taking care not to contaminate the inner surface of the collection container or inside portion of the container lid. Collect at least 10 mL of midstream urine. Pour the urine into a sterile transport container, cap the container securely, and invert to dissolve the preservative tablet.

Timed Urine Specimen Collection

- Specimens are collected over a specific period. Collection may take 2 hours or as long as 24 to 48 hours. Because substances excreted by the kidney are not excreted at the same rate or in the same amounts during different periods of the day and night, a random urine specimen may not give an accurate picture of the metabolic processes taking place over a 24-hour period. For measurement of total urine protein, creatinine, electrolytes, and other substances, more accurate information is obtained from urine collected over a 24-hour period.
- The 24-hour collection involves collecting the urine specimen into a suitable receptacle that contains an added preservative or keeping it refrigerated (or both) until transport to the laboratory. Explain the procedure to the patient carefully and provide written instructions if possible. The *total* urine specimen must be collected for the designated time period. If any part of the specimen is lost, the entire collection process must start over; otherwise, the results will be inaccurate.
- Emphasize dietary, drug, or activity restrictions. Some of these apply for several days before the test.
- Use the appropriate collection container for the test. Some tests require preservatives or specimen refrigeration. Label the container properly. Include the times the test begins and ends.
A sign that warns "SAVE ALL URINE" signals everyone that a specimen collection is in progress.
- The patient is asked to void immediately before beginning the timed collection. Discard this urine and record this time. From this time forward, collect all urine for the designated time period. Transfer it to the proper container after each voiding. The time the collection begins and ends should be noted on the container. It may be helpful to post a sign above the toilet stating that urine collection is in progress with the beginning and end times noted. At the end of the specified period, the patient should void the last collected specimen to complete the collection process.

The 24-Hour Urine Collection

Most 24-hour urine collections start in the early morning. Instruct the patient to do the following:

* Empty the bladder completely on awakening and discard this urine specimen. Record the time this voided specimen is discarded. This is the time when the test begins. All urine voided during the next 24 hours is collected into a large container (usually glass or polyethylene) and labeled with the patient's name, time frame for collection, test ordered, and other pertinent information. It is not necessary to measure the volume of individual voidings unless specifically requested.

* A urinal, wide-mouth container, special toilet catch basin (device), bedpan, or the collection container itself can be used to catch urine. It is probably easier for women to void into another wide-mouth receptacle first and then to carefully transfer the entire specimen to the collection bottle. Men may find it simpler to void directly into the collection container.

* To conclude the process, the patient voids 24 hours after the first voiding or as close to the end time as possible. This specimen must be added to the container.

* If indicated, the container should be refrigerated or placed in ice for the duration of the test and until it can be transferred to the laboratory.

* Test results are calculated on the basis of a 24-hour output. Unless *all* the urine is saved, results will be inaccurate. Because these tests are usually expensive and complicated to process, care should be taken to comply with instructions and to ensure the patient and others involved in the process understand the activities necessary for this test. Specific written instructions for patients are highly recommended because they lessen the risk of misinterpreting directions.

* In a health care facility, nonrefrigerated samples may be kept in a specified area, usually the patient's bathroom. If refrigeration is necessary, refrigerate the urine specimen immediately in a designated refrigerator, or place the collection bottle into an iced container and renew the ice as necessary. At home, the same focus may be adapted to that environment, with attention to childproofing the area if necessary.

* In a health care facility, assign the responsibility for collecting urine specimens to designated individuals on each shift.

* Do not predate and pretime requisitions for serial collections. It is difficult for some patients to void at specific times. Instead, mark actual times of collection on containers.

- Documenting the exact times the specimens are obtained is crucial to many urine tests.
- When a preservative is added to the collection container, the patient must be instructed to take precautions against spilling the contents. A caution sign should be placed on the specimen container to warn the patient of caustic or toxic substances present and to explain how accidental spillage should be handled. The container should be placed in a child-proof area.
- The preservative used is determined by the urine substance to be tested. The laboratory usually provides the container and proper preservative. If in doubt, verify this with the laboratory personnel.

Posttest Care

- Observe standard precautions when handling specimens. Wear gloves and wash hands according to protocols. Document the type of specimen; test ordered; disposition of the specimen; color, amount, odor, and appearance of urine; and time collected. Transfer specimens to the laboratory. If unable to do so immediately, refrigerate the specimen (unless contraindicated) until transfer occurs.
- If appropriate, use a transport kit. Many laboratories require the person who collects the specimen to pour the urine into a special transport tube containing a tablet or substance designed to prevent alterations of formed elements (eg, casts, cells) and chemical properties due to bacterial overgrowth. Cap the tube securely and invert to dissolve preservatives (if so instructed). Clean the outside of the receptacle (if soiled) and place it in a biohazard bag.

Pediatric Specimens

- For infants, essentially the same basic collection procedures are used for all types of urine specimens. Thoroughly clean and dry the urethral area with the infant in the supine position, with the hips externally rotated and abducted and the knees bent (ie, frog position). Then apply the urine collection bag.
- For boys, apply the device over the penis and scrotum and press the flaps of the collection bag closely against perineum to ensure a tight fit.
- For girls, apply the device to the perineal area by starting at the point between anus and vagina and working toward the pubic area.
- Loosely cover the collection bag with a diaper to prevent dislodging. If possible, elevate the infant's upper body to facilitate drainage into the collection bag.

Suprapubic Aspiration

- Suprapubic urine aspiration is done when a sample free of extraneous contamination is needed. This method is often used with infants and young children when it is difficult to obtain a sterile specimen for microbiologic examination or cytologic analysis.
- If possible, the patient should not void before this test and should drink sufficient fluids to ensure urine in the bladder.
- The skin over the suprapubic area is cleaned with an antiseptic agent and draped with sterile drapes. A local anesthetic can be injected around the area through which aspiration is planned.
- Using sterile technique, a sterile needle is inserted through the abdominal wall above the symphysis pubis and advanced into the full bladder.
- A syringe is used to aspirate at least 1 mL of the sterile urine.
- The specimen is transferred to a sterile urine culture container and the needle is removed.
- A sterile dressing is applied to the site and the area is observed for leakage, bleeding, inflammation, or any other abnormal drainage. A small amount of urine leakage is normal for 24 hours.

Collection of Urine From a Catheter

- Follow agency protocols for a one-time catheterization. Allow a few milliliters of urine to drain out of the catheter before collecting the specimen (at least 1 mL) into a sterile container. If an indwelling catheter is in place, clamp the catheter for 30 minutes before collection unless contraindicated (eg, after bladder surgery). Wipe the sample port of the catheter with an alcohol swab, insert an adaptor into the port, aspirate the urine sample with a syringe, and transfer the sample to a sterile specimen container.
- If the catheter is self-sealing rubber (never with silicone or plastic), the process used is the same, except that the catheter is pierced near the area where it attaches to the collection bag.
- *Important:* Unclamp the catheter after the specimen is collected, unless it was specifically ordered to be clamped.

Urine Collection for Drug Investigation

- Urine is collected for suspected substance use or abuse to identify certain classifications of ingested drugs, including sedatives, depressants, stimulants, and hallucinogens, that can be detected in urine. Urine testing is preferred over blood testing because most drugs (except alcohol, blood testing is preferred) are detectable in urine for longer periods. Urine tests can also confirm clinical or after-death diagnoses and identify ethanol abuse, trauma, the presence of other drugs, or underlying psychosis. They are used as a basis for hemodialysis, to test for drug abuse in the workplace, for pre-employment screening, and to test prisoners and parolees. This is an economical, noninvasive procedure, the specimen is relatively easily obtained, and the test is easily done.

- When urine is collected for suspected drug use or abuse, the patient must be informed that the collection must be witnessed. The reporting protocol for test results and their possible implications should be addressed at the same time.

CLINICAL ALERT

National Institute for Drug Abuse (NIDA)-approved laboratory standards have stringent requirements. At the collection site (eg, bathroom), place toilet bluing markers in the toilet tank and use tamper-proof tape on water faucet and soap dispensers to prevent water access for specimen dilution.

A signed informed consent and photo identification of the subject are required. Extra outer garments need to be removed and left outside the bathroom. Provisions are made for personal privacy during specimen procurement.

Direct the subject to void a random sample of 60 to 100 mL of urine into the clean specimen cup. The toilet may not be flushed at any time.

On receipt of the voided specimen from the subject, the witness transfers the contents of the cup into the laboratory specimen bottle. The subject is present during the entire transfer procedure (viewing this and the following procedure).

Check and record any visible signs of contamination (eg, sediment, discoloration).

The entire procedure must be witnessed by a trained, designated individual who is legally responsible to ensure that the 50-mL specimen has been obtained from the correct patient.

Affix a temperature-sensing strip to the specimen bottle and read and record the temperature within 4 minutes of specimen collection. Temperature strips and collection containers must be at room temperature (urine temperature must be between 90°F and 98°F).

Very firmly screw down the cap onto the laboratory specimen bottle to seal it. The rim of the specimen bottle should be dry.

Affix one end of the tamper-evident tape to the side of the specimen bottle. Record the date collected and have the donor initial the evidence tape. Wrap the tamper-evident tape across the top of the bottle and overlap the free end of the tape with the other end to discourage tampering with the specimen.

Seal the specimen bottle in a zip-lock bag with absorbent material.

After sealing, have the subject sign and date the Drug Screen Request Form in the space provided. The collector then signs, dates, and provides a telephone number on the Drug Screen Request Form, indicating that all of the above steps have been followed. Every person who handles the sample thereafter must also sign the form (ie, chain-of-custody procedure).

Put the original and the first copy of the Drug Screen Request Form and the sealed laboratory specimen bottle into the shipping container and seal it. Place tamper-evident tape across the seal.

Retain the third copy of the form for agency records.

Give the fourth copy of the form to the subject, or send it to the company or place of employment, as required.

The foregoing procedure is an example of the chain of custody. A chain-of-custody document is originated at the time the sample is collected. The subject and the individual who witnessed specimen collection must sign and date the document, as does *every* person who handles the sample thereafter. The sealed chain-of-custody specimen bag remains in the possession and control of the collector or is kept in a secured area until shipment to the testing facility. Sealed collections are placed in large shipping cartons or specially designated bags.

After initial and confirmatory testing, the sample is resealed in a labeled bag and securely stored for 30 days or longer. All records of tests done on the sample and the chain-of-custody report must be carefully maintained.

The test results should be released only to predesignated, authorized persons to lessen the risk of false or speculative information being communicated to inappropriate persons.

Several factors may interfere with accurate outcomes and could cause incorrect or false-positive or false-negative results: higher or lower pH than normal; presence of blood, sodium chloride, detergents, or other contaminants; or low specific gravity.

Nursing Protocols for Stool Specimen Collection

Stool examination is often done for evaluation of gastrointestinal disorders such as bleeding, gastrointestinal obstruction, obstructive jaundice, parasitic disease, dysentery, ulcerative colitis, and increased fat excretion (see Stool Analysis in Chapter 3).

Stool Testing

Stool analysis determines various stool properties for diagnostic purposes. Some of the more frequently ordered fecal tests include those for leukocytes, blood, fat, ova and parasites, and pathogens. Stool is also examined in the laboratory by *chromatographic analysis* for the presence of gallstones. The recovery of a gallstone from feces may provide the only proof that a common bile duct stone has been dislodged and excreted. Stool testing also screens for colon cancer and asymptomatic ulcerations or other gastrointestinal tract masses and evaluates for gastrointestinal diseases in the presence of diarrhea or constipation. Stool testing is done in immunocompromised persons to test for parasitic diseases. Fat analysis is the gold standard to diagnose malabsorption syndrome.

Collection of stool for fecal studies is usually a one-time, random specimen collection. However, some studies may require more extensive samples (eg, occult blood or fat).

Nursing Interventions

Pretest Care

- Explain the purpose, procedure, and interfering factors related to stool specimen collection. Because the specimen cannot be obtained on demand, it is important to provide detailed written and verbal instructions before the test so that the specimen is collected when the opportunity presents itself.
- Assess for interfering factors. Ingesting certain foods (eg, red meat) may alter occult blood test results. Barium sulfate or certain medications such as tetracyclines, antidiarrheal agents, bismuth, oil, iron, or magnesium affect parasite detection and may interfere with accurate results. Certain disease states such as malabsorption syndrome can also affect accurate test outcomes. Specimen contamination with urine or toilet tissue (especially paper towels or toilet tissue containing bismuth) or not procuring a representative sample of the entire stool may result in inaccurate test results. Lifestyle, personal habits, travel, working patterns, home environment, and bathroom accessibility are other factors that may interfere with proper sample procurement.

Intratest Care

- The type of stool analysis ordered determines the collection process. Observe standard precautions when procuring and handling fecal specimens to avoid contact with pathogens (eg, hepatitis A virus,

Salmonella, Shigella) (see Appendix). Patients need to be instructed in proper hand-washing techniques. Provide for and respect the patient's privacy.

- Provide the proper container and other supplies. Collect feces in a dry, clean, urine-free container that has a properly fitting cover.
- Stool may be evacuated into a clean, wide-mouth container or a clean, dry bedpan. At home, any clean, disposable plastic container may be used, such as food item containers that have been thoroughly washed and dried. The specimen should not be contaminated with urine, water, toilet tissue, toilet bowl cleanser, or body secretions such as menstrual blood. Do not collect stool from the toilet bowl. Stool can be collected from the diaper of an infant or incontinent adult. Samples can also be collected from ostomy bags. If the patient has diarrhea, a large plastic bag attached by adhesive tape to the toilet seat may be helpful in the collection process. After defecation, the bag can be placed into a gallon container.
- Specimens for most tests can also be produced by the use of a warm saline enema or Fleet Phospho-Soda enema.
- Post signs in bathrooms that say "SAVE STOOL" to serve as reminders that fecal specimen collection is in progress.
- Observe standard precautions while transferring the entire specimen to a container with a clean tongue blade or similar object. Inaccurate test results may occur if the sample is not representative of the entire stool evacuated. One inch or 1 oz of liquid stool may be sufficient for some tests. Other tests may require the first, middle, and last parts of the stool. Include blood, pus, mucus, and any other unusual-appearing parts of the sample. Dispose of remaining stool and supplies in the usual manner.
- For best results, cover the specimens, label them properly, and seal the container in a biohazard bag. Deliver the specimen to the laboratory as soon as possible after collection. Depending on the examination to be performed, the specimen should be refrigerated or kept warm. If unsure of handling procedures, contact the laboratory for detailed instructions concerning the disposition of the fecal specimen before collection is even begun.
- Document information about stool appearance characteristics, tests ordered on the specimen, and other relevant information in the health care record.

CLINICAL ALERT

- Rejection of the stool specimen and false-negative or false-positive results may result from inadequate specimen sampling; improper specimen collection; patient noncompliance in following pretest instructions; ingestion of certain medications (eg, laxatives, antidiarrheals, antibiotics, barium); specimen contamination with water, urine, toilet tissue, or menstrual blood; or delay in transporting the specimen for analysis.

- Certain stool specimen collection and transport protocols may require strict adherence to procedures. If clarification is necessary, contact laboratory personnel before collection begins. Stool containing enteric pathogens or ova and parasites is highly infectious. It is important to wear gloves, follow proper hand-washing techniques, and observe standard precautions (see Appendix). Instruct patients in proper hand-washing techniques to be used after each bathroom visit.

- Collect stool specimens for enteric pathogens before initiating antibiotic therapy and as early in the course of the disease as possible. A diarrheal stool usually gives accurate results.

- If mucus or blood is present in the stool, it should definitely be included with the specimen because pathogens are more likely to be present. If only a small amount of stool is available, a walnut-sized specimen is usually adequate.

- For the best pathogen preservation and transport, Cary-Blair solution vials should be used.

- Refrigerate the specimen immediately (unless specifically prohibited) because some coliform bacilli produce antibiotic-like substances that destroy existing enteric pathogens.

- Collect a *warm* stool specimen for identifying suspected ova and parasites. *Do not refrigerate* the specimen. Because of the cyclic life cycle of parasites, three separate, random stool specimens should be submitted for analysis. Special vials containing 10% formalin and polyvinyl alcohol (PVA) fixative may also be used for ova and parasite stool samples. In this case, maintaining a warm specimen storage temperature is not critical to the test process.

- Use the Scotch® (clear cellulose) tape method for suspected pinworm eggs. The procedure must be followed exactly. The specimen is best obtained a few hours after the patient has retired for the evening, or early in the morning before defecation. Clear Scotch® tape (nontransparent tape produces unsatisfactory results) is placed around the perianal area to trap the eggs, which are laid at night by the female pinworm.

- Collection of ova and parasite cultures for enteric pathogen tests may be ordered together. In this case, the specimen should be divided into two samples: one portion refrigerated for culture testing and the other portion kept at room temperature for ova and parasite testing. Commercial collection kits for divided specimens are available.

Posttest Care
- Provide the patient the opportunity to clean his or her hands and perianal area. Assist if necessary.
- Pretest medications and diet may be resumed as prescribed.
- Inform the patient when he or she may reasonably expect test result reports. This time depends on prescribed tests and the location of testing facility.
- Inform the patient that testing may need to be done and treatment ordered (especially for ova and parasites) for other family members or significant others to eradicate the disease.

Nursing Protocols for Collecting Microbiologic Specimens

Overview of Microbiologic Studies
Diagnostic Testing and Microbes
In diagnostic testing, microorganisms are referred to as *pathogens*. The word *pathogenic* is usually defined as causing infectious disease, but organisms that are pathogenic under one set of conditions may under other conditions reside within or on the surface of the body without causing disease. When these organisms are present but do not cause harm to the host, they are called *commensals*. When they begin to multiply and cause tissue damage, they are considered pathogens, with the potential for causing or expanding a pathogenic process. Many newly discovered organisms have clinical relevance. Some organisms that were formerly considered as insignificant contaminants or commensals have taken on the roles of causative agents for opportunistic diseases in patients with HIV infection, other immunodeficiency syndromes, and other diseases associated with a compromised health state. Consequently, virtually any organism recovered in pure culture from a body site must be considered a *potential pathogen*.

Sources of Specimens
Microbiologic specimens are collected from many sources, such as blood, pus, or wound exudates or drainage, urine, sputum, feces, genital

discharges or secretions, cerebrospinal fluid, and eye or ear drainage. During specimen collection, specimens should be labeled properly with the following information (institutional requirements may vary):

- Patient's name, age, sex, address, hospital identification numbers, date and time, and prescribing physician's full name
- Exact specimen source (eg, throat, conjunctiva)
- Times when the collection was begun and was completed
- Specific studies ordered
- Clinical diagnosis and suspected microorganisms
- Patient's history
- Patient's immune status
- Previous and current infections
- Previous or current antibiotic therapy
- Isolation status—state type of isolation (eg, respiratory, wound)
- Other pertinent information

During specimen collection, maintain aseptic or sterile technique to avoid contaminating the specimen. Assemble special supplies such as sterile specimen containers and specifically designated kits. Several precautions apply:

- Maintain clean container outer surfaces.
- Use appropriately fitting covers or plugs for specimen tubes and bottles.
- Replace contaminated plugs and caps with sterile ones.
- Observe standard precautions.
- Deliver specimens to the laboratory as soon as possible.

Many specimens may be refrigerated (not frozen) for a few hours without any adverse effects. Several precautions apply:

- Urine culture samples must be *refrigerated.*
- Cerebrospinal fluid specimens should be transported to the laboratory as soon as possible. If this is problematic, the culture should be *incubated* at 37°C (ie, body temperature); a suspected meningococcal organism cannot withstand refrigeration.
- Specimens should be promptly transported to the laboratory to preserve the integrity of the specimen. For anaerobic microbe cultures, no more than 10 minutes should elapse between the time of collection and start of the culture process. Anaerobic specimens should be placed into a butyl-rubber–stoppered, gassed-out glass tube or CO_2-containing transport medium. Fecal specimens suspected of harboring *Salmonella* or *Shigella* organisms should be placed in a special transport medium, such as buffered glycerol with saline, if there will be a delay in culturing of the specimens.

- Obtain the correct quantity of specimen. With few exceptions, this quantity should be as large as possible. When a very small quantity is available, the sterile swabs used should be moistened with sterile saline just before collection, especially for nasopharyngeal cultures.
- Time the specimen collection correctly. If possible, specimens should be collected before antibiotic regimens are instituted. For example, complete all blood culture sampling before starting antibiotic therapy.
- Specimen collection times must also be matched to the onset of symptoms such as fever. The practitioner should become familiar with the clinical course of the suspected disease and its implications for specimen collection.

Basics of Infectious Disease

Infectious diseases cause pathologic conditions. There are observable physiologic and other human responses to the invasion and multiplication of the offending microorganisms. After an infectious disease is suspected, appropriate cultures should be done, or nonculture techniques, such as serologic testing for antigens and antibodies, monoclonal antibodies, and DNA probes, should be used. Proper specimen collection and other appropriate tests are necessary to detect and diagnose the presence of the microorganism.

Nursing Interventions

Pretest Care

Explain the need for testing and its relation to the treatment of infectious disease. The opportunity for infection to occur depends on host resistance, organism volumes, the ability of the organisms to find a portal of entry into the host, and the ability of the microbes to overcome host defenses, to invade tissues, and to produce toxins. Organisms may become seated through inhalation, ingestion, direct contact, inoculation, breaks in natural skin or mucous membrane barriers, changes in organism volumes, alterations in normal flora balances, or changes in other host defense mechanisms.

Assess for factors that influence the development of an infectious disease such as the patient's general health, normal defense mechanisms, previous contact with the offending organism, clinical history, and the type and location of infected tissue. Mechanisms of host defense and resistance are detailed in the following sections.

Primary Host Defenses

- *Anatomic barriers* include intact skin surfaces, nose hairs, respiratory tract cilia, coughing, flow of respiratory tract fluids and mucus, swallowing, and gastrointestinal tract peristalsis.

- *Physiologic barriers* include high or low pH and oxygen tension (ie, prevents proliferation of organisms), chemical inhibitors to bacterial growth such as protease, bile acids, active lysozymes in saliva and tears, and fatty acids on skin surfaces.

Secondary Host Defenses
- *Physiologic barriers* include the responses of complement, lysozymes, opsonins, and secretions; phagocytosis; IgA, IgG, and IgM antibody formation; and cell-mediated immune responses.

Decreased Host Resistance Factors
- Age; the very young and very old are more susceptible; the presence of chronic diseases such as cancer, cardiovascular disease, HIV infection, and diabetes
- Current or previous use of select therapeutic modalities such as irradiation, chemotherapy, corticosteroids, antibiotics, or immunosuppressants
- Presence of toxins, including alcohol, street drugs, legitimate therapeutic drugs, and venom or toxic secretions from reptiles, insects, or other nonhuman bites or punctures
- Other factors such as excessive physical or emotional stress, foreign material at the site, or altered nutritional status

Intratest Care
- Specimens obtained for bacterial culture should be representative of the disease process taking place. Collect sufficient material to ensure an accurate analysis. If a purulent sputum specimen cannot be produced to aid in the diagnosis of pneumonia, laboratory evaluations from blood cultures, pleural fluid specimens, and bronchoalveolar lavage (BAL) specimens are also acceptable.
- Material must be collected where the suspected organism is most likely to be found and with as little outside contamination as possible.
- Culture the specimen for specific pathogens only, not for normal flora present in the area.
- Collect fluids, tissues, skin scrapings, and urine in sterile containers with tight-fitting lids.
- Place specimens in a biohazard bag.
- Observe standard precautions.

Posttest Care
Posttest care includes the transport or mailing of microspecimens. Several kits containing transport media are available when there is a significant delay between collection and culturing. Culturette swabs

(Becton-Dickinson Microbiology Systems, Franklin Lakes, NJ) are available for bacterial, viral, and anaerobic specimen collections. Some laboratories provide Cary-Blair and PVA fixative transport vials for the collection of stool samples used for culture and ova and parasite examination. Some specimens may have to be shipped in a Styrofoam box with refrigerant packs. This is especially true for those used for viral examination. If in doubt, prudence dictates consultation with the reference laboratory where specimens will be sent to ensure proper collection and shipment.

According to the Code of Federal Regulations, a viable organism or its toxin or a diagnostic specimen (volume less than 50 mL) must be placed in a secure, closed, water-tight container that is then enclosed in a second, secure, water-tight container. Biohazard labels should be placed on the outside of the containers.

Specimens that are to be transported within an institution should be placed in a biohazard resealable bag. Ideally, the requisition should accompany the specimen but should not be sealed inside the bag.

Nursing Protocols for Hair, Nails, Saliva, and Breath Specimen Collection

Samples of clean hair and nails can be analyzed for evidence of fungal infections, abnormal concentrates of toxic and nutrient minerals, heavy metals, therapeutic drugs, and illegal drugs. High levels of some elements are caused by exposure to industrial wastes and by contaminated drinking water. The limit of detection of most drugs in hair is 0.1 ng/mL or higher.

Saliva specimens may be used to identify high levels of immunoglobulin G (IgG) in gingival crevices or systemic alcohol levels. Exhaled breath specimens are obtained to identify *Heliobacter pylori* infections, to detect alcohol, and to monitor hormones and other byproducts of abnormal metabolism.

Indications for Testing

- As a marker of toxin exposure
- To monitor parolees and probationers
- To validate drug self-reporting
- To identify in utero drug use
- To assess pattern of drug use (at 1-month intervals)
- To aid in drug treatment programs
- To screen employees in the workplace
- To evaluate parents' drug use in child custody cases

- As forensic evidence after death
- To verify compliance with nonpsychotropic regimens for months to years

Nursing Interventions
Pretest Care
- Assess and document signs and symptoms of drug presence or toxic exposure. Include the geographic location, water supply sources and quality, pesticide use, industrial waste exposure, food contaminants, and current medications.
- Explain how keratin is laid down in bone, hair, and nails and how this relates to the test purpose.
- Explain how mycotic organisms (eg, ringworm) attack the keratin.
- If testing is done for illicit or improperly used drugs, follow chain-of-custody protocols.

Intratest Care
- For hair sampling, use extreme care in obtaining hair samples. Wear gloves and follow established protocols. Hair should be shampooed and free of oil, conditioners, hair spray, and gels. Clip the hair close to the scalp. Color-treated hair is usually acceptable. Pubic hair is preferred.
- Obtain hairs from the correct sites: beard, mustache, axilla, genital area, and scalp. Inform the patient not to use any deodorant, powder, or lotion after shampooing or bathing until sampling is done. Use sterile scissors or instruments when cutting hair or nails.
- For nail sampling, clip nails close to the cuticle; toenails are preferred. Before clipping, thoroughly wash and dry toenails or fingernails.
- For saliva sampling, wear gloves, and using the special testing kit, follow the established procedure. Place the specially treated cotton pad between the lower cheek and gum and rub it back and forth until moistened. Allow the pad to remain in the mouth for 2 to 5 minutes before removing and inserting it into the specimen vial.
- For breath testing, wear gloves, and using a breath alcohol–testing device, follow the instructions to obtain a proper breath sample.
- Transfer specimens to the laboratory in a special envelope with a biohazard label or a metal-free, screw-top plastic container.
- Document the type and amount of specimen, site of hair or nail sampling, tests ordered, disposition of specimen, hair color (also include if chemically treated), condition of nails (eg, soft, gangrenous), appearance of follicle at hair shaft, time of collection, and the relevant skin conditions (eg, scaling, dermatitis, inflamed, reddened).

Nursing Protocols for Sputum Collection ─────────

Sputum specimens are examined to identify pathogens or conditions related to the respiratory system. Pertinent symptoms may include cough with or without sputum production, fever, chest pain, shortness of breath, and fatigue. Sputum specimens can also provide clues about antibiotic or drug sensitivity, the best course of treatment, and the effectiveness of treatment.

Interfering Factors

Unsatisfactory sputum samples include "dry" specimens (ie, saliva samples without actual sputum) or contaminated specimens.

Nursing Interventions

Pretest Care

- Explain the purpose and procedure of sputum specimen collection. An early morning specimen produces the best organism-concentrated sputum sample of deeply located pulmonary secretions.
- Obtain a sputum collection kit and supplies.
- Instruct the patient about all aspects of collection.
- Inform the patient not to touch the inside of the sputum container.

Intratest Care

- Sputum specimens must come from the bronchi. Postnasal secretions or saliva is unacceptable. Expectoration, ultrasonic nebulization, chest physiotherapy, nasotracheal or tracheal suctioning, and bronchoscopy are methods used to obtain sputum and bronchial specimens.
- Instruct the patient to remove dentures, rinse the mouth with water, and gargle, if possible.
- The patient should first clear the nose and throat, take three or four deep breaths, perform a series of short coughs, and then inhale deeply and cough forcefully to raise a sputum specimen.
- The sputum should be expectorated into a sterile container with the proper preservative if indicated. A 2- to 3-mL sample is adequate. Place the sealed container into a leak-proof biohazard bag, and transfer it to the laboratory after labeling properly.
- Sputum specimens are usually not refrigerated and should be taken to the laboratory as soon as possible. Include the pertinent information, such as type of specimen, appearance, preservative, tests ordered, date and time of collection, and disposition of specimen.
- Document the specimen appearance and the patient's response to the procedure.

Posttest Care
- Evaluate patient outcomes, and counsel appropriately about treatment and self-care for respiratory illness.
- Monitor the respiratory status as necessary, and intervene appropriately when indicated.

CLINICAL ALERT

Ultrasonic nebulizers may be used for sputum induction when the cough is not productive. If this is the case, proper cleaning and disinfection of the nebulizer must be done.

Do not obtain a suctioned sample without first consulting the physician.

Document when a patient is neutropenic (ie, very low white blood cell count and low or absent neutrophils). In this instance, no white blood cells are seen in the specimen and this may be interpreted as an unacceptable specimen.

Nursing Protocols for Evidentiary Specimen Collection in Criminal or Forensic Cases

Important evidentiary specimens are collected from the living and the deceased and can include blood, tissue, hair, nails, body fluids (eg, urine, semen, saliva, vaginal fluid, gastric fluid), and evidence generated by diagnostic procedures such as computed tomography (CT) scans, angiograms, and electrocardiograms. Collaboration with other professionals is mandatory.

Indications
- To obtain evidence from the victim or subject, including victims of physical and sexual assault, homicide, and child, elder, and spousal abuse. Specimens may be obtained from the patient, the deceased person, the perpetrator, the suspect, the accused or falsely accused, or the public in general.
- To retrieve evidentiary items during diagnostic and therapeutic procedures (eg, headshot projections and shotgun wadding that is often recovered from the victim or suspect's clothing or the sheets on which the victim is transported)
- To collect victim's clothing that may contain the victim's or perpetrator's fluid and tissue
- To obtain trace evidentiary specimens, such as traces of soot as in gunshot wound

- To record and have a witnessed record (ie, by a record person) of narcotics, dangerous drugs, and money (ie, two people count)
- To collect evidential material required by law enforcement, the medical examiner, and participants in the scientific investigation of death and criminal injury

Nursing Interventions
Pretest Care
- Use standard precautions to collect specimens.
- Prepare to institute a witnessed chain-of-custody procedure and follow these policies throughout when obtaining, handling, and preserving specimens.

Intratest Care
- Items that are wet (eg, bloody clothing) are first dried and then placed in thick paper bags (*not plastic*) and then labeled as a biohazard.
- Each specimen is to be labeled and packaged separately.

Posttest Care
- Follow chain of custody when turning over evidentiary specimens.
- Record all actions regarding specimen retrieval, including photographs and expected and unexpected samples (eg, bullets, drugs).

> **CLINICAL ALERT**
>
> - Specimens of newborn cord blood and meconium may be examined for evidence of the mother's drug use during pregnancy.

Sexual Assault Evidence Collection
The Sexual Assault Evidence Collection Kit contains the items needed to collect samples as required by the area crime laboratory for alleged sexual assault cases. Samples can be obtained with the kit from males and females, victims, and suspects.

A normal finding is less than 10 units/L of acid phosphatase, whereas a level that is 50 units/L or higher indicates a positive result for semen. Although the acid phosphatase levels of prostatic fluid can still be elevated in about 10% of women 72 hours after intercourse, low levels do not exclude recent intercourse. In cases of rape, samples should also be obtained for the identification of sexually transmitted diseases (STDs).

Interfering Factors
Samples should ideally be collected immediately after an alleged assault, because 66% of women examined within 6 hours of the

incident do not show motile sperm. Consequently, estimating the time of assault may be hampered. Bathing can wash away evidence.

Pretest Care

Explain the purpose and procedure of procuring samples, as they relate to the alleged incident. Check to see whether informed consent must be signed before obtaining specimens. Ensure that all forms are completed accurately and signed by the victim or suspect.

Intratest Procedure

Provide information on a form enclosed in the kit and have the individual and the examining medical professional sign and date the form.

- *Clothing samples:* Have the individual stand on a clean piece of examination paper and remove clothing, placing each article into a new, clean paper bag. Then fold the examination paper, placing it also into a clean paper bag. Date, seal, and initial each bag.
- *Vaginal swab:* Using the four swabs in the kit, thoroughly swab the vagina. Prepare a smear using the four swabs; allow the swabs and smear to air dry. Place the swabs in a swab box, return the smear to the cardboard slide holder, and tape it shut. Seal and complete the information requested on the envelope provided.
- *Cervical swab:* Using two swabs, thoroughly swab the cervix and immediately prepare a smear. Allow the swabs and smear to thoroughly air dry, return the swabs to the swab box, and return the smear to the cardboard slide holder. Seal and complete the information requested on the envelope provided.
- *Penile swab:* Using a single swab, moisten it with sterile water, and thoroughly swab the external area of the entire penis. Allow the swab to air dry, place it in the envelope, and seal and label it.
- *Blood sample for DNA testing:* Perform a venipuncture and collect at least 5 mL of blood in the lavender-stoppered (EDTA) blood tube provided in the kit. Label the tube with the individual's name and the date. From this tube, withdraw 1 mL of blood and fill each of the four printed circles on the DNA Stain Card. Allow the card to air dry, write the individual's name on the card, place it in the envelope, seal it, and complete the information requested. The blood tube should be placed in the Styrofoam blood tube holder. Seal the holder with the evidence tape, supply the information requested, and place the unit in the resealable bag provided.

After all samples have been collected, place all specimens (except blood tube) back into the kit. The blood tube should be refrigerated and the kit kept at room temperature until picked up by the police.

Posttest Care

Evaluate patient outcomes and monitor and counsel the patient appropriately.

✐ Nursing Protocols for Transdermal Collection ——————

Transdermal testing using reverse iontophoresis is a noninvasive method for extracting substances within or below the skin surface. Electrodes are applied to the skin surface, typically on the inner surface of the forearm, and a small electric current is applied (4 mA). Using specialized equipment and collection devices, specimens are collected for chemical analyses.

✐ Nursing Protocols for Specimen Collection in Chemical Poisoning or Terrorism ——————

Samples of blood and urine can be analyzed for evidence of exposure to chemical agents or toxins and as a part of managing hazardous chemical emergencies. Exposure can be either unintentional (eg, a chemical spill) or intentional (eg, an act of terrorism). Chemical agents can be classified as either toxins (produced by living organisms, for example, ricin from the castor bean plant or abrin from the rosary pea or jequirity pea) or toxicants (produced synthetically, for example, sarin, a nerve agent, or organophosphate pesticides).

Indications

- Collect specimens from every person who may have been exposed or potentially exposed to a chemical poisoning or terrorism agent (eg, ammonia, arsenic, or nerve gas).
- Identification of the chemical toxin or toxicant (eg, chlorine, cyanide).
- Aid in the management of emergencies, in the recognition of illness and toxic syndromes, and in defining chemical poisonings (eg, mercury).

Nursing Interventions

Pretest

- Assess and document signs and symptoms (blisters, dyspnea, skin discoloration, choking, bleeding, incapacitation, vomiting, diarrhea, muscle pain, weakness) of chemical poisoning, toxic exposure, and the location of incident.

- Explain the purpose and procedure of sampling for the presence of toxic chemical agents.

Intratest
- Obtain required urine cups and blood tubes.
- Collect 25 mL of urine in a screw-top container for all patients. For pediatric patients, collect urine only.
- Collect blood using three purple-top tubes (EDTA) and one gray- or green-top tube, in that order.
- Label so that when the tubes or cups are upright, the bar code looks like a ladder.
- Date, time, and initial the tube of the cup so that your initials are half on the tube or cup and half on the forensic evidence (waterproof) tape that you have placed on the top of the tube or cup.
- Prepare containers for shipment—tubes and cups are packaged and shipped separately on dry ice, as is done for diagnostic specimens.
- Dispose of your contaminated clothing.

Posttest
- Report results to patients.
- Counsel and begin treatment (eg, chelation therapy, supplemental oxygen).
- Monitor all systems (eg, respiratory, circulatory).
- If there has been unintentional chemical exposure, notification of local authorities may be all that is required.
- If there has been suspected or intentional chemical exposure, the local poison-control center, law enforcement and state health officials, and the CDC should be notified. The CDC has established a Laboratory Response Network (LRN) that includes a network of three (3) laboratory levels. Level 3 laboratories work with hospitals in their jurisdiction to coordinate proper specimen collection, transport, chain of custody (if applicable), and recognition of health effects of exposure to chemical agents. The Level 2 laboratory includes all activities associated with Level 3; however, there is increased training of personnel to detect exposure to a limited number of toxic chemicals. In the Level 1 laboratory, all activities of Level 3 and 2 laboratories are included in addition to more advanced training of laboratory personnel and specimen analyses.

Alphabetical List of Laboratory Tests of Body Fluids, Imaging Procedures, and Special Studies of Body Functions

☞ The Nurse's Role

Nursing Practice Standard

Nurses need a specialized knowledge base to provide safe, effective care; to manage outcomes; and to visualize their unique caring role during diagnostic testing. The nurse applies this knowledge and the nursing process model to all phases of testing to achieve the proper test results and expected patient outcomes. The information provided about each test, as well as the guidelines presented in Chapters 1 and 2, is part of this knowledge base.

Safe Practices for Procedures

The nurse has the required knowledge and skills to safely perform or assist with procedures; follows approved standards; educates patients about both invasive and noninvasive examinations; obtains informed consent; identifies patients at risk for adverse events, especially when barium, iodine, or radiopharmaceuticals are used; allows family presence as needed; and monitors the patient through all phases of care: pre-, intra-, and posttest.

Endoscopic Procedures

These examinations use an endoscope (a fiber-optic instrument with a lighted lens system) for direct visual examination of body organs and cavities. Pretest preparations are usually required to include patient compliance. A contrast agent may be instilled via an IV line, moderate/procedural sedation or analgesia may be given, topical anesthetics may be applied, and/or other medications may be given, depending upon the type of examination. Although the most common risks are perforation and infection, depending upon the site of the exam, other side effects can include sore throat after a bronchoscopic procedure or anal irritation following a colonoscopy. A consent form needs to be signed. Virtual colonoscopy and GI endoscopy are performed without an endoscope.

Nuclear Scan Procedures

These examinations use enhancement agents (radiopharmaceuticals), which are administered by IV or oral route. These radiopharmaceutical substances (not dyes or contrast agents as in X-rays) distribute throughout the organ or tissue to be studied. Viewed through special cameras, diseased tissue appears in a manner different from normal tissue as evidenced by areas of reduced activity or uptake (cold spots) or by increased activity or uptake (hot spots). The radiopharmaceutical dissipates over time and is eliminated in urine, feces, and/or other body fluids. These procedures can be performed on adults as well as pediatric patients. Risks include reaction to the radiopharmaceutical, including hives, rash, itching, flushing, fever, dyspnea, bronchospasm, and anaphylaxis. These reactions may occur immediately or 2 to 24 hours after the injection, as in bone scans. Nuclear scans are contraindicated in pregnancy. Positron emission tomography (PET) scans are often combined with CAT scans for monitoring cancer progression. A consent form needs to be signed.

Prenatal Tests

These tests assess maternal health, fetal well-being, and fetus at risk for intrauterine asphyxia. Fetal well-being depends on maternal health. Maternal fetal testing during pregnancy can be divided into the first trimester, second trimester, integrated screening from first and second trimesters, and third trimester tests. Prenatal testing usually includes maternal blood testing for CBC, hemoglobin, hematocrit, Rh type, ABO blood group, red blood cell antibody screen, rubella immunity status, glucose challenge, maternal serum alpha-fetoprotein (MS-AFP) or maternal triple screen, hepatitis B, test culture for STDs, group B streptococci (infection), urinalysis, ultrasound, amniocentesis (developmental abnormalities), fluoroscopy, CVS (fetal genetics or biochemical disorders), and sometimes MRI (fetal abnormalities).

Ultrasound and Doppler Procedures

These examinations, also known as echograms or sonograms, use a noninvasive method for visualizing soft tissue structures of the body. High-frequency sound waves produce a computerized "echo map" to characterize the position, size, form, and nature of soft tissue organs and demonstrate motion (fetus and heart). The Doppler effect, a phenomenon that accompanies movement, can be combined with ultrasound imagery for duplex scans. After a gel is applied, transducers are placed on the skin over a special body part; they can also be introduced in the vagina (gynecologic anatomy) or rectum (prostate exam), or placed on catheters (transesophageal echocardiography). Ultrasound cannot appropriately image air-filled structures such as the lungs. Ultrasound may be combined with other procedures, such as CAT scans and endoscopic examinations. There are no known risks.

Radiographic Procedures

These examinations, recorded on film or in a digital format, use electromagnetic rays (radiation) capable of penetrating through air but not dense substances. CAT scans of head, neck, and body are commonly performed. Contrast agents (eg, iodine and barium) can be injected, instilled, or swallowed, depending on the area to be studied. Side effects of contrast agents may include an allergic reaction or constipation. Whenever the body is exposed to radiation, exposures are cumulative—there is a risk of tissue damage, genetic defects, reddened skin, or cancer. Lead aprons and other protective gear must be worn by all staff members.

Special Study Procedures

Tests in this category may include skin, hair, saliva, sputum, gastric fluid, and breath sample collection to analyze for infections, toxins, and DNA identification. Gloves, special kits, and collection equipment are needed. Special diagnostic studies of the eye, brain, nervous system, and heart are of great value in identifying disease and disorders of these organ systems and used to rule out disorders, for example, tumors or cognitive defects. Sleep-and-awake studies incorporate various technologies such as EEG, EOG, EMG, and ECG. The application of skin, scalp, or chest electrodes, pulse oximeter, and airflow sensors, with subsequent awake or nocturnal recordings, provide evidence of pathology. Postmortem tests include autopsy and after-death donation of organs.

Tests, Procedures, and Special Studies, A Through X

The title of each test includes common and alternate names, abbreviations, specimen sources, and types of procedures. Titles of combined tests, such as those for electrolytes, also include the names of all substances measured, such as calcium, magnesium, potassium, chloride, and phosphate. Examples of combined tests include adrenal function, amniotic fluid analysis, antinuclear antibodies, arterial blood gases (ABGs), bioterrorism agents, diabetes tests, cardiac markers, coagulation tests, cerebrospinal fluid analysis, cholesterol tests, complete blood count (CBC), duplex scans, fetal well-being, hepatitis, kidney function, liver function, newborn screening panels, pancreatic function, protein analysis, pulmonary function, routine urinalysis, stool analysis, thyroid function, and tumor markers, among others.

ABDOMINAL ULTRASOUND-ABDOMEN SONOGRAM, AORTIC SONOGRAM, UPPER ABDOMINAL ECHOGRAM

Ultrasound Imaging: Gallbladder, Liver, Spleen, Pancreas, Kidney, Vessels

This noninvasive procedure visualizes all solid upper abdominal organs, including the liver, bile ducts, gallbladder, appendix, pancreas, kidneys, adrenals, spleen, and the abdominal aorta and vena cava. Some diagnostic laboratories may perform organ-specific studies, such as renal or hepatobiliary ultrasound scans, together with abdominal ultrasound scanning. Specific large vessels (such as the renal and mesenteric artery and portal vein) may be evaluated using Doppler analysis.

Indications

- Evaluate abdominal pathologies associated with abdominal pain, increased abdominal girth, obstructions, fluid collections, infections with fever, weight loss, and generalized ill health.
- Characterize known or suspected masses and determine cause of jaundice.
- Screen for abdominal aortic aneurysms and stage known carcinomas.
- Provide guidance during biopsy, cyst aspiration, and other invasive procedures.

Reference Values

Normal

- Normal position and appearance of the liver, gallbladder, bile ducts, pancreas, kidneys, adrenals, and spleen, as well as the abdominal aorta, inferior vena cava, and their major tributaries.
- Sizes of organs:

  Gallbladder: Length, diameter, and wall thickness within normal limits

  Liver: Anteroposterior (AP) diameter at the midclavicular line (ie, transverse) and length of the maximum right lobe (ie, sagittal) within normal limits

  Spleen: Width and length within normal limits

  Pancreas: Diameter of head and tail within normal limits

  Kidney: No more than a 1.5-cm difference between the sizes of the two functional kidneys

Clinical Implications

- Presence of space-occupying lesions: cysts, pancreatic cysts, solid masses, hematomas, abscesses, ascites, aneurysms, obstructions, arteriosclerotic changes to blood vessels, and abnormal blood flow patterns.
- Organ size, location, or structural abnormalities.
- Biliary tract obstruction, dilation, calculi, or hydronephrosis.
- One or more than two kidneys.

Interfering Factors

- Retained barium from prior x-ray studies may compromise the study.
- Intestinal gas overlying the area of interest interferes with sonographic visualization.
- Obesity adversely affects tissue visualization.

Procedure

- A liberal coating of coupling agent (ie, gel) is applied to the skin so that there is no air between the skin and the transducer, which promotes sound transmission. The coupling agent also allows easy movement of the transducer over the skin.
- In most laboratories, a handheld transducer is slowly moved across the skin of the area that is to be examined.
- The patient is asked to lie quietly on an examination table and control breathing pattern. Scans are generally performed with the patient in the supine and decubitus positions.
- The patient may hear a "swishing" sound during Doppler analysis.
- Total examination time is about 20 to 60 minutes.

Nursing Interventions

▸*Pretest*

- Explain the test purpose and procedure. Assure the patient that no radiation is employed and that the test is painless.
- Instruct the patient to avoid oral intake (remain NPO) for a minimum of 8 hours before the examination to fully dilate the gallbladder and to improve the visualization of all structures.
- Special attention is necessary for diabetic patients. Because of pretest fasting, the administration of insulin or oral hypoglycemic agents may be contraindicated. Check with the x-ray department for specific instructions. Schedule the test early in the day, if possible.
- Administer enemas if ordered.
- Explain that a coupling gel will be applied to the skin and that a sensation of warmth or wetness may be felt. Although the couplant

does not stain, advise the patient to avoid wearing nonwashable clothing.

 Intratest

• Explain to the patient that it is necessary to regulate the breathing pattern as instructed.
• Provide support and assure the patient that the test is proceeding normally.
• Instruct the patient that it is necessary to lie quietly during test, even though it may be uncomfortable.

Posttest

• Remove any residual gel from the skin.
• Normal diet and fluids may be resumed, unless contraindicated by the test results.
• Evaluate the outcomes and counsel the patient appropriately regarding further tests or possible treatments.

CLINICAL ALERT

• Scans cannot be performed over open wounds or through dressings.
• This examination must be performed before radiographic studies involving barium. If such scheduling is not possible, at least 24 hours must elapse between the barium procedure and the sonogram.
• Not fasting results in inadequate visualization of the gallbladder.
• Some laboratories administer a noniodine, nonionic oral contrast to aid in the delineation of upper abdominal structures (particularly the pancreas).

 ADRENAL FUNCTION TESTS

Blood, Saliva, and Urine, 24-Hour Endocrine

Cortisol, Cortisol Suppression or Dexamethasone Suppression Test (DST), Cortisol Stimulation or Cosyntropin Stimulation, and Corticotropin (ACTH)-Releasing Hormone (CRH) Stimulation

These tests measure adrenal hormone function, insufficiency, and hyperfunction; insufficiency is more common than Cushing's disease. The adrenal gland produces mineral corticosteroids, catecholamines, and combined sex steroids and glucosteroids. DHEA-S in urine or plasma is the major androgen produced by the adrenals.

Indications

- Evaluate adrenal diseases: hyperplasia, adrenal carcinoma, Addison's disease, Cushing's syndrome, amenorrhea, and hypertension.
- DST identifies persons most likely to respond to therapy for clinical depression.
- Measurement of plasma ACTH differentiates primary from secondary adrenal insufficiency.
- Because single measurements of plasma or urine cortisol are difficult to interpret, suppressor tests (DST), using agents that affect the hypothalamic-pituitary-adrenal axis, identify the source of the problem.
- Stimulation tests localize source of dysfunction and evaluate adrenal insufficiency.
- DHEA-S determines adrenal sources of androgens, cause of hirsutism, virilization, and polycystic ovary disease.

Reference Values

Normal

SERUM CORTISOL

Adult
8:00 AM: 8–25 μg/dL or 221–690 nmol/L
4:00 PM: 3–16 μg/dL or 83–441 nmol/L
Midnight: <7.5 μg/dL or 207 nmol/L
Newborns: 2.0–11 μg/dL or 55–304 nmol/L
Maternal (at birth): 51.2–57.4 μg/dL or 1413–1584 nmol/L

After first week of life, cortisol levels attain adult values.

SALIVARY CORTISOL

11:00 PM to midnight: <0.15 μg/dL or <4.2 nmol/L

CORTISOL SUPPRESSION DEXAMETHASONE SUPPRESSION TEST (DST)

Morning after dexamethasone administered: <5 μg/dL or <138 nmol/L

COSYNTROPIN-STIMULATED SERUM CORTISOL

Baseline at 8:00 AM: 8–25 μg/dL or 221–690 nmol/L
30 minutes postcosyntropin iv: >18 μg/dL or 499 nmol/L

CLINICAL ALERT

- Increased cortisol levels correlate with acute illness (eg, severe inflammation).

Clinical Implications

- *Cortisol levels increase* with oat-cell cancer, hyperthyroidism, adrenal adenoma, and Cushing's syndrome (adrenal adenoma, Cushing's disease, and overproduction of adrenocorticotropic hormone [ACTH]).
- *Cortisol levels decrease* with liver disease, adrenal insufficiency (Addison's disease, anterior pituitary hyposecretion and destruction), hypothyroidism, and steroid therapy.
- The overnight DST result is abnormal above 5 μg/dL (138 nmol/L); no suppression in stress states, and in renal failure.
- *No cortisol suppression* (DST) or diurnal variation (due to melatonin) is seen with Cushing's disease or with clinical depression.
- *No cortisol stimulation or a blunted response* occurs with adrenal insufficiency, hypopituitarism, and prolonged steroid therapy.

Interfering Factors

- Cortisol elevations occur during obesity, pregnancy, in newborns, and with some drugs (eg, spironolactone, oral contraceptives).
- Cortisol is falsely low in renal disease and in patients with low plasma albumin (eg, albumin).
- A false-positive result occurs for cortisol suppression if the patient fails to take dexamethasone; with alcohol; with some drugs (eg, Dilantin [phenytoin], estrogen); in newborns; and in cases of anorexia, stress, trauma, dehydration, fever, and uncontrolled diabetes.

Procedure

- *Cortisol:* Serum (5-mL) samples are obtained by venipuncture at 8:00 AM and 4:00 PM, using a red-marbled–top tube. Heparin anticoagulant may be used. Salivary cortisol is obtained between 11:00 PM and midnight. Obtain a 24-hour urine specimen.
- *Cortisol (dexamethasone) suppression (DST):* Venous serum (5-mL) samples are obtained the day after oral administration of 1.0 mg of dexamethasone at 11:00 PM. Plasma is acceptable.
- *Cortisol stimulation:* Fasting serum (5 mL) is obtained by venipuncture using red-top tube. Then collect additional 4-mL specimens 30 and 60 minutes after IV administration of 250 μg of cosyntropin (Cortrosyn).

> ### CLINICAL ALERT
>
> - Other tests for depression include the following:
>   Thyrotropin-releasing hormone (TRH) stimulation test
>   Prolactin response to TRH
>   3-Methoxy-4-hydroxyphenylglycol (MHPG) in urine
>   Platelet monamine oxidase (MAO) activity
>   Phenylacetic acid (PAA) in urine
> - Psychiatric manifestations are associated with conditions such as
>   hyperthyroidism, hypothyroidism, primary hyperparathyroidism,
>   Cushing's syndrome, acute intermittent porphyria (AIP), and vitamin
> B_{12} deficiency.

Nursing Interventions

▶ Pretest

- Explain the purpose and procedure of the study; assess the
  patient's knowledge of the test and symptoms. Remind the patient
  about fasting for the stimulant and suppression tests. Weigh
  patient.
- Check with the physician and discontinue drugs, especially glucocorticoids, aldosterones, estrogens, birth control medications,
  tetracycline, and anticonvulsants, for 24 to 48 hours before the
  study. Ensure that no radiopharmaceuticals are administered 1 day
  before the cortisol test and 1 week before suppression.

▶ Posttest

- Evaluate the outcome and counsel the patient appropriately about
  the effects of hormone dysfunction.
- Dysfunction occurs in Addison's disease, Cushing's syndrome,
  acute illness, and malignant tumors producing ACTH and is present with metabolic acidosis and hyperglycemia.

ADRENAL GLAND SCAN (MIBG)

Nuclear Medicine Scan, Endocrine System Imaging

This procedure is used to identify certain tumors of the adrenal
medulla that produce excessive amounts of catecholamines:
pheochromocytomas and adrenal and extra-adrenal paraganglions.
It is especially useful for detecting ectopic sites and metastatic
lesions.

Indications

- Diagnose adrenal and extra-adrenal paraganglions.
- Locate pheochromocytoma sites before surgery.
- Determine the nature of a particular nodule and whether tissue is functioning or nonfunctioning.
- Evaluate the patient with multiple pheochromocytomas.

Reference Values

Normal

- No evidence of tumors or a hypersecreting hormone site.
- Normal salivary glands, liver, and heart.

Clinical Implications

- Abnormal concentrations reveal pheochromocytomas and give substance to the rough rule of 10. This means that 10% of tumors are in children, 10% are familial, 10% are bilateral in the adrenals, 10% are malignant, 10% are multiple (in addition to bilateral tumors), and 10% are enterorenal.
- Two or more pheochromocytomas usually indicate malignant disease. *Multiple extra-adrenal* pheochromocytomas are often malignant.

Interfering Factors

- Presence of barium from previous procedures.

Procedure

- Lugol's solution or supersaturated potassium iodide (SSKI), which is administered before the test (1 day before is typical) and after injection (6–10 days is typical) to prevent thyroid uptake of radioactive iodine.
- Radiopharmaceutical iobenguane (^{131}I-metaiodobenzylguanidine [MIBG]) is injected intravenously. Whole-body images will be taken at 24 hours postinjection. The nuclear medicine physician may request imaging at 48, 72, and 96 hours postinjection. Imaging time is 1 hour each day.

Nursing Interventions

▶*Pretest*

- Specific drug protocols involving SSKI must be followed: 1 drop of SSKI (1 g/mL) 1 day before and 6 days after ^{131}I-MIBG administration.
- Explain the test purpose and procedure. Weigh patient.
- Exclude pregnant and breast-feeding women.

- Reassure the patient regarding the safety of the nuclear scan.
- No bowel preparation is necessary.
- Obtain an accurate medication history 4 to 6 weeks prior to the procedure. The patient should be off all tricyclic antidepressants, reserpine, cocaine, over-the-counter Sudafed, and imipramine. The patient should discontinue labetalol for 3 days to 2 weeks before the study and should not be taking amphetamines, nasal decongestants, or diet-control pills.

CLINICAL ALERT

- Obtain informed consent, if needed.
- Schedule this test before x-ray studies using iodine contrast agents and before thyroid- or iodine-containing drugs are given.

▸Intratest
- Provide support and reassurance during serial imaging each day.
- The patient may eat and drink normally between scans.

▸Posttest
- Evaluate posttest outcomes and counsel the patient appropriately about the need for possible follow-up testing, which may include kidney (renogram) and bone nuclear scans, CT scans, pelvic ultrasound of tumor-producing urinary symptoms, and possible treatment (eg, surgical removal of tumor).
- Monitor the site of radiopharmaceutical injection for infection and infiltration.
- Routinely dispose of body fluids and secretions.
- Document any patient problems (eg, vomiting) that may have occurred during the procedure.

ALCOHOL, ETHANOL (ETOH)

Blood, Breath, Saliva

This test measures the presence of alcohol in the blood, breath, or saliva as an indication of intoxication or overdose. Upon consuming an alcoholic beverage, the alcohol is absorbed by the stomach and duodenum and enters the bloodstream. Distribution of the alcohol is fairly rapid (about 20–30 minutes) and uniform throughout body water. Because of this, alcohol concentration can be measured in the blood, breath (a portion of the alcohol is eliminated via the lungs), or saliva (used as a screening value).

Indications
- U.S. Department of Transportation (U.S. DOT) mandates (eg, performing safety-sensitive duties, following vehicular accident).
- Assess levels for alcohol influence and alcohol intoxication.
- Routine trauma protocol for seizure victims.

Reference Values

Normal
- None detected; negative.

Clinical Implications
- Alcohol levels <50 mg/dL (<10.8 mmol/L) generally will not affect individuals, although some studies suggest that levels as low as 10–30 mg/dL (2.17–6.51 mmol/L) can impair one's ability to perform fine motor skills.
- Levels between 50 and 100 mg/dL (10.8–21.7 mmol/L) can result in decreased inhibitions, impaired judgment, interference with motor skills, and increased reaction times.
- At levels >100 mg/dL (>21.7 mmol/L), individuals will become uncoordinated and disoriented with loss of memory and critical judgment skills.
- Death has been associated with levels >400 mg/dL (>86.8 mmol/L).

Interfering Factors
- Residual mouth alcohol (recent ingestion of an alcoholic beverage or mouthwash containing alcohol) or gastric reflux can falsely elevate the reading if the appropriate waiting time before obtaining a saliva or breath sample is not followed.
- Isopropanol, *n*-propanol, acetone, and ascorbic acid may interfere with the measurement.
- Increased blood ketones, eg, as in diabetic ketoacidosis, can falsely elevate test results.

Procedure
Blood Alcohol
- The state provides a kit that contains the necessary items for procuring a blood sample as well as appropriate forms for chain of custody if necessary.

• A venipuncture is performed and two (5-mL) gray-top tubes of blood are obtained. One tube is used for immediate analysis and the other tube is retained for future repeat analysis for evidentiary purposes.

Breath Alcohol
• A 15-minute waiting period is observed prior to collection of the sample to ensure residual mouth alcohol will not be an interfering factor.
• The individual is then instructed to take a deep breath, and, inserting the mouthpiece into his or her mouth, blow forcefully for approximately 6 seconds.

Salivary Alcohol
• A 15-minute waiting period is observed prior to collection of the sample to ensure residual mouth alcohol will not be an interfering factor.
• If a cotton or foam swab is used, it is placed into the individual's mouth; the inside of the cheeks, the underside of the tongue, and the gums are swabbed for approximately 10–60 seconds or until the swab is thoroughly soaked. The swab is then inserted into the entry port of the salivary measuring device for measurement of alcohol content.

Nursing Interventions
▸*Pretest*
• Explain the test's purpose and procedure as proof of alcohol-related impaired ability to perform certain safety-sensitive duties, operate a motor vehicle, intoxication, or validation of alcohol-free status. Check to see if informed consent must be signed before obtaining a specimen.

▸*Posttest*
• Evaluate patient outcomes and monitor and counsel appropriately regarding state mandates.

ALDOSTERONE

Blood, Urine

Aldosterone is a mineralocorticoid hormone produced in the adrenal zona glomerulosa under complex control by the renin-angiotensin system. This test is useful in detecting primary or secondary aldosteronism. Patients with primary aldosteronism characteristically have hypertension, muscular pain and cramps, weakness, tetany, paralysis, and polyuria. It is also used to evaluate causes of hypertension (found in 1% of hypertension cases).

Note: A random aldosterone test is of no diagnostic value unless a plasma renin activity is performed at the same time.

Indications
- Detect primary or secondary aldosteronism
- Check for adrenal tumors
- Investigate causes of hypertension or low blood potassium levels

Reference Values

Normal
In upright position
- Adults: 7–30 ng/dL or 0.19–0.83 nmol/L
- Adolescents: 4–48 ng/dL or 0.11–1.33 nmol/L
- Children: 5–80 mg/dL or 0.14–2.22 nmol/L

In supine position
- Adults: 3–16 ng/dL or 0.08–0.44 nmol/L
- Adolescents: 2–22 ng/dL or 0.06–0.61 nmol/L
- Children: 3–35 mg/dL or 0.08–0.97 nmol/L
- Low-sodium diet: values 3–5 times higher
- 24-Hour Urine: 5–24 mg/day or 14–66 mmol/day

Procedure
- Obtain a 5-mL venous blood specimen in a heparinized or EDTA Vacutainer tube. Serum, EDTA, or heparinized blood may be used. The cells must be separated from plasma immediately. Blood should be drawn with patient in a sitting position. Observe standard precautions.
- Specify patient position (upright or supine), site of puncture, and time of the venipuncture. Circadian rhythm exists in normal subjects, with levels of aldosterone peaking in the morning.
- A 24-hour urine specimen with boric acid preservative may also be ordered. Refrigerate immediately following collection.
- Patient should follow a normal sodium diet 2–4 weeks before test.

Clinical Implications
- *Elevated levels of aldosterone (primary aldosteronism)* occur in the following conditions:
    - Aldosterone-producing adenoma (Conn's disease)
    - Adrenocortical hyperplasia (pseudoprimary aldosteronism)

- Indeterminate hyperaldosteronism
- Glucocorticoid-remediable hyperaldosteronism
- *Secondary aldosteronism*, in which aldosterone output is elevated because of external stimuli or greater activity in the renin-angiotensin system, occurs in the following conditions:
  - Salt depletion
  - Potassium loading
  - Laxative abuse
  - Cardiac failure
  - Cirrhosis of liver with ascites
  - Nephrotic syndrome
  - Bartter's syndrome
  - Diuretic abuse
  - Hypovolemia and hemorrhage
  - After 10 days of starvation
  - Toxemia of pregnancy
- *Decreased aldosterone levels* are found in the following conditions:
  - Aldosterone deficiency
  - Addison's disease
  - Syndrome of renin deficiency (very rare)
  - Low aldosterone levels associated with hypertension are found in Turner's syndrome, diabetes mellitus, and alcohol intoxication

Interfering Factors

- Values are increased by upright posture.
- Recently administered radioactive medications affect test outcomes.
- Heparin therapy causes levels to fall.
- Thermal stress, late pregnancy, and starvation cause levels to rise.
- Aldosterone levels decrease with age.
- Many drugs—diuretics, antihypertensives, progestogens, estrogens, and licorice—should be terminated 2–4 weeks before the test.

 CLINICAL ALERT

Potassium deficiency should be corrected before testing for aldosterone.

Nursing Interventions
▶*Pretest*

- Explain test purpose and procedures. Assess for history of diuretic or laxative abuse.
- Discontinue diuretic agents, progestational agents, estrogens, and black licorice for 2 weeks before the test.

- Ensure that the patient's diet for 2 weeks before the test is normal (other than the previously listed restrictions) and should include 3 g/day (135 mEq/L/day) of sodium. Check with your laboratory for special protocols.
- Follow guidelines in Chapter 1 for safe, effective, informed *pretest* care.

▸*Posttest*
- Have patient resume normal activities and diet.
- Interpret test results and monitor appropriately for aldosteronism and aldosterone deficiency.
- Follow guidelines in Chapter 1 for safe, effective, informed *posttest* care.

ALPHA₁-ANTITRYPSIN (AAT)

Blood, Inflammation, Fasting per Order, Liver, Lung

This test measures alpha₁-antitrypsin (AAT), which is a protein produced by the liver. Deficiency is associated with pulmonary emphysema, liver disease, and other metabolic disorders. The prevalence of ATT deficiency is about 1:3,000 in the U.S.

Indications
- Evaluate respiratory disease and liver cirrhosis.
- Screen for genetic AAT deficiency with family history of emphysema.
- Nonspecific diagnosis of inflammation, severe infection, and necrosis.

Reference Values

Normal
- AAT level of 100–200 mg/dL or 1.1–2.0 g/L

Clinical Implications
- *Elevated AAT levels* occur with inflammatory or hematologic disorders, cancer, and acute hepatitis.
- *Decreased AAT levels* indicate adult early-onset chronic pulmonary emphysema, liver cirrhosis in infants and children, as well as severe liver damage, nephrotic syndrome, and malnutrition. Patients with serum levels less than 70 mg/dL (0.7 g/L) are likely to have a homozygous deficiency and are at risk for early lung disease.

Interfering Factors

- Any inflammatory process elevates serum levels. Exercise stress increases AAT levels.
- Serum levels may normally increase by 100% in pregnancy. Some drugs (eg, estrogens, oral contraceptives, tamoxifen) increase serum levels.

Procedure

- Serum (7 mL) is obtained by venipuncture using a red-top tube.
- Fasting is required if the patient has elevated cholesterol or triglyceride levels.

Nursing Interventions

▸ *Pretest*

- Explain the purpose of the test and instruct patient about fasting, if necessary.

▸ *Posttest*

- Evaluate test outcomes and provide appropriate counseling. Genetic counseling may be indicated because AAT deficiencies are inherited.
- Advise the patients with decreased AAT levels to avoid smoking and, if possible, occupational hazards such as dust, fumes, and other respiratory pollutants.
- Explain to the patient that further testing may be necessary if the level of this protein is decreased. This involves phenotyping the serum specimen to assess a significant risk of related disease such as pulmonary emphysema, liver cirrhosis in children, severe liver damage, and nephrotic syndrome.
- Augmentation therapy (infusions of human purified AAT) may be indicated in some cases.

ALPHA-FETOPROTEIN (AFP)

Blood, Maternal

Maternal Serum Alpha-Fetoprotein (MS-AFP)

The measurement of maternal serum AFP usually is done at 16 weeks' gestation when AFP concentration rises dramatically. About 90% of infants with neural tube defects are born to parents who have no recognized risk factors for the disorder. Maternal triple screen (MoM [multiples of the median]: AFP, hCG, and E_3) aids in identifying Down's syndrome risk (see alphabetical listing for maternal triple test). The test also detects complications of pregnancy, and AFP serves as a tumor marker in nonpregnant women.

Indications
- Maternal AFP is routinely offered between 16 and 18 weeks' gestation to all pregnant women in order to screen for fetal abnormalities and neural tube defects.
- Diagnose and monitor hepatocellular, testicular, ovarian, and malignant liver diseases.
- Detect pregnancy complications, such as intrauterine growth retardation, fetal distress, and fetal demise.

Reference Values

Normal
- At 15 to 18 weeks' gestation: 10–150 ng/mL or 10–150 μg/L
- Normal adult level: <10 ng/mL or <10 μg/L
- MoM: 0.5–2.5 (calculated by dividing patient's AFP by median AFP for a normal pregnancy at the same gestational age)

Clinical Implications
- Elevated maternal AFP level can indicate a neural tube defect, anencephaly, underestimation of gestational age, multiple gestation, threatened abortion, Rh incompatibility disease, and congenital abnormalities. In the third trimester, an elevated AFP level can be the result of esophageal atresia, tetralogy of Fallot, hydranencephaly, Rh isoimmunization, and gastrointestinal tract obstruction.
- Low maternal AFP levels may indicate trophoblastic neoplasia, Down's syndrome, or other chromosomal abnormalities (ie, trisomy 13, 18, or 21, or second-trimester fetal wastage).
- Elevated levels occur with cancer of the liver, pancreas, stomach, bile ducts, and gonads and with hepatitis, cirrhosis, and liver injury.

Interfering Factors
- Obesity causes low maternal serum AFP (MS-AFP) levels.
- Insulin-dependent diabetes results in low MS-AFP levels.
- Race is a factor. MS-AFP is 10% to 15% higher in African Americans and lower in Asians than in Caucasians.

Procedure
- Obtain 10 mL of venous blood; use a red-top tube. Plan the first screening at 15 to 18 weeks. If the result is normal, no further screening is necessary.

- Include for the laboratory information about duration of pregnancy, mother's weight, ethnicity, and presence of diabetes.

Nursing Interventions

▶Pretest
- Determine the gestational age from the last menstrual period.
- Explain the AFP procedure to the patient.

▶Posttest
- Collaborate with the physician to interpret the outcome and counsel the patient about the results.
- Explain the possible need for future testing.
- Elevated maternal AFP levels should be followed by a second screening or ultrasound studies for fetal age.
- Low maternal AFP levels should be followed by ultrasound studies and then by amniocentesis.

CLINICAL ALERT

- The incidence of neural tube defect is 1 case per 1000 births in the United States and 1 case per 5000 births in England.
- Knowledge of the precise gestational age is paramount for the accuracy of this test.
- If the MS-AFP level is elevated and no fetal defect is demonstrated (ie, by ultrasound or amniocentesis), the pregnancy is at an increased risk for a poor outcome (eg, premature birth, low-weight infant, fetal death).

AMNIOTIC FLUID ANALYSIS

Amniotic Fluid

Color, Volume, Alpha-Fetoprotein (AFP), Creatinine, Lecithin-Sphingomyelin (LS) Ratio, Bilirubin, Fern Test

Amniotic fluid is examined *early* in pregnancy to study genetic makeup of the fetus and determine developmental abnormalities. Testing in the third trimester is done to determine fetal age and well-being, to study blood groups, and to detect amnionitis.

Indications
- Offer prenatal diagnosis to high-risk parents in order to detect an abnormal fetus.

- Evaluate hematologic disease, fetal infections, inborn metabolic disorders, and fetal distress.
- Diagnose sex-linked disorders, chromosomal abnormalities, and neural tube defects.
- Determine presence of amniotic fluid in the vagina by sterile speculum examination to diagnose rupture of the membranes.

Reference Values

Normal

- Clear or pale yellow fluid, with volumes of 30 to 1500 mL, depending on the stage of gestation.
- AFP level is age dependent; the peak at 12 to 16 weeks is 14.5 μg/mL or 196 pmol/L.
- The creatinine level gradually declines to 1.5 to 2.0 mg/dL (133–177 μmol/L) at fetal maturity.
- Lecithin-sphingomyelin (LS) ratio of 2:1 or greater indicates pulmonary maturity; a 1:2 dilution (shake test) indicates lung maturity.
- A bilirubin optical density of <0.02 mg/dL or <0.34 μmol/L indicates maturity.
- A positive fern test result shows a fern pattern, indicating amniotic fluid rather than urine.
- A negative fern test result shows no fern pattern, indicating urine.

Clinical Implications

- Abnormal colors are associated with fetal distress, death, a missed abortion, a chromosomally abnormal fetus, anencephaly, and blood incompatibility.
- Increased volume in polyhydramnios is often associated with congenital abnormalities such as esophageal atresia, anencephaly, Rh disorder, and diabetes.
- Decreased volume occurs with abnormal kidney function, premature rupture of membranes, and intrauterine growth retardation.
- Creatinine levels decrease with prematurity.
- Increased bilirubin levels indicate impending fetal death.
- Elevated AFP levels indicate possible neural tube defects.
- Decreased AFP levels indicate fetal trisomy 21.
- Sickle cell anemia and thalassemia are detected by fibroblast DNA examination.
- The LS ratio is decreased with pulmonary immaturity and respiratory distress syndrome.

CLINICAL ALERT

- Consider RhoGAM injection for Rh-negative women after amniocentesis unless previously sensitized, especially if fluid is bloody or a significant number of fetal cells are found in the fluid.
- A maternal (AFP) blood test can be done.
- Fetal position, viability, number, and pockets of fluid are assessed by ultrasound before an amniotic tap.

Procedure

- Insert a special needle through the abdominal wall into the amniotic sac. Obtain a 20- to 30-mL specimen and apply a dressing to the needle site.
- Perform a sterile speculum examination, obtain a sample of vaginal or cervical secretions with a sterile cotton swab, and place it on a glass slide. Let it dry and then inspect the slide under the microscope for fern or urine formation.

Nursing Interventions

▸ *Pretest*

- Genetic counseling, including both parents, should include the risk of a positive result and decision making regarding the risks during pregnancy, birth, and support systems in place for affected families after birth, as well as decision making regarding an elective abortion, including the psychologic effects of this choice.
- Explain the purpose and risks of prenatal diagnosis procedure and assess for contraindications: premature labor history, incompetent cervix, placenta previa, or abruptio placentae.
- Obtain the baseline blood pressure (BP), pulse, respiration, and fetal heart rate.
- The patient should empty her bladder before the procedure.

▸ *Intratest*

- Provide support and reassurance during the procedure.
- Nausea, vertigo, and mild cramps may occur.

▸ *Posttest*

- Evaluate test outcomes and counsel the patient appropriately in collaboration with the physician.
- Monitor for complications: spontaneous abortion, fetal injury, hemorrhage, infection, and Rh sensitivity if fetal blood enters the mother's circulation.

- Assess for signs of labor by palpation of the uterine fundus for tightening and use of an external fetal monitor to assess for contractions and fetal well-being.
- Administer RhoGAM injection to the Rh-negative woman who has not been previously sensitized.

ANDROSTENEDIONE

Blood

Androstenedione is one of the major androgens produced by the ovaries in females and to a lesser extent in the adrenal gland in both genders.

Indications
- Evaluate hirsutism (abnormal or increased hair growth) and virilization.

Reference Values

Normal
- Newborns: 20–290 ng/dL or 0.7–10.1 mmol/L
- Prepubescents: 8–50 ng/dL or 0.3–1.7 mmol/L
- Women: 75–205 ng/dL or 2.6–7.2 mmol/L
- Men: 85–275 ng/dL or 3.0–9.6 mmol/L
- Postmenopausal women: <10 ng/dL or 0.35 mmol/L (abrupt decline at menopause)

Procedure
- Obtain a 5-mL venous blood sample in the morning and place on ice. Serum or EDTA can be used.
- In women, collect this specimen 1 week before or after the menstrual period. Record date of last menstrual period on the laboratory form.

Clinical Implications
- *Increased androstenedione values* are associated with the following conditions:
    - Stein-Leventhal syndrome
    - Cushing's syndrome
    - Certain ovarian tumors (polycystic ovarian syndrome)

- Ectopic ACTH-producing tumor
- Late-onset congenital adrenal hyperplasia
- Ovarian stromal hyperplasia
- Osteoporosis in females
- *Decreased androstenedione values* are found in the following conditions:
    - Sickle cell anemia
    - Adrenal and ovarian failure

Nursing Interventions
▶*Pretest*
- Explain purpose of test and blood-drawing procedure. Obtain pertinent history of signs and symptoms (eg, excessive hair growth and infertility).
- Ensure that patient is fasting and that blood is drawn at peak production (7:00 AM or 0700 hours).
- Collect specimen 1 week before the menstrual period in women.
- Follow guidelines in Chapter 1 for safe, effective, informed *pretest* care.

▶*Posttest*
- Have patient resume normal activities.
- Interpret test results and counsel appropriately for ovarian and adrenal dysfunction.
- Follow guidelines in Chapter 1 for safe, effective, informed *posttest* care.

ANTIBODY TO HUMAN IMMUNODEFICIENCY VIRUS (HIV-1 AND -2); ACQUIRED IMMUNODEFICIENCY SYNDROME (AIDS) TEST; HIV GROUP O, HUMAN IMMUNODEFICIENCY VIRUS (HIV-1/2)

Blood, Saliva, Urine Testing

This test is done to determine the presence of antibody to human immunodeficiency viruses types 1 and 2 (HIV-1, HIV-2), the etiologic agents of acquired immunodeficiency syndrome (AIDS). An HIV infection is described as a continuum of stages that include the acute, transient, mononucleosis-like syndrome associated with seroconversion; asymptomatic HIV infection; symptomatic HIV infection; and AIDS. AIDS is *end-stage* HIV infection.

Indications

- Evaluate suspected HIV infection and assessment of patients with a history of exposure to HIV-infected persons through sexual or parenteral activities.
- Screen persons whose blood, plasma products, tissues, and organs are being donated for transfusion and transplantation.
- Test pregnant women and infants born to infected women.
- Test sexual partners of HIV-infected persons.
- Test after needlestick exposure or bite by infected person.

Reference Values

Normal

- Negative: nonreactive for antibody to HIV-1 and HIV-2 using enzyme-linked immunosorbent assay (ELISA), Western blot (WB), and immunofixation (IFA) methods
- HIV proviral RNA: not reactive or negative by PCR
- HIV proviral DNA: not reactive or negative
- HIV core P24 antigen: not reactive or negative
- Nucleic acid test (NAT): low viral load

Clinical Implications

- A positive test result should be repeated and confirmed by other tests.
- An ELISA test is used as a screening procedure and, if positive, must be followed by a Western blot to confirm the presence of antibody to HIV.
- A positive ELISA result may occur in noninfected persons because of unknown factors.
- A negative test result tends to rule out AIDS as a diagnosis for high-risk patients who do not have a characteristic opportunistic infection or tumor.
- False-negative results occur for 6% to 20% of tests.

Interfering Factors

- Nonreactive HIV test results occur during the acute stage of infection, when virus is present but antibody development is not sufficient to be detected. Virus may be present for up to 6 months before the antibody can be detected. During this stage, the test for HIV antigen may confirm an HIV infection.
- Nonspecific reactions may occur with prior pregnancy, blood transfusions, or use of HIV test kits that are extremely sensitive.

Procedure

- Serum (7 mL) (red-top tube) or plasma (lavender-top tube) is obtained by venipuncture. Place the specimen in a biohazard bag for transport.
- Home HIV test users should obtain a fingerstick blood sample with a lancet provided by the manufacturer; the sample is placed on a test card and mailed to a certified laboratory.
- Saliva or oral specimens may be obtained using a special commercial testing kit. The kit's components usually consist of a specially treated cotton pad on a nylon stick and a vial containing preservative solution. Place the pad between the lower cheeks and gum, rub it back and forth until moistened, and leave it in place for 2 minutes. Remove the specially treated pad and place it in the vial of special antimicrobial preservative solution. Place the specimen container in a biohazard bag and transport it to the laboratory.
- A urine specimen may also be used for testing.

Nursing Interventions

▶Pretest

- Assess the patient's knowledge about the HIV test, false-positive factors, accuracy of the test, and the test procedure.
- Assess the frequency and intensity of symptoms: increased temperature, diarrhea, neuropathy, nausea, depression, and fatigue.
- Provide pretest counseling, which is essential.
- Be supportive and sensitive to the patient's fear and anxiety.

CLINICAL ALERT

- An informed consent must be signed by any person who is being tested for HIV/AIDS. The consent must accompany the specimen to the laboratory, or if the patient goes to the laboratory for venipuncture, consent must accompany the patient.
- Issues of confidentiality surround HIV testing. The test should not be performed without the subject's knowledge.
- The professional ordering the test must sign a legal form stating that patient has been informed of the risks of testing.

▶Posttest

- Evaluate outcomes along with $CD4^+$ lymphocyte cell counts and explain significance and accuracy of the test results to the patient. Describe behavioral modifications (eg, sexual contacts, shared needles, blood transfusions).

- A person who has antibodies to HIV is presumed to be infected with the virus and appropriate counseling and medical evaluation (treatment with potent antiviral drugs and protease inhibitors) should be offered.

ANTIDIURETIC HORMONE (ADH); ARGININE VASOPRESSIN HORMONE

Blood

Antidiuretic hormone (ADH) is excreted by the posterior pituitary gland. Its major physiologic function is regulation of body water. In the dehydrated state, ADH release results in decreased urine excretion and conservation of water. Additionally, ADH increases blood pressure.

Indications
- Provide a differential diagnosis of polyuric and hyponatremic states.
- Aid in diagnosis of diabetes insipidus and psychogenic water intoxication.

Reference Values

Normal
- <2.5 pg/mL or <2.3 pmol/L

Clinical Implications
- *Increased secretion of ADH* is associated with the following conditions:
  - Syndrome of inappropriate antidiuretic hormone (SIADH) (with respect to plasma osmolality)
  - Ectopic ADH production (systemic neoplasm)
  - Nephrogenic diabetes insipidus
  - Acute intermittent porphyria
  - Guillain-Barré syndrome
  - Brain tumor, diseases, injury, neurosurgery
  - Pulmonary diseases (tuberculosis)
- *Decreased secretion of ADH* occurs in the following conditions:
  - Central diabetes insipidus (hypothalamic or neurogenic)
  - Psychogenic polydipsia (water intoxication)
  - Nephrotic syndrome

Interfering Factors
- Recently administered radioisotopes cause spurious results.
- Many drugs affect results (eg, thiazide diuretics, oral hypoglycemic agents, and narcotics).

Procedure

- Draw venous blood samples (5 mL) into prechilled tubes and put on ice. Plasma with EDTA anticoagulant is needed. Observe standard precautions. Place specimen in a biohazard bag.
- Ensure that patient is in a sitting position and calm during blood collection.

Nursing Interventions

▸ Pretest

- Explain test purpose and procedure.
- Encourage relaxation before and during blood-drawing procedure.
- Follow guidelines in Chapter 1 for safe, effective, informed *pretest* care.

▸ Posttest

- Resume normal activities.
- Interpret test results and counsel appropriately for urine concentration disorders and polyuria.
- Follow guidelines in Chapter 1 for safe, effective, informed *posttest* care.

ANTINUCLEAR ANTIBODY (ANA) TITER, ANTI-DOUBLE-STRANDED–DNA (ANTI-DS-DNA) ANTIBODY (IMMUNOGLOBULIN G [IGG])

Blood for Systemic Rheumatic Disease (SRD)

ANA tests are the most commonly performed screening tests for patients suspected of having systemic rheumatic disease (SRD). These tests measure and differentiate autoantibodies associated with certain autoimmune diseases and related connective tissue diseases.

Indications

- Screen for systemic rheumatic diseases, systemic lupus erythematosus (SLE), Sjögren's syndrome, systemic scleroses, and mixed immune disease.
- Monitor disease activity and therapy.

Reference Values

Normal

- Negative for ELISA and IFA method; if positive, pattern is reported and serum is titered.

• Anti-ds-DNA antibody IgG: negative if <25 IU by ELISA method, borderline if 25–30 IU, positive if 31–200 IU, and strongly positive if >200 IU.

Clinical Implications

• Positive test results point to a number of clinical disorders, as shown in TABLE 3.1.

Interfering Factors

• Age, smoking, female gender, and several drugs cause positive results for ANA testing. Patients receiving anticonvulsants, oral contraceptives, procainamide, or hydralazine, for example, may develop increased titers of even ANAs, though they may not exhibit any clinical features of SLE.

Procedure

• Serum (7 mL) is obtained by venipuncture, using a red-top tube. Place the specimen in a biohazard bag.

Nursing Interventions

▶Pretest

• Assess the patient's knowledge of the test and cardiac medication usage, such as procainamide and hydralazine, which cause SLE-like symptoms.

• Explain that the purpose of blood test is to determine the presence of connective tissue disorder. No fasting is required.

▶Posttest

• Evaluate outcomes, and monitor and counsel the patient appropriately about possible treatment (eg, use of nonsteroidal anti-inflammatory drugs [NSAIDs], prednisone).

• Prepare for the possibility of repeat testing (ie, anti-ds-DNA increases or decreases according to disease activity and response to therapy). Additional tests include assays for anti-RNP, anti-Sm, anti-SSA (anti-Ro), anti-SSB (anti-La), antiscleroderma (Scl-70), and CREST antibody.

• Observe the venipuncture site for signs of infection. Patients with autoimmune disease have compromised immune systems.

• Patient education plays a major role in the prevention of infection. Infection resulting from immunosuppressive treatment is a leading cause of death in SLE patients (DISPLAYS 3.1 and 3.2).

(text continues on page 126)

TABLE 3.1 CORRELATION OF POSITIVE TEST RESULTS AND CLINICAL DISORDERS

CLINICAL DISEASE	SIGNS AND SYMPTOMS	PROPORTIONS OF PEOPLE WITH A POSITIVE TEST (SENSITIVITY)
Systemic lupus erythematosus (SLE)	Systemic autoimmune disease characterized by skin eruptions, arthritis, arthralgias, renal involvement, neurologic changes, serositis, hematologic abnormalities, and other findings.	>95%
Sjögren's syndrome	Autoimmune disease, dry eyes and mouth, arthritis, arthralgia.	50%–60%
Systemic sclerosis, diffuse	Diffuse multiorgan fibrosis, often involving the skin, heart, lung, kidney, and esophagus.	90%
Systemic sclerosis, limited cutaneous involvement (CREST)	A limited form of systemic sclerosis characterized by subcutaneous calcium deposits, Raynaud's phenomenon, esophageal dysmotility, sclerodactyly (ie, tissue fibrosis of the fingers), and telangiectasia (ie, dilation of groups of small blood vessels that give a characteristic skin finding).	90%
Mixed connective tissue disease (MCTD)	Has features of SLE, systemic sclerosis, and polymyositis in combination with Raynaud's phenomenon and/or swelling of the hands.	>95%
Dermatomyositis or polymyositis	Muscle weakness and fatigue are associated with chronic inflammation of skeletal muscle and chronically elevated serum creatine kinase. In dermatomyositis, characteristic rashes are also present.	20%
Rheumatoid arthritis	Systemic immune complex disease with primary manifestations in the joints and characterized by diffuse joint inflammation, erosive changes to cartilage and bone, and eventual joint destruction	25%–30%

Adapted from Astin, M. J., Waner, M. H., & Hutchinson, K. (2000). Auto-antibody testing. *Clinical Laboratory News*, 8, 32.

DISPLAY 3.1 Autoantibodies Used in the Diagnosis of Clinical Disorders

Diseases	*Autoantibodies**
Systemic lupus erythematosus	dsDNA, histones, Sm, RNP, SS-A/Ro, SS/B/La, ribosomal P
Sjögren's syndrome	SS-A/Ro, SS-B/La, Sjögren's syndrome antigen A or B
Rheumatoid arthritis	Fc portion of IgG
Mixed connective tissue disease	RNP (ribonuclear protein)
Systemic sclerosis, diffuse cutaneous involvement	Scl-70 (DNA topoisomerase)
Systemic sclerosis, limited cutaneous involvement (CREST syndrome)	Centromere proteins
Dermatomyositis/polymyositis	Jo-1 (histidine transfer RNA synthetase)

Vasculitis

Wegener's granulomatosis	Proteinase-3, myeloperoxidase†
Microscopic polyangiitis	Myeloperoxidase

Organ-specific autoimmune diseases

Thyroid: Hashimoto's thyroiditis Thyroid peroxidase (anti-Graves' disease thyroid microsomal antibodies),‡ thyroglobulin	
Liver: type 1 autoimmune hepatitis	Smooth muscle antigens§
Liver: type 2 autoimmune hepatitis	Liver kidney microsomes (LKM)
Liver: primary biliary cirrhosis	Mitochondrial antigens
Celiac disease	Tissue transglutaminase?‖ (anti-endomysial antibodies); gliadin
Goodpasture's syndrome	Glomerular basement membrane antigens
Pernicious anemia	Gastric proton-ATPase¶intrinsic factor

CREST, calcinosis, Raynaud's phenomenon, esophageal dysmotility, sclerodactyly, telangiectasia; dsDNA, double-stranded DNA; Sm, Smith; SSA, Sjögren's syndrome antigen A; SSB, Sjögren's syndrome antigen B; RNP, ribonucleoprotein.

*The autoantibodies are listed by their target antigens.

†Autoantibodies to myeloperoxidase, proteinase-3, and a variety of other antigens are known as antineutrophil cytoplasmic antibodies (ANCA), based on the IFA detection method that uses neutrophils as a substrate.

‡Autoantibodies to thyroid peroxidase are also known as antithyroid microsomal antibodies.

§Autoantibodies to smooth muscle are often directed against actin.

‖Autoantibodies to tissue transglutaminase are also known as antiendomysial antibodies.

¶Autoantibodies to gastric proton-ATPase are also known as antiparietal cell antibodies.

DISPLAY 3.2 **Autoantibodies and Common Diagnostic Tests**

Clinical Condition	Autoantibody Test
Systemic rheumatic diseases	ANA screening test
	dsDNA
	Histones
	Sm, RNP, SS-A/Ro, SS-B/La, Scl-70, Jo-1
	Centromere proteins
	Ribosomal P
Vasculitis: Wegener's granulomatosis, microscopic polycytosis	Proteinase-3, myeloperoxidase
Organ-specific autoimmune diseases:	
Thyroid: Hashimoto's thyroiditis, Graves' disease	Thyroid peroxidase thyroglobulin
Liver: type 2 autoimmune hepatitis (LKM)	Liver kidney microsomes
	Mitochondrial antigens
Liver: primary biliary cirrhosis	
Celiac disease	Tissue transglutaminase gliadin
Goodpasture's syndrome	Glomerular basement membrane antigens
Pernicious anemia	Gastric proton-ATPase

ARTERIAL BLOOD GASES (ABGS), BLOOD GASES

Blood

Arterial blood is analyzed to assess the adequacy of oxygenation, ventilation, and acid-base status. It furnishes accurate, rapid information about how well lungs and kidneys are working.

Indications
- Evaluate ventilatory processes, acid-base disturbances, and effectiveness of therapy.
- Qualify a patient for home-oxygen use.

Reference Values

Normal

pH adults: 7.35–7.45; children: 7.36–7.44
$Paco_2$: 35–45 mm Hg (4.6–5.9 kPa)

HCO_3^-: 22–26 mEq/L or mmol/L
Sao_2: oxygen saturation >95% (>0.95)
Pao_2: >80–100 mm Hg (12.6–13.3 kPa) (normal value decreases with age; subtract 1 mm Hg from 80 mm Hg for every year for patients older than 60 years up to 90 years)
Base excess (BE) or deficit: ±2 mEq/L or mmol/L

Clinical Implications

Blood gas values outside of the previously stated ranges can be grouped into two primary and four underlying disturbances for interpretive basis.

	pH	$Paco_2$	HCO_3^-	BE
VENTILATORY DISTURBANCE				
Respiratory acidosis	Decrease	Increase	Normal	Normal
Compensated	Normal	Increase	Increase	Increase
Respiratory alkalosis	Increase	Decrease	Normal	Normal
Compensated	Normal	Decrease	Decrease	Decrease
ACID-BASE DISTURBANCE				
Metabolic acidosis	Decrease	Normal	Decrease	Decrease
Compensated	Normal	Decrease	Decrease	Decrease
Metabolic alkalosis	Increase	Normal	Increase	Increase
Compensated	Normal	Increase	Increase	Increase

Critical Values

pH: <7.20 or >7.60
$Paco_2$: <20 or >70 mm Hg (<2.7 or >9.4 kPa)
Pao_2: <40 mm Hg (<5.4 kPa)
HCO_3^-: <10 or >40 mEq/L (<10 or >40 mmol/L)

> ## CLINICAL ALERT
>
> - Although there are four basic disturbances, a combined disturbance is generally the case. Uncompensated disturbances are referred to as *acute* and compensated disturbances as *chronic*. The terms "metabolic" and "nonrespiratory" are often used interchangeably.
> - A decrease in the Pao_2 is referred to as *hypoxemia*.
> - An increase in the $Paco_2$ is referred to as *hypercapnia*.

Interfering Factors

- Recent smoking can increase the carboxyhemoglobin level, thereby decreasing the SaO_2 with little to no effect on the PaO_2.
- Although supplemental oxygen increases the PaO_2, it can also cause CO_2 retention because of a decrease in ventilatory drive by means of the hypoxic stimulus.

Procedure

- Obtain an arterial blood specimen (3–5 mL) in a heparinized syringe. See the specimen collection guidelines in Chapter 2.
- Label the syringe with the patient's name, identification number, date, time, whether on room air or oxygen, and rate of flow.
- Report and compare the results against established laboratory or clinical ranges.

CLINICAL ALERT

- If sample cannot be analyzed within 10 minutes, place it on ice. An iced blood gas sample should be analyzed within 1 hour. Longer delays can result in changes in oxygen, carbon dioxide, and pH levels.

Nursing Interventions

▶ Pretest

- Explain the ABG purpose and procedure.
- Assure the patient that arterial puncture is similar to other blood tests, although a local anesthetic (1% lidocaine) can be used if desired.

▶ Intratest

- During the procedure, if the patient experiences a dull or sharp pain radiating up the arm, the needle should be withdrawn slightly and repositioned. If repositioning does not alleviate the pain, the needle should be completely withdrawn.
- Some patients may experience lightheadedness, nausea, and, in some cases, vasovagal syncope; be ready to respond appropriately.

▶ Posttest

- Observe frequently for bleeding. Apply pressure to the site for 5 minutes and then use a pressure dressing.
- Evaluate outcomes and assess and monitor the patient appropriately for hypoxemia and for ventilatory and acid-base disturbances.

ARTERIOGRAPHY: ARTERIES; ANGIOGRAPHY: ANTERIOR HEART AND ADJACENT VESSELS; VENOGRAPHY: PERIPHERAL AND VENTRAL VEINS; ARTERIOGRAPHY: THORACIC, ABDOMINAL, AND LUMBAR AORTA; DIGITAL VASCULAR IMAGING; DIGITAL SUBTRACTION ANGIOGRAPHY (DSA), AND TRANSVENOUS DIGITAL SUBTRACTION VASCULAR RADIOGRAPHY

Invasive X-ray Blood Vessel Imaging with Contrast; Interventional Procedures

An arteriogram is an x-ray procedure requiring catheterization of certain vessels that can be used to demonstrate the vascular anatomy of specific areas in the body. Aortic, renal, carotid or vertebral, and femoral arteriograms are commonly performed. Venograms of the cavae, extremity veins, and veins of the abdomen are also performed. Interventional procedures include angioplasty, stent placement, abscess drainage, venous filter placement, tube placement, and tumor embolizations (eg, liver metastases, uterine fibroids).

Indications
- Assess vessel patency.
- Determine presence of an aneurysm or arteriovenous shunting.
- Assess vascularity of a known neoplasm.
- Ensure vena cava filter placement.
- Provide preoperative and postoperative evaluation for vascular and tumor surgery.
- Provide nonsurgical intervention for known pathologies.

Reference Values

Normal
- Normal vascular anatomy, with no evidence of stenosis, aneurysm, or other arteriovenous malformation
- Normal carotid arteries, vertebral arteries, and abdominal aorta and its branches; normal renal and peripheral arteries

Clinical Implications

Abnormal findings indicate the following:

- Stenosis or occlusion of vessels, aneurysm, arteriovenous malformations, incorrect placement of vena cava filter

- Intravascular or extravascular tumors or other masses
- Pulmonary emboli and ulcerative plaque

Interfering Factors

- Metallic objects that overlie the area of interest interfere with visualization of anatomy.
- Patient motion interferes with image quality.
- Severe obesity adversely affects image quality.

Procedure

- The patient is positioned on an operating table and IV access is maintained. Typically, ECG and a pulse oximeter are applied. Procedural/moderate sedation is administered.
- Using sterile techniques and standard precautions, a local anesthetic is injected in the tissues surrounding the selected catheterization site.
- Various guide wires and catheters are introduced into the blood vessel and directed under fluoroscopic guidance. An iodinated contrast agent is introduced into the blood vessel of choice while x-ray imaging is performed. When iodine contrast agents are contraindicated, some labs use sterile CO_2 as an alternative.
- Procedure time depends on the complexity of the examination and the patient's condition. One hour is typical.
- When the catheter is removed at the end of the exam, pressure is applied over the site.

Nursing Interventions

▸ Pretest

- Assess for test contraindications such as pregnancy, sensitivity to iodine or latex, and evidence of renal failure.
- Most x-ray laboratories require that current creatinine, prothrombin time (PT), partial thromboplastin time (PTT), and platelet levels be available.
- Assess for a history of anticoagulation therapy (eg, Persantine [dipyridamole], Coumadin, aspirin).
- The patient must fast for a minimum of 6 to 8 hours before the procedure to minimize vomiting if an iodine contrast reaction occurs.
- Explain the examination purpose and procedure. Make certain that jewelry and metallic objects are removed from the area of study.

▸ Intratest

- Provide support during the procedure.
- The patient must be coherent and cooperative, able to hold his or her breath, and remain absolutely still when so instructed.
- Some discomfort is to be expected; administer medications as directed. Monitor vital signs.

▶*Posttest*
- Monitor vital signs and report and document unstable signs.
- Check the catheterization site for signs of infection, hemorrhage, or hematoma.
- Monitor the neuromuscular status of the extremity.
- Instruct the patient to increase fluid intake to at least 2000 mL for the 24 hours after the procedure to facilitate excretion of the iodine contrast agent and to avoid strenuous physical activity for at least 12 hours postprocedure.
- Order a follow-up blood test for kidney function.

CLINICAL ALERT

- Diabetic patients who take the oral drug metformin (Glucophage) require preprocedure and postprocedure modifications because of the potential for renal failure with lactic acidosis when contrast is used. Check with the radiology department or the physician regarding diabetes control medications.

ARTHROGRAM, ARTHROGRAPHY

X-ray Imaging with Joint Contrast

An arthrogram involves multiple x-ray examinations of encapsulated synovial joint structures after injection of contrast agents into the joint capsular space. Knee, ankle, shoulder, hip, elbow, temporomandibular joint, and wrist arthrograms are commonly performed under local anesthesia.

Indications
- Evaluate persistent, unexplained joint pain.
- Evaluate cartilage, tendons, and ligaments.

Reference Values

Normal
- Normal filling of joint space, bursae, ligaments, articular cartilage, menisci, and tendons

Clinical Implications

- Narrowing of joint space, dislocation, ligament tear or rotator cuff rupture, ligaments, cartilage, tendons, cysts, or synovial abnormalities

Interfering Factors

- Metallic objects that overlie the area of interest interfere with organ visualization.
- Severe obesity adversely affects image quality.

Procedure

- A local anesthetic is injected in the surrounding tissues. A needle is placed into the joint space (ie, knee, shoulder, ankle, hip, elbow, wrist, or metacarpophalangeal joints). Fluid from the joint may be aspirated. An iodinated contrast agent or a negative contrast agent such as air is introduced into the joint space. After needle removal, the joint is manipulated to distribute the contrast material. X-ray films of the joint are taken in several positions.
- Local anesthetic or procedural/conscious sedation may be used.
- The procedure time is generally less than 1 hour.

Nursing Interventions

▸Pretest

- Assess for test contraindications such as pregnancy and sensitivity to iodine.
- Explain the procedure and use of sedation and local anesthesia. Some discomfort is expected during contrast agent injection and joint manipulation.
- Instruct the patient to remove jewelry and metallic objects from the joint to be examined.

▸Intratest

- Provide support during needle placement. Some discomfort is to be expected.
- Encourage the patient to follow positional instructions during contrast manipulation and x-ray exposures.

▸Posttest

- Evaluate outcomes and monitor the patient appropriately for extreme swelling, pain, and signs of infection.
- An elastic bandage may be applied to the joint for several days and ice packs or analgesics may be used to alleviate pain.
- Check for complications at the injection site.

- Cracking or clicking noises may be heard in the joint for 1 to 2 days after the procedure. This is normal. Notify the physician if this noise persists or if increased pain, swelling, or redness occurs.

ARTHROSCOPY

Endoscopic Joint Imaging

Arthroscopy is a visual examination of a joint with a fiber-optic endoscope and is frequently associated with a surgical procedure.

Indications
- Detect and diagnose diseases and injuries of the meniscus, patella, condyle, extrasynovial area, and synovium.
- Differentiate degenerative processes from injuries.
- Assess response to treatment.

Reference Values

Normal
- Normal joints, vasculature, and color of synovium, capsule, menisci, tendons, ligaments, and articular cartilage

Clinical Implications
- Torn or displaced meniscus or cartilage, trapped synovium, loose fragments of joint components, torn or ruptured ligaments, necrosis, nerve entrapment, fractures, nonunion of fractures, and subluxation
- Degenerative disease, osteochondritis, osteoarthritis, inflammatory arthritis, osteochondritis desiccans (ie, cartilage and bone detach from the articular surface), chondromalacia, cysts, ganglions, and infections
- Chondromalacia of femoral condyle (ie, wearing down of back of knee cap, producing a grinding sensation)

Interfering Factors
- Ankylosis, fibrosis, sepsis, or contrast medium from previous arthrogram may be present in the joint

Procedure
- Under general, local, or spinal anesthesia, an arthroscope is inserted into the joint through a small incision after a tourniquet is applied to the area. After the joint is aspirated, continuous irrigation

flushes the joint during the procedure. Specimens are retrieved from the flush solution.
- Photographs and videotapes are frequently obtained during the process.
- The joint is compressed as instruments are withdrawn to expel the irrigant. Steroids or local anesthetics may be injected into the joint at end of the procedure.
- The wound is closed and dressed. Splints or immobilizers may be applied.

Nursing Interventions
▶Pretest
- Explain the test purpose and procedure.
- The patient should fast from midnight before the procedure, unless otherwise ordered.

▶Intratest
- Follow the usual protocols for arthroscopic procedures in the operative environment.

▶Posttest
- Apply ice immediately after the procedure.
- Manage the patient's recovery according to protocols. Check the neurovascular status of the affected extremity (eg, color, temperature, motion, sensation, pulses, and capillary refill times).
- Administer pain medication as needed or ordered, and ice and elevate the affected area if ordered.
- Instruct the patient to report numbness, tingling, coldness, duskiness (ie, bluish color), swelling, bleeding, fever, or abnormally severe pain to the physician immediately. Mild soreness and a mild grinding sensation for a few days are normal.
- No drugs or alcohol are permitted for 24 hours after the procedure.

CLINICAL ALERT

- On elevating the leg, make sure the *entire* leg is elevated in a straight position.
- Signs of thrombophlebitis include calf tenderness, pain, and warmth. Instruct the patient to report these symptoms immediately. *Note:* Do not massage the area.
- Compartment syndrome is a musculoskeletal complication that occurs most frequently in the forearm or leg. This is an emergency situation and usually requires surgical intervention to release the pressure.

AUTOPSY AND POSTMORTEM PROCEDURES, INCLUDING ORGAN AND TISSUE DONATION

Organs, Tissues, Fluids

Autopsy is a procedure used to determine the cause and manner of death by detailed examination of internal and external body structures and by specific postmortem laboratory tests and procedures. Organs and tissues for transplantation may be procured with special family consent before and during an autopsy.

CLINICAL ALERT

- All deaths, whether from a natural sequence of events, during medical treatment, in unexplained circumstances, or criminally related, need to be investigated for the cause and manner of death so that the legal death certificate is accurately completed, signed, and recorded.
- *Natural death* is the cessation of cardiorespiratory function from a disease process (eg, metastatic cancer, myocardial infarction, cerebrovascular accident, pneumonia) or from the natural progression of life events (ie, old age).
- *Medicolegal death* results from some unnatural, unexpected, unusual, or suspicious event such as homicide, suicide, accident, or untoward outcome of a medical procedure.
- Consent from the family is required unless autopsy is ordered by the coroner or medical examiner.

Indications

- Mandatory or routine in sudden, suspicious, or unexplained death.
- Investigate accidental and work-related deaths.
- Identify and track disease prevalence, incidence, and traumas associated with certain lifestyle changes and with environmental and occupational influences.
- Provide evidence for civil or criminal suits and for insurance settlements.

Reference Values

Normal

- External and internal findings are within normal limits or demonstrate no significant pathology related to the cause of death.

- Gross and microscopic findings are within normal limits, or abnormalities are related to the cause of death.
- No drugs, alcohol, or other toxic substances are present in blood, bile, urine, and ocular fluids or detected by toxicology screens.
- No evidence of inherited metabolic disorders on metabolic autopsy.

Clinical Implications

In autopsies and postmortem procedures, causes of death are categorized as natural and unnatural.

The most common natural causes include the following:

- Cardiovascular
- Brain related
- Respiratory
- Gastrointestinal
- Other (eg, hemorrhage, sepsis)

The most common unnatural causes include the following:

- Trauma
- Sudden infant death syndrome (SIDS)
- Fire or smoke inhalation
- Drowning
- Electrocution
- Hyperthermia (heat)
- Hypothermia (cold)
- Embolism
- Homicide

CLINICAL ALERT

- Observe standard precautions during these procedures.
- Indicate location of wounds, skin lesions or abrasions, and other abnormal markings on a diagram.
- Process toxicologic specimens if indicated. Specimens for toxicologic analysis include the following: all ocular fluid from both eyes, blood with sodium fluoride preservative (50 mL), blood with sodium fluoride preservative (retainer tube, 10 mL), liver tissue (3 g), bile fluid (10 mL), urine (50 mL), and stomach and bowel contents.
- Store specimens and fragments in paper envelopes or bags; never use plastic, which allows mold and fungus to grow.

Procedure

- Obtain a signed consent from the family unless the autopsy is ordered by the coroner or medical examiner.
- The body is identified and tagged; weigh and measure the height; map, measure, and record in detail distinguishing features, markings, and colors from head to toe, front, back, sides, extremities, and all surface features. Particularly note injuries, wounds, and bruises (individual and patterns). Fingerprints are made (fingertips of children) only in criminal cases.
- Photograph and obtain x-ray films for wounds, fractures, and foreign bodies (ie, two views in criminal cases). The head and chest are photographed in nonhospital deaths.
- Clean the body and record the features again. Photograph as needed.
- The autopsy proceeds in an orderly manner. Complete dissection of the major body cavities (thoracic and abdominal, including removal and sectioning of all major body organs), head, and neck is performed.
- Section all major organs. Save sections (entire organs in some cases) for microscope slide preparation for further examination and as evidence. Retain organs and slides as required.

CLINICAL ALERT

- If an external examination is done in lieu of an autopsy, collect blood from the subclavian vessel and vitreous humor from the eyes.
- On completion of autopsy, return organs (not saved for slides or evidence) to body cavity and suture the body cavity.
- Release the body immediately to a funeral home for burial or cremation according to the family's wishes. If there are legal questions, the body may be kept for some time.
- Specific blood tests are sent to a qualified laboratory for toxicology tests as ordered by the pathologist, medical examiner, or law enforcement officials.
- Toxicology screens are used. Alcohol screens determine the levels of various alcohols; acid-neutral screens detect barbiturates and salicylates; basic screens detect tranquilizers, synthetic narcotics, local anesthetics, antihistamines, antidepressants, and alkaloids. Higher-volatile screens use gas chromatography to detect substances such as toluene, benzene, trichloroethane, and trichloroethylene; and cannabis screens detect the presence of marijuana.

Procedure for Postmortem Cultures

- Sometimes, it is necessary to collect specimens for culture. Most internal organs of previously uninfected persons remain sterile for about 20 hours after death.
- Use sterile instruments and gloves when obtaining specimens for culture. Clean the area with a povidone-iodine 5-minute scrub, followed by a 70% alcohol 5-minute scrub.
- For sample collection, aspirate body fluid samples and transfer them to a sterile tube, or swab the area with sterile swabs.
- Obtain blood culture specimens from the right ventricle of the heart.
- Collect peritoneal fluid immediately after entering the peritoneal cavity.
- Collect bladder urine directly from the bladder with a syringe and needle.
- Sample pericardial or pleural cavity fluid on a swab or with a syringe and needle.
- Sear the external surface of an abscess to dryness with a red-hot spatula; collect pus with a syringe and needle (if possible), or use a swab.

> ### CLINICAL ALERT
>
> - Evidence, which may include clothing, a toothbrush, eyeglasses, and other items, should be transported to the proper laboratory as quickly as possible.
>   *From hands:* Automobile armrest, baseball cap brim, bottle cap, chocolate bar (the handled end), dime, doorbell, electrical cord, ignition switch, keys, pen, seat-belt buckle, shoelaces, wiener.
>   *From mouth and nose:* Bite mark, chicken wing, envelope, glass rim, lipstick, peach strudel, ski coat collar, telephone receiver, welding goggles.
>   *From eyes:* Contact lens fragments in vacuum cleaner, tears on a tissue, eyeglasses.
>   *From the body in general:* Burned remains, hair comb, automobile headrest, razor, shirt underarms, socks, and urine in snow.
> - Chapter 2 describes methods for collection of evidentiary specimens.

*DNA Evidence Procedure and Collection
of Specimens for Criminal Evidence*

DNA extracted from the victim or related evidence is compared with samples taken from a suspect. Scientists can be more certain when they are eliminating suspects.

Special Procedures

Drug Overdose Procedure

Photograph evidence suggesting drug abuse, such as injection sites on body; presence of drug paraphernalia or drugs; and drug residue on lips, face, teeth, oral cavity, tongue, nose, or hands. Assess the mouth area and body for bite marks and "fall" injuries (ie, suggests seizure activity associated with drug ingestion). Check the lymph nodes, spleen, and liver (ie, abnormal in an intravenous drug abuser).

Special Battery Procedure

If sexual assault is suspected, the following evaluations are done *in order.* With the body supine (ie, face up), obtain scalp and pubic hair, oral samples, and semen from inner thighs. With the body prone (ie, face down), obtain an anal specimen first and then a vaginal specimen. Collect fingernail evidence. Collect 25 pubic hairs from entire vulvar area. Collect 25 head hairs from affected area. Obtain oral, anal, and cervical specimens and obtain specimens from other areas suspected of containing DNA (ie, blood, saliva, bite marks, and semen).

Child Abuse and SIDS Procedure

Obtain radiographs and photographs of the entire body. For SIDS procedure, obtain bile and blood-dried spot specimens to detect inherited metabolic disease as cause of death. Perform external examination of the conjunctival petechiae, fingertip bruises, torso and shoulders (front and back), frenulum, and back; the posterior thighs and buttocks may be incised (from buckles or other sharp objects). Perform an internal examination for hematomas (due to direct injury); if present and there is no evidence of head trauma, remove the eyes and examine the retinas (ie, they show characteristic signs in presence of SIDS). Document recent or healed fractures and the estimated time of injury.

Procedure for Time of Death

Although the time of death is usually not a major issue, determination of this time is important in natural deaths (ie, insurance and other death benefits) and unnatural deaths (ie, unwitnessed or when body parts have been intentionally altered to conceal an individual's distinguishing features). The time of death estimate is based on the presence of *rigor mortis,* or stiffening of the body. Rigidity appears instantly or up to 6 to 12 hours after death. *Livor mortis* is a reddish purple color caused by settling of blood in dependent body parts because of gravity; onset is immediate. *Algor mortis* is cooling of the body; body temperature interpretation is based on cocaine use, presence of infections, or fever before death. *Decomposition* is the chemical breakdown of cells and organs by intracellular enzymes and putrefaction from bacterial action. *Gastric emptying* is the movement of food from stomach; digestion and stomach emptying vary in life and death. *Chemical changes* occur after death; for example, the potassium concentration increases in the vitreous fluid of the eye. *Insect activity* is used to time the death; flies and other insects are associated with decomposed bodies, but any attempts to fix time of death using insect evidence should be done with the aid of an entomologist.

CLINICAL ALERT

The time of death is expressed as an estimate of the time range during which a death could have occurred. Witnesses and a history of decedent's activities or environment assist in the time of death determination.

Organ and Tissue Donation

Organs and tissues for transplantation are procured before and during autopsy. Tissues that can be donated at or after death include the eyes and various other tissues that remain viable for up to 24 hours: cornea (several days), heart valves, bones, tendons, fascia, veins, and arteries.

CLINICAL ALERT

- Organs and tissues for transplantation are procured before and during autopsy.
- A special consent form must be signed by a responsible adult and witnessed by a health care professional.
- Life-saving organs (eg, kidneys, lungs, heart, pancreas, liver, intestines) are harvested before autopsy.
- Other tissues and organs (eg, eyes, bones, connective tissues, joints, ligament, heart valves, and veins) are harvested simultaneously with autopsy procedures or after autopsy.
- A request for organ donation is made in any hospital or medical examiner death (in many states), and the request and answer report are documented in the deceased person's chart or record.

Indications for Organ Donor Testing

- Determining history of cancer and the exposure to infectious disease (eg, viral hepatitis B and C, possibly TT virus in the future, HIV-1, HIV-2, human T-cell lymphotrophic virus [HTLV-1 and -2], cytomegalovirus [CMV], syphilis, other sexually transmitted diseases) to possibly exclude the organ.
- Matching donor and recipient.
- Establishing blood-type compatibility, ABO and Rh, for all transplant donors and recipients.
- Testing postmortem specimens for hepatitis B and HIV.
- Cadaver donor blood specimens are usually obtained before death, except in postmortem specimens for corneal transplantation, which may not be procured until days after death.

Procedure

- Obtain common blood and urine samples for initial testing and evaluation of the potential organ donor.

Nursing Interventions

▸*Pretest*

- Discuss potential tissue and organ donation with grieving family members.
- Determine if the possible donor is suitable for eye and tissue donation.
- Be sensitive. Allow family members to have as much time as needed to see their loved one.
- See the Transplant Testing section.

▸*Intratest*

- Preparing the body for tissue donation after consent has been given includes applying saline drops to the eyes, paper taping the eyes closed, placing eye pads over the brow, and placing the body in a refrigerated morgue if possible (DISPLAY 3.3).
- Type human leukocyte antigens (HLAs) on lymphocytes and determine compatibility before kidney and pancreas transplantation. A strong reaction in compatibility testing predicts rapid transplant rejection and is a contraindication.

DISPLAY 3.3 **Laboratory Tests for Organ Transplants**	
Organ Transplant	*Test*
For all	Complete blood count (CBC), white blood cell count, creatinine, blood urea nitrogen, electrolytes, prothrombin time, partial thromboplastin time
Kidney	Urinalysis
Liver	Bilirubin (direct and indirect), alanine aminotransferase (ALT), aspartate aminotransferase (AST), gamma-glutamyl transpeptidase (GGT), alkaline phosphatase, lactate dehydrogenase
Pancreas	Glucose, amylase, lipase
Intestine	Bilirubin (direct and indirect)
Heart	Arterial blood gases (ABGs), creatinine kinase (CK), CK-MB
Lung	ABGs

Adapted from Phillips, M. G., & Malinin, T. (1996). Donor evaluation for organ and tissue procurement. In Phillips, M. G. (Ed.), *Organ procurement, preservation and distribution in transplantation* (pp. 67–79). Richmond, VA: UNOS.

CLINICAL ALERT

• Toxins that can be found in transplanted organs.

TOXIN	ORGANS TRANSPLANTED
Acetaminophen	Heart, cornea, kidney
Carbon monoxide	Heart, liver, kidney, pancreas
Barbiturate	Liver, heart, kidney
Ethanol	Kidney
Cocaine	Liver, kidney
Cyanide	Cornea, skin, bone, heart, liver, kidney, pancreas
Methaqualone	Liver
Benzodiazepines	Kidney, heart, liver
Tricyclic antidepressants	Kidney
Methanol	Kidney
Insulin	Kidney, heart, pancreas (islet cells)

CLINICAL ALERT

- Victims of poisoning may be organ donors, especially in cases determined by brain death status:

Toxin	Optimal Condition for Transplant
Ethylene glycol, methanol	Acidosis corrected; serum alcohol level low or absent
Cyanide	Shock corrected; serum cyanide level <8 mEq/L or mmol/L

Nursing Interventions
▶Pretest: Family Preparation

- Explain the rationale for procedures after death and for donation of tissue or organ. Concern and respect for the deceased and significant others can reduce anxiety and objections to or misinterpretation of after-death testing. Obtain a signed, witnessed consent form for the autopsy and donation.
- If family members are undecided about an autopsy, they may wish to consider it as an option when no firm medical diagnosis has been established; in the event of an unexpected or mysterious death of apparent natural causes or suspected exposure to environmental or other hazards; or to identify hereditary, genetic, or contagious diseases. The cause of death could affect insurance settlements and other legal matters if the death was associated with unexpected medical or obstetric complications, occurred during the use of experimental drugs, or occurred as the result of certain dental, invasive, surgical, or diagnostic procedures.
- Consider the family's cultural habits and practices. Human response to the death of a loved one varies among different societies, religions, cultures, and races, and postmortem examination and organ donation may be offensive to some groups.
- Assure family members that nothing will be done without their permission, except as required by law. If fear of mutilation or delay in release of body for burial is a concern, provide clear and concise information to help with decision making. The autopsy procedure itself does not preclude a normal funeral, including viewing the body. In case of religious dilemmas, facilitate counseling and communication with clergy.
- Conflict may occur when the statutory authority is at odds with the family's wishes. Explanations may help with conflict resolution. Use team approach of medical examiner, clergy, funeral director, and law enforcement.

▸ *Posttest: Family Aftercare*
- Interpret death investigation results and counsel the family about the findings. Counsel families about organs and tissue procured for donation.
- After the investigated life events and death scene, autopsy, and laboratory tests are completed, data from all sources are scrutinized and analyzed. Findings are then documented and certified on the death certificate, where they become a matter of public record. This information may be shared with the decedent's immediate family, become a part of a court deposition process, or both.

CLINICAL ALERT

- If HIV status of decedent is not directly related to the cause of death, the decedent's HIV status need not be recorded.
- Cancer is reported when it is first discovered or confirmed upon autopsy.
- High risks for examiners and participants in postmortem procedures are the transmission of tuberculosis, hepatitis B, AIDS, and Jakob-Creutzfeldt disease.

BARIUM ENEMA (BE), DEFECOGRAPHY (DEF), COLON X-RAY, AIR-CONTRAST STUDY, ANUS AND RECTUM, EVACUATIVE PORTOGRAPHY

Air-Contrast Study, X-ray with Barium, Contrast Enema

The examination uses x-ray and fluoroscopic studies to demonstrate the anatomy of the large intestine (colon) and allows visualization of the filling and movement of contrast through the colon. DEF and evacuative portography are contrast studies of anus and rectum function during evacuation (used in young patients).

Indications

- Exclude obstruction, polyps, diverticula or other masses, fistula, and inflammatory changes.
- Evaluate bowel changes and abdominal pain.
- Provide treatment of intussusception.

Reference Values

Normal
- Normal position, contour, filling, movement time, patency of the large bowel and colon, and appendix size and position.

Clinical Implications
- Congenital deformities, bowel obstruction, stenosis, or megacolon
- Benign lesions such as diverticula, polyps, tumors, fistulas, and hernia
- Inflammatory changes such as colitis, appendicitis, chronic ulcerative colitis, and intussusception
- Carcinoma

Interfering Factors
- Retained fecal material caused by poor or inadequate bowel cleansing.
- Inability of the patient to maintain contrast-filled colon long enough to allow complete examination.
- Severe obesity adversely affecting image quality.

Procedure
- The patient lies on his or her side on the exam table and is given a contrast agent (usually barium) in the form of an enema through the rectum (ie, up through the sigmoid, descending, transverse, and ascending colon) or through a stoma. Under fluoroscopy, the colon is completely filled to the ileocecal junction. For a satisfactory examination, the contrast-filled colon must be maintained for several minutes while x-ray films are taken. In most instances, air is also introduced into the colon (ie, air-contrast or double-contrast enema).
- The patient is instructed to retain barium while spot films are taken with the patient in a variety of positions. A postevacuation film can also be taken to document colon emptying. Total examination time is approximately 30 minutes.
- Defecography requires the patient to evacuate into a specially designed commode while being evaluated fluoroscopically.

Nursing Interventions
▶Pretest
- Assess for test contraindications (usually pregnancy). Explain the examination purpose and procedure.
- No food or beverage is allowed for approximately 6 to 8 hours before the study. Make certain that jewelry and metallic objects are removed from abdominal area.
- Special attention is necessary for diabetic patients. Because of the pretest fasting, the administration of insulin or some oral hypoglycemic agents may be contraindicated for the day of and several days after the test.

- Bowel preparation routines vary (usually a three-step process) over 1 to 2 days and may involve any combination of diet restrictions preceding the test, mechanical cleaning with enemas and physiologic stool softeners, or cleaning with laxatives.

▶*Posttest*
- Provide fluids, food, and rest after study. Administer laxatives for 1 to 2 days or until the stool returns to normal.
- Observe and record stool color and consistency to determine if all barium has been eliminated from the bowel.
- Evaluate outcomes and provide the patient with support and counseling about further tests and possible treatment.

CLINICAL ALERT

- The use of barium is contraindicated when bowel perforation is suspected. A water-soluble, iodinated contrast is substituted for barium in this instance.
- Multiple enemas given before the procedure, especially to a person at risk for electrolyte imbalances, could rapidly induce hypokalemia.
- Caution should guide the administration of cathartics or enemas in the presence of acute abdominal pain, active bleeding, ulcerative colitis, or obstruction.
- Strong cathartics administered in the presence of obstructive lesions or acute ulcerative colitis can produce hazardous or life-threatening situations.
- Complications can occur when barium sulfate or other contrast media are introduced into the gastrointestinal tract.
- Fasting orders include oral medications except when specified otherwise.
- Determine whether the patient is allergic to latex or barium and inform the radiology department.

BIOTERRORISM: INFECTIOUS AGENTS AND DISEASES

Blood, Sputum, Tissue, Stool, Urine, Gastric Contents, Lymph Node Samples

Bioterrorism: Infectious diseases that may arise in a bioterrorism context include botulism, anthrax, smallpox, hemorrhagic fever, Hantaan virus, Ebola virus, yellow fever, plague, bubonic plague, and primary septicemic plague.

Botulism

Botulism is caused by *Clostridium botulinum* (seven types) and results when the toxin is absorbed by a mucosal surface (eg, GI tract or lung) or a wound into the circulation system. Botulinus toxin is the most poisonous substance known. The organism is found in undercooked food that is not kept hot (eg, foil-wrapped baked potatoes held at room temperature, contaminated condiments, sautéed onions, or cheese sauce).

Reference Values

Normal

- Absence of botulinus toxin.
- Absence of incremental response to repetitive nerve stimulation on electromyogram.

Clinical Implications

- Botulism paralyzes muscles, and untreated patients die quickly because they cannot breathe.

Anthrax

Anthrax is caused by *Bacillus anthracis* and can be contracted cutaneously, through the GI tract, and by inhalation. The organism is contracted by handling or consuming undercooked meat from infected animals, contact with inhalants from animal products (eg, wool), or intentional release of spores.

Reference Values

Normal

- Negative for the *B. anthracis* organism (appears as two to four cells, encapsulated).

Clinical Implications

- The isolation of *B. anthracis* rods confirms the diagnosis of anthrax.

Hemorrhagic Fever (HF) and Yellow Fever

Hemorrhagic fever (HF), hemorrhagic fever with renal symptoms (HFRS), and yellow fever associated with hepatitis are endemic threats in the United States and are caused by Hantaan virus, Ebola virus, and 17 other viruses that cause HF in rodents or deer mice. Hantavirus sin nombre (no name) virus causes hantavirus pulmonary syndrome (HPS). The organisms are found in rodent vectors in HF and mosquitoes in yellow fever.

Reference Values

Normal

- No evidence of Hantaan virus, Ebola virus, or the 17 other viruses that cause HF in rodents or deer mice.

Clinical Implications

- Growth of Hantaan, Ebola, or 17 other causative viruses in cultures or the presence of hantavirus antigens is evidence of disease.
- Thrombocytopenia is present in blood samples.

Plague, Bubonic Plague, and Primary Septicemic Plague

Plague, bubonic plague, and primary septicemic plague are caused by *Yersinia pestis*. Plague is an enzootic infection of rats, squirrels, prairie dogs, and other rodents.

Reference Values

Normal

- Negative for the presence of *Y. pestis*.

Clinical Implications

- A positive test for *Y. pestis* is evidence of disease; treatment (eg, streptomycin, tetracycline, doxycycline) should begin immediately. Isolation is not necessary, as person-to-person transmission has not been identified.

Smallpox

Smallpox is caused by variola virus, a DNA virus; only a few virions are required for transmission. Smallpox takes two principal forms: variola minor and variola major. Two other forms, hemorrhagic and malignant, are difficult to recognize. Smallpox is transmitted from person to person by means of coughing, direct contact, or contaminated clothing or bedding.

Reference Values

Normal

- No Guarnieri bodies isolated in scrapings of skin lesions. Absence of brick-shaped virions (ie, variola virus) confirmed by electron microscopy. Low levels of neutralizing, hemagglutination-inhibiting factor or complement-fixing antibodies.

Clinical Implications

- Evidence of virions or Guarnieri bodies indicates the presence of smallpox. High levels of antibodies indicate infection.

Tularemia

Tularemia is caused by *Francisella tularensis*. Two subspecies exist: type A, *F. tularensis* biovar *tularensis*, which is highly virulent in humans, and type B, *F. tularensis* biovar *palaearctica*, which is relatively avirulent. This intracellular parasitic disease spreads to humans by infected animals or contaminated water, soil, and vegetation. Mice, squirrels, and rabbits become infected through tick, fly, or mosquito bites. Humans contract the disease through the skin, mucous membranes, lungs, and GI tract.

Reference Values

Normal
- Absence of the *F. tularensis* organism.
- Negative serum antibody titers.

Clinical Implications
- Identification of *F. tularensis* and increased antibody titers indicate the presence of tularemia.

Procedure

General procedures for all bioterrorism infections or disease include the following:

- Specimens should be processed in a Biological Safety Level 2 (BSL2) microbiological laboratory or Biological Safety Level 3 (BSL3) laboratory if there is a high potential for aerosolization (eg, from centrifugation procedures).
- Surfaces should be decontaminated, using household bleach solutions (5.25% hypochlorite) diluted 1:10. Contaminated clothing or linens should be disinfected per standard precaution protocols, which usually include washing in soap and water, transporting laundry or waste in biohazard bags, and autoclaving before laundering or incineration. For contaminated instruments, autoclave following immersion in decontaminated solution.

    Specific procedural requirements for each infection or disease specimen collection include the following.

Botulism
- Specimens are obtained from blood, stool, gastric aspirates or vomitus, and, if available, suspected food. All samples are examined for the presence of botulinus toxin and should be refrigerated.
- At least 30 mL of venous blood should be obtained in a red-top Vacutainer.

- If the patient is constipated, an enema (with sterile water) can be used to obtain an adequate fecal sample. Saline **should not** be used for enemas, as it will interfere with the bioassay.
- The use of anticholinesterases (eg, physostigmine salicylate or pralidoxime chloride) by the patient can interfere with the bioassay.

CLINICAL ALERT

- In some cases, an electromyogram is performed to differentiate cause of acute flaccid paralysis.

Anthrax

- For GI anthrax, samples of gastric aspirate, feces, or food should be collected, along with three blood samples for culture.
- For inhalation anthrax, a sputum specimen or, in the later stages, a blood sample should be used.
- For cutaneous anthrax, two dry, sterile swabs should be soaked in vesicular fluid (in a previously unopened vesicle).
- For the analysis of samples, a certified Class II biological safety cabinet (BSC) should be used.

Hemorrhagic Fever and Yellow Fever

- Specimens of blood, sputum, tissue, and possibly urine should be obtained.

Plague, Bubonic Plague, and Primary Septicemic Plague

- Specimens of blood, sputum, or lymph node aspirate should be obtained.
- No rapid diagnosis exists for plague. Cultures take about 24 to 48 hours to complete.

Smallpox

- Specimen collection and examination should be performed by laboratory personnel who have recently been vaccinated.
- Skin lesions are opened with a blunt instrument (eg, blunt edge of a scalpel) and the vesicular or pustular fluid collected on a cotton swab.
- Scabs can also be used as specimens and should be removed with a forceps.
- Specimens are placed in a Vacutainer tube, restoppered, and sealed with adhesive tape.

- The Vacutainer tube is then placed in a durable, watertight container for transport.
- Specimens for virus cell culture can also be obtained from the oral cavity or oropharynx by use of a cotton swab.
- A Biosafety Level 4 (BSL4) laboratory is required.

Tularemia
- Specimens of respiratory secretions (ie, sputum), blood, lymph node biopsies, or scrapings from infected ulcers are obtained.
- Sputum samples are collected after a forced deep cough and placed in a sterile, screw-top container.
- For blood samples, obtain 5–7 mL in a Vacutainer by venipuncture.
- From an infected ulcer, obtain a skin scraping at the leading edge of a lesion and place in a clean, screw-top tube.
- Presumptive identification of *F. tularensis* should be done in a BSL2 laboratory.
- Confirmation of the organism should be done in a BSL3 laboratory.
- Laboratory personnel who may have had a potential infective exposure should be given prophylactic antibiotics if the risk of infection is high (eg, needlestick).
- Postexposure prophylactic antibiotic treatment of persons in close contact with the infected patient is not recommended except for pregnant women, considering person-to-person transmission has not been documented.

Nursing Interventions
▸*Pretest*
- Explain the necessity, purpose, procedure for testing, and risks of obtaining specimens (eg, with anthrax).
- Obtain a history of occupations (eg, handling infected animal carcasses), community settings, (eg, rural or urban), and living accommodations and circumstances (eg, recent heavy rains, mosquitoes, tropical climate, port city, near military warfare [bioterrorism]).
- Obtain a pertinent history of signs and symptoms related to the specific infection or disease; that is, botulism (paralysis of chest muscles and sudden inability to breathe); anthrax (fever, dyspnea, coughing, chest pain, heavy perspiration, and bluish skin caused by lack of oxygen); hemorrhagic fever and yellow fever (pneumonia, fever, muscular pain, jaundice, renal failure, hemorrhage from nose and GI tract, facial swelling); plague (sudden-onset fever; chills; general weakness; and swollen, tender lymph nodes, usually in groin, axilla, or cervical areas); smallpox (chills, fever,

backache, pustules that become a pockmark); and tularemia (bloody sputum, coughing, infected cutaneous ulcers, enlarged lymph glands).

‣*Posttest*

- Interpret test results, counsel and provide supportive care, and monitor for signs and symptoms of specific infection.
- If disease is contagious and transmitted from person to person, isolate the patient immediately according to infection control standards (eg, as in smallpox).
- Monitor treatment of specific infection, that is, botulism (administer an antitoxin [equine antitoxin] in a timely manner to minimize subsequent nerve damage); anthrax (administer antibiotics); hemorrhagic and yellow fever (administer antibiotics for secondary bacterial infections, correct dehydration, treat acidosis and blood cell abnormalities, and monitor close and high-risk contacts for 21 days); plague (provide postexposure antibiotic prophylaxis for 7 days for persons having close contact [≤2 m] with an infected individual); and tularemia (postexposure treatment includes antibiotics [treat pregnant women with ciprofloxacin because rare cases of fetal nerve damage, deafness, and renal damage have been reported with some of the aminoglycosides]).
- Report diseases to official government agencies as applicable.

BLOOD CULTURE

Blood Infection

Normally, blood is considered sterile. A blood culture is done to identify the specific aerobic or anaerobic microorganism that is causing a clinical infection. Ideally, two to three cultures (1 hour apart) are adequate to identify bacteria causing septicemia.

Indications

- Evaluate for bacteremia, septicemia, meningitis, and endocarditis in debilitated patients receiving antibiotics, steroids, or immunosuppressants.
- Investigate unexplained postoperative shock, chills, hyperventilation, and fever of more than several days' duration (eg, UTIs, infected burns, sepsis).

Reference Values

Normal

• Negative cultures for pathogens; no growth after 5–7 days.

Clinical Implications

• Positive cultures and identification of pathogens, the most common of which are *Staphylococcus aureus*, *Escherichia coli*, *Enterococcus* (*Streptococcus* D), *Streptococcus pneumoniae*, *Klebsiella pneumoniae*, *Corynebacteria* group JK, and anaerobes (*Bacteroides* sp., *Clostridium* sp., *Peptostreptococcus*, and *Actinomyces israeli*), *Streptococcus pyogenes* (*Streptococcus* A), *Pseudomonas*, and *Candida albicans*.

Interfering Factors

• Contamination of the specimen by skin bacteria.
• Transient bacteremia caused by teeth brushing or bowel movements.

Procedure

• Using the appropriate tube, blood (20–30 mL) is obtained by venipuncture using careful skin preparation and antiseptic techniques following the specimen collection guidelines in Chapter 2.
• Scrub the puncture site with Betadine (povidone-iodine solution), allow to dry, and then clean the area with 70% alcohol.
• Collect two to three cultures at least 30 to 60 minutes apart (if possible) per 24-hour period.
• In iodine-sensitive patients, a double-alcohol, green soap or acetone-alcohol prep may be used.

Nursing Interventions

▸*Pretest*

• Assess the patient's knowledge about the test, signs and symptoms of infection (eg, chills, fever, shock), and medication use (specifically, antibiotics).
• Explain the purpose and timing of the blood test procedure.

▸*Posttest*

• Send the specimen to the laboratory immediately. Label with the patient's name, age, date and time, number of the culture, notation of the patient's isolation category, and whether the patient is on antibiotics.
• Counsel the patient regarding results, possible need for further testing to identify where the infection is located in the body, and treatment (eg, triple antibiotic therapy).

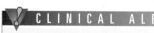

CLINICAL ALERT

• Critical value: positive culture. Notify the physician.

BLOOD GROUPS (ABO GROUPS)

Blood, Saliva, Tissue

Tests before Transfusion or Transplantation

Human blood is grouped according to the presence or the absence of specific blood group antigens (ABO). These antigens, found on the surface of red blood cells (RBCs), can induce the body to produce antibodies. Compatibility of the ABO group is the foundation for all other pretransfusion testing.

BLOOD GROUP	ABO ANTIGENS	ANTIGENS PRESENT ON RED BLOOD CELLS	ANTIBODIES PRESENT IN SERUM
A	A	A	Anti-B
B	B	B	Anti-A
AB	A and B	AB	None
O	Neither A nor B	None	Anti-A, Anti-B

Blood group O is called the universal donor for red blood cells; because no antigens are present on red blood cells, a person with blood group O can donate blood to all blood groups.

Blood group AB is called the universal recipient for red blood cells; because no serum antibodies are present, a person with blood group AB can receive blood from all blood groups. Blood group AB is also called the universal donor for fresh frozen plasma; because no serum antibodies are present, a person with blood group AB can donate plasma to all blood groups.

In general, patients are transfused or receive transplants with blood or tissue of their own ABO group because antibodies against the other blood antigens may be present in the blood serum. These antibodies are designated anti-A or anti-B, based on the antigen they act against.

Indications

• To prevent incompatibility reactions before blood transfusion (donor and recipient).

- Before tissue or organ transplantation (donor and recipient).
- Performed as part of prenatal testing.

CLINICAL ALERT

- A transfusion reaction could be extremely serious and potentially fatal. The blood group must be determined in vitro before any blood is transfused into an individual.
- Before blood administration, two professionals (physicians or nurses) must check the recipient's blood group and type with the donor group and type to ensure compatibility.
- A blood group change or suppression may be induced by cancer, leukemia, or infection.

Reference Values

Normal
- Group A, B, AB, or O (DISPLAY 3.4)

Clinical Implications

ANTIGEN PRESENT ON RED BLOOD CELLS	ANTIBODIES PRESENT IN SERUM	MAJOR BLOOD GROUP DESIGNATION	DISTRIBUTION IN THE UNITED STATES
None	Anti-A, Anti-B	O (universal donor)*	O—46%
A	Anti-B	A	A—41%
B	Anti-A	B	B—9%
AB	None	AB (universal recipient)†	AB—4%

*Named universal donor because no antigens are present on red blood cells; therefore, the person can donate blood to all blood groups.
†Named universal recipient because no serum antibodies are present; therefore, the person can receive blood from all blood groups.

Procedure
- Obtain a 7-mL, venous, clotted blood sample in a red-top Vacutainer tube.
- Test for saliva or tissue if ordered.

DISPLAY 3.4   **Incidence and Frequency of Blood Group and Rh Type**

Blood Group and Rh Type	Incidence	Frequency of Occurrence
O Rh-positive	1 of 3	37.4%
O Rh-negative	1 of 15	6.6%
A Rh-positive	1 of 3	35.7%
A Rh-negative	1 of 16	6.3%
B Rh-positive	1 of 12	8.5%
B Rh-negative	1 of 67	1.5%
AB Rh-positive	1 of 29	3.4%
AB Rh-negative	1 of 167	0.6%

Follow Chapter 1 guidelines for safe, effective, informed *posttest* care.

Nursing Interventions

▸*Pretest*
- Explain the test purpose and procedure.

▸*Posttest*
- Inform the patient about his or her blood group and interpret the meaning. Rh type may have implications for the pregnant woman and the fetus.
- Maintain confidentiality of the results, especially in legal situations.

BONE MARROW ASPIRATION OR BIOPSY

Bone Marrow from Cancellous/Long Bones

A bone marrow specimen is obtained through aspiration biopsy or needle biopsy to fully evaluate blood cell formation (ie, hematopoiesis).

Indications

- Diagnose hemolytic blood disorders by analyzing cell number appearance, development, presence of infection, and deficiency states of vitamin B_{12}, folic acid, iron, and pyridoxine.
- Diagnose primary and metastatic tumors, infectious diseases, and certain granulomas.
- Help the diagnosis and staging process of solid malignancies and leukemias.

- Isolate bacteria or other pathogenic agents by culture.
- Evaluate effectiveness of chemotherapy/therapy and monitor myelosuppression.

Reference Values

Normal
- Different types of formed cell elements in given numbers, ratios, and stages of maturation are identified.

Clinical Implications
- Abnormal cell patterns, leukemia, Hodgkin's disease, multiple myeloma, anemia, agranulocytosis, polycythemia vera, and myelofibrosis
- Infection, rheumatic fever, mononucleosis, chronic inflammatory disease, and many others
- Lipid or glycogen storage disease
- Deficiency of body iron stores, microcytic anemia
- Platelet dysfunction

Procedure
- Inject a local anesthetic (eg, procaine or lidocaine). Cleanse as in any minor surgical sterile procedure. The preferred site is the posterior iliac crest.
- Using sterile technique, aspirate a fluid specimen (0.5 mL) that contains suspended marrow pustule from the bone marrow. During *needle biopsy*, a core of actual marrow cells (not fluid) is removed. A small incision is made before the introduction of special needle.
- Label the specimen properly and promptly deliver it to laboratory.

Nursing Interventions
▶Pretest
- Instruct the patient about the procedure and purpose.
- Administer moderate sedation/analgesia, if ordered.
- Sites used for bone marrow aspiration or biopsy affect pretest, intratest, and posttest care. Sites used include the posterior superior iliac crest; anterior iliac crest (if the patient is very obese); sternum (not used as often with children because cavity is too shallow; danger of mediastinal and cardiac perforation is too great; and observation of procedure is associated with apprehension and lack of cooperation); vertebral spinous processes T10 through L4 and ribs; tibia (often in children); and ribs.

- Assess for contraindications, such as severe bleeding disorders (eg, hemophilia).

▶ *Intratest*
- Position according to the site selected and assist in preparing the local anesthetic (ie, procaine or lidocaine) for injection.

▶ *Posttest*
- Monitor vital signs until stable and assess the site for excess drainage or bleeding.
- Evaluate discomfort and administer analgesics or sedatives as necessary.
- Osteomyelitis or injury to the heart or great vessels is rare but can occur in a sternal site. Fever, headache, unusual pain, or tissue redness or abscess at biopsy site may indicate infection (may be a later event). Instruct the patient to report unusual symptoms to the physician immediately.

BONE MINERAL DENSITY, BONE DENSITOMETRY (DEXA) OSTEOPOROSIS SCAN PROCEDURES

Special Bone Density Imaging

Bone densitometry helps diagnose osteoporosis or osteopenia, often before fractures occur, by measuring bone mineral density. X-ray absorptiometry for measuring bone mineral density (BMD) includes the following special modalities:

- Dual-energy absorptiometry (DEXA or DXA) to measure spine, hip, and forearm density.
- Peripheral dual-energy absorptiometry (pDXA) to measure forearm density.
- Single-energy x-ray absorptiometry (SXA) to measure the heel and forearm density.

Indications
- Determine bone mineral content and density to detect osteoporosis and osteopenia.
- Diagnose osteoporosis related to early premenopausal oophorectomy or estrogen deficiency syndrome or in postmenopausal women.

- Evaluate osteoporosis that may be related to unexplained or multiple fractures, multiple myeloma, anorexia, prolonged immobility, gastrointestinal malabsorption, and chronic renal diseases.
- Detect vertebral abnormalities.
- Evaluate the results of x-ray films that indicate osteopenia.
- Differentiate the causes associated with osteopenia such as endocrinopathies (eg, hyperparathyroidism, prolactinoma, Cushing's syndrome, and male hypogonadism and hyperthyroidism) and treatment-related osteopenia (eg, long-term heparin, anticonvulsant, or steroid therapy).
- Monitor osteoporosis treatment such as hormone replacement therapy, exercise, calcitonin analog, vitamin D, and calcium supplements.
- Aid in making an informed decision at the onset of menopause regarding the risks and benefits of hormone replacement therapy.

Reference Values

Normal

- The absence of osteoporosis or osteopenia when assessing BMD
- Normal T score of -1.0 or above
- Osteopenia: below -1.0 to -2.5
- Osteoporosis: below -2.5

Clinical Implications

- Abnormal scans may be associated with estrogen deficiency in postmenopausal women, vertebral abnormalities, osteoporosis diagnosed from x-ray films, hyperparathyroidism, and long-term corticosteroid therapy.

Interfering Factors

- False readings may occur with the following:
  Nuclear medicine scans in the previous 72 hours.
  Barium studies in the previous 7 to 10 days.
- Calcified abdominal aortic aneurysm may increase the BMD of the spine.
- Prosthetic devices or metallic clips surgically implanted in areas of interest falsely increase the BMD of these bones.

Procedure

- The patient is positioned in such a way as to keep the scanned area immobile. Jewelry or other objects overlying bone and previous bone fractures should be removed.

- A foam block is placed under both knees during the spine scan, and a leg brace immobilizer is used during the femur scan; an arm brace is used when scanning the forearm.

Nursing Interventions

▶ *Pretest*

- Instruct the patient about the BMD scan purpose; the procedure for measuring spine, hip, and forearm; benefits; and the patient's involvement.
- Inform the patient that no special preparation such as fasting or sedation is needed.
- Encourage the patient to wear cotton garments, free of plastic or metal.
- Ask the patient to remove all metallic objects (eg, jewelry, belts, buckles, zippers, coins, keys) before the test.

▶ *Intratest*

- Reassure the patient that the test is proceeding normally.
- The BMD study takes about 35 to 45 minutes, and no pain is associated with the procedure.
- This test does not involve radiopharmaceuticals.

▶ *Posttest*

- Serial studies may be ordered to measure the effectiveness of treatment.
- If outcomes indicate osteoporosis, advise weight-bearing exercise, strength training, prescribed medications, and calcium and magnesium supplements.

BONE SCAN IMAGING

Nuclear Medicine, Skeletal Imaging

This procedure involves injecting a bone-seeking radiopharmaceutical to visualize the skeleton. It is done primarily to evaluate and monitor patients with known or suspected metastatic disease to the bone.

Indications

- Evaluate unexplained skeletal pain, trauma, or frostbite.
- Assess infection sites and rule out osteomyelitis versus cellulitis.
- Diagnose, stage, and follow up on metastatic diseases.
- Evaluate patients with primary bone tumors, fractures, and compression fractures of the vertebral column.

- Evaluate pediatric patients with hip pain to assess possible child abuse, bone growth plates, and age of traumatic injuries and infections.

Reference Values

Normal
- Symmetrical concentration of radiopharmaceutical in axial skeleton (head and trunk) and slightly less uptake in limbs
- Regression of metastasis after treatment

Clinical Implications
Abnormal concentrations indicate the following:
- Any process increasing calcium turnover rate is reflected by increased uptake in the bones, including early bone disease and healing and metastatic bone disease (multiple focal areas in axial skeleton are common).
- Extraskeletal, abnormal intense uptake may occur rarely in the myocardium, brain, spleen, and gastrointestinal tract.
- Primary and secondary cancers, multiple myeloma, osteomyelitis, arthritis, necrosis, child abuse, bone graft viability imaging.

Interfering Factors
- False-negative bone imaging may occur in patients with multiple myeloma of the bone and follicular thyroid cancer.

Procedure
Bone Imaging
- ^{99}Tc-MDP, a radioactive phosphate, is injected intravenously.
- A 2- to 3-hour waiting period is necessary for the radiopharmaceutical to concentrate in the bone. During this time, the patient drinks four to six glasses of water.
- Before imaging, the patient must empty the bladder because a full bladder obscures pelvic bones. The scan takes about 30 to 60 minutes to complete.
- Whole-body images and single-photon emission computerized tomography (SPECT) may be performed.

Nursing Interventions
▶ *Pretest*
- Instruct the patient about the purpose and procedure of bone imaging.
- Assess for incontinence and urine elimination problems and notify the nuclear medicine department of potential concerns.

- If the patient is in pain or debilitated, assist him or her to void before the test.
- Pain medication may be necessary for any patient who may have difficulty lying still during the imaging.
- The test should be deferred for pregnant or breast-feeding women.

▶*Intratest*
- Avoid urine contamination of the patient, the patient's clothing, or the imaging table or bedding.
- The patient must lie still during the examination.

▶*Posttest*
- Assess the outcomes and counsel the patient regarding the possible need for follow-up bone images. The flare phenomenon occurs in patients with metastatic disease who are receiving a new therapy. It is caused by a healing response in prostate and breast cancers within the first few months of a new treatment. These lesions should show marked improvement on scans 3 to 4 months later.
- Urge fluids and frequent urination to promote excretion of the radionuclide.
- Monitor the injection site for signs of infection and extravasation of the radiopharmaceutical agent.
- Observe and treat mild reactions with medications: pruritus, rashes, and flushing reactions 2 to 24 hours after injection; sometimes nausea and vomiting may occur.

BRAIN AND CEREBRAL BLOOD FLOW IMAGING

Nuclear Medicine Scan, Neurologic Imaging

The imaging uses several different radiopharmaceuticals that can cross the blood-brain barrier (BBB) and provide information about brain perfusion and function.

Indications
- Evaluate stroke, dementia, abscess, seizure disorders, Alzheimer's disease, Huntington's disease, epilepsy, Parkinson's disease, and schizophrenia.
- Detect brain trauma and tumors in adults and children.
- Determine brain death by documenting absent intracerebral perfusion.
- Evaluate encephalitis in adults and children.
- Determine presence or absence of intracranial blood flow.

- Assess children with hydrocephalus, locate epileptic foci, assess metabolic activity, and assess childhood development disorders.
- Assess adults with early-onset dementia for whom a diagnosis of normal pressure hydrocephalus is possible.
- Evaluate infectious disease (eg, encephalitis, Lyme disease, toxoplasmosis, lupus, and CNS lymphoma) and psychiatric disorders.

Reference Values

Normal

- Normal extracranial and intracranial blood flow, normal distribution and symmetry with highest uptake in the gray matter, basal ganglia, thalamus, and peripheral cortex, and less activity in the central white matter and ventricles.

Clinical Implications

- Abnormally decreased radionuclide distribution occurs in certain brain diseases (eg, Alzheimer's, dementia), seizure disorders, epilepsy, Parkinson's disease, mental disorders, and in recent stroke.
- The cerebral blood flow in the presence of brain death shows a distinct image of no tracer uptake in the anterior or middle cerebral artery or the cerebral hemisphere and the presence of uptake in the scalp.

Interfering Factors

- Any patient motion (eg, coughing, leg movement) can alter cerebral alignment, as well as sudden reaction to loud noises.
- Sedation may affect brain activity.

Procedure

- The radionuclide technetium ^{99m}Tc bicisate (ECD)/Neurolite or ^{99m}Tc exametazime/ceretec is injected intravenously, and imaging usually begins within half an hour of administration and takes about 1 hour to complete.
- With the patient in the supine position, SPECT images are obtained around the circumference of the head.

Nursing Interventions

▸*Pretest*

- Explain the brain imaging purpose and procedure.
- Because precise head alignment is crucial, advise the patient to remain quiet and still.

▸*Intratest*

- Provide support and assure the patient that the test is proceeding normally.

▶*Posttest*
- Evaluate outcomes and counsel the patient appropriately regarding further tests and possible treatment.
- Monitor the intravenous injection site for infection, extravasation, or hematoma.

BREAST BIOPSY AND PROGNOSTIC MARKERS

Cells and Tissue

Breast tissue and cells are examined to determine surgical margins, presence or absence of vascular invasion, and tumor type, staging, and grading. Secondary studies relevant to survival may include imaging procedures, along with estrogen and progesterone hormone receptors (ER and PR) and DNA ploidy.

Indications for Biopsy
- Establish the presence of breast disease, diagnose histopathology, and classify the process.
- Confirm and characterize calcifications noted in prebiopsy mammogram and abnormal ultrasound.

Reference Values

Normal
Negative for malignant or abnormal cells/tissues.
No vascular invasion.
Negative or of no significance for following prognostic markers:

- *S-phase fraction* (SPF): low levels of SPF appear to correlate with longer survival and a reduced chance of relapse.
- *Cathepsin D:* may promote tumor spread.
- *Epidural growth factor receptor* (EGFR): correlates with ER-negative tumors, aneuploid tumors, and lymph node metastases.
- *TP53 gene:* tumor suppression gene regulates cell cycles.
- *HER2 oncogen:* used to predict response to chemotherapy.

Clinical Implications
- Favorable prognostic indicators include tumor size of less than 1 cm, a low histologic grade, tumor-negative axillary lymph nodes, and ER- and PR)- positive tumors.

- Fibroplasia and fibroadenoplasia are benign conditions.
- High levels of HER2 in recurrent metastatic breast cancers are associated with a poor response to conventional chemotherapy.

Procedure
- Breast tissue specimens may be obtained by open surgical technique, x-ray–guided core biopsy, or needle biopsy. Place the specimen in a biohazard bag. These specimens are taken directly to the laboratory and given to the pathologist or histotechnologist.
- The breast tissue is examined and the extent of the tumor is determined. Reaction margins are evaluated and the grade and stage of disease are identified.

Nursing Interventions
▶Pretest
- Explain the biopsy purpose and procedure. Obtain and record relevant family or personal history, prior biopsy, trauma, recent or current pregnancy, nipple discharge, location of lump, and how the lesion was detected.
- Open-breast biopsies are performed under local or general anesthesia. Procedural or moderate sedation may be used with local anesthesia. NPO status is required when general anesthesia is used.
- Provide information and support, recognizing the fear the patient experiences about the procedure and outcome.

▶Posttest
- If general anesthesia is used, follow the recovery protocols.
- Interpret the biopsy outcome and counsel the patient appropriately about possible further testing and treatment (eg, surgery, chemotherapy, hormone therapy).
- TCH (docetaxel [Taxotere] and carboplatin combined with trastuzumab [Herceptin]) regimen has recently been approved in the treatment of HER2-positive early breast cancer.

BREAST IMAGING OF BREAST MASSES (SCINTIMAMMOGRAPHY)

Nuclear Medicine, Tumor Imaging

This scan can visualize breast masses using a radiopharmaceutical specific to breast tumors. Scintimammography is used in conjunction with indeterminate mammography. This test aids in decreasing the number of unnecessary breast biopsies.

Indications

- Differentiate between benign and malignant lesions; more specific than x-ray mammography.
- Monitor after breast biopsy surgery, radiation therapy, and chemotherapy.
- Detect axillary lymph node involvement by breast cancer.
- Assess the lymphatic drainage of tumor and metastatic spread to vulva, uterus, penis, head, or neck.

Reference Values

Normal

- Uniform distribution of radiopharmaceutical uptake in the breasts without focal areas of concentration.
- No focal uptake in lymphatic tissue.
- No abnormal lymph node (indicated by obstruction to tracer).

Clinical Implications

- Abnormal increased focal uptake is found in cases of fibroadenoma and adenocarcinoma.
- Nonuniform increased diffuse uptake of activity in fibrous dysplasia, which may be unilateral or bilateral.
- Several areas of increased focal uptake are often seen in cases of multifocal breast cancer.
- Axillary metastasis is detected as focal areas of increased uptake in the axillary nodes.
- Abnormal nodes show leaks into adjacent tissue and unusual collateral lymph drainage pathways.
- The first lymph node to drain the tumor invariably contains the tumor.

Interfering Factors

- Detectable radioactivity from a previous nuclear procedure.
- To eliminate a false-positive appearance, the patient is injected on the opposite side of a known lymphatic lesion or in the foot.
- Extravasation of the radiopharmaceutical can result in "hot spots" of radioactivity in the location of the axillary lymph nodes.

Procedure

- The radiopharmaceutical, ^{99m}Tc sestamibi, is injected intravenously in the opposite arm from the breast that is of concern or in the foot. For lymph node imagery, the tracer is injected intradermally or subcutaneously.
- The patient lies in the prone position on a special cutout table that allows the breasts to hang through the table unobstructed. For

lymph node exam, special positioning is required (see sentinel node testing, under alphabetical listing).

- The patient is also placed in the supine position with the arms raised (for obtaining images of the axillary lymph nodes).
- The total time for breast scans is approximately 45–60 minutes; for lymph node scans, images are obtained immediately and 2–4 hours after injection.
- An optional SPECT examination may be requested by the nuclear medicine physician. This examination may take an additional 30 to 40 minutes.

Nursing Interventions

▶Pretest
- Instruct the patient about the breast and lymph node scan purposes, procedures, benefits, risks, and patient involvement.
- There are no dietary or medication restrictions.
- Remove all clothing and jewelry from the waist up.
- Defer the test for breast-feeding women. The test is contraindicated during pregnancy.

▶Intratest
- Reassure the patient that the test is proceeding normally.
- Provide privacy during the procedure and respect the patient's rights.

▶Posttest
- Assess outcomes and counsel the patient appropriately.
- Monitor the injection site for signs of infection, extravasation, or bleeding.
- Observe and treat mild reactions, including pruritus, rash, and flushing, 2 to 24 hours after injection. Patients sometimes have nausea and vomiting.

BREAST ULTRASOUND-BREAST SONOGRAM, BREAST ECHOGRAM, SONOMAMMOGRAPHY

Ultrasound Imaging

This noninvasive study is useful for differentiating the nature of breast masses identified by palpation or x-ray mammography.

Indications
- Differentiate a cystic lesion from a solid breast lesion.
- Perform imaging of male, very young, pregnant, very dense, augmented, or lactating breasts, or silicone breast implants.
- Guide during biopsy or cyst aspiration.

Reference Values

Normal
- Symmetrical echo patterns in both breasts, including subcutaneous, mammary, and retromammary layers.

Clinical Implications
- Presence of space-occupying lesions: cysts, solid masses, hematomas, abscesses, duct dilation, calcifications, lymph and muscle metastasis, enlarged lymph nodes.

Procedure
- A coupling medium, usually a gel, is applied to exposed breast to promote transmission of sound.
- A handheld transducer is slowly moved across the breast.
- Total examination time is approximately 15 to 25 minutes.

Nursing Interventions
▸*Pretest*
- Explain the breast ultrasound examination purpose and procedure. Because no radiation is used, breast ultrasound is effectively used in very young or pregnant patients.
- Explain that a coupling gel will be applied to skin. Although the couplant does not stain, advise the patient to avoid wearing nonwashable clothing.

▸*Posttest*
- Remove or instruct the patient to remove any residual gel or glue from skin.
- Evaluate outcomes and provide the patient with support and counseling about further testing (eg, biopsy).

BRONCHOSCOPY

Endoscopic Respiratory Tract Interventional Imaging

This invasive examination is done to view, diagnose, and treat disorders of the trachea, bronchi, and selected bronchioles with a flexible fiberoptic bronchoscope.

Indications
- Diagnose tumors, stage lung cancer, determine surgical resectability, and locate hemorrhage site.

- Evaluate trauma, nerve paralysis, and inflammation.
- Assess the patient before and after lung transplantation.
- Remove foreign bodies (eg, teeth, food).
- Assess intubation damage.
- Place large-airway stents.
- Use bronchoscopy aspirates to diagnose *Mycobacterium tuberculosis* infections, pathogenic fungi, *Legionella*, and *Nocardia* species.
- Perform transbronchial needle biopsy in suspected cases of lung cancer.

Reference Values

Normal
- Normal trachea, bronchi, nasopharynx, pharynx, and select peripheral airways.

Clinical Implications
- Abnormal findings indicate fibrosis, bronchogenic cancer, tumors, fractured airway, upper-airway obstruction after smoke inhalation, signs of nonresectability, and inflammatory and infectious processes.

Procedure
- A local anesthetic is applied to the tongue, pharynx, and epiglottis. The bronchoscope is inserted through the mouth, nose, endotracheal tube, or tracheostomy and advanced into the pulmonary system.
- Sputum, biopsies, and bronchial brushings specimens may be collected for cytology, culture, and sensitivity test.
- Continuous pulse oximetry readings indicate levels of oxygen saturation before, during, and after the procedure.
- Moderate sedation/analgesia (eg, midazolam) is often used.
- Bronchoalveolar lavage with 20-mL aliquots of normal saline (up to 100–120 mL) may be done to obtain alveolar infiltrates.
- Typically, bronchoscopy is performed under fluoroscopic guidance during lung biopsy.

Nursing Interventions
▶Pretest
- Reinforce information related to the purpose, procedure, equipment, and sensations.
- Explain that local anesthetic is bitter and that numbness occurs rapidly. Feelings of a thickened tongue and sensation of something in the back of the throat pass within a few hours. Gag, cough, and swallowing reflexes are blocked.

- Explain NPO restrictions for at least 6 hours before the procedure to reduce risk of aspiration.
- Instruct the patient to remove hairpieces, nail polish, makeup, dentures, jewelry, and contact lenses before examination.

▸Intratest

- Use relaxation techniques to help the patient relax and breathe normally during procedure.
- Administer intravenous procedural sedation according to protocols and watch for untoward reactions.
- Monitor vital signs and oxygen saturation (via continuous pulse oximetry). Report abnormal values immediately.
- Collect specimens if ordered.

▸Posttest

- Monitor breathing patterns, lung sounds, and vital signs. Have resuscitation equipment and a tracheotomy setup available. Continue pulse oximeter monitoring and O_2 administration if indicated.
- A semi-Fowler position is used for conscious patients, and a side-lying position is used for sedated or unconscious patients.
- Do not administer oral food or fluids until the gag reflex returns (about 2 hours after the test).
- Instruct the patient to spit out saliva rather than swallow it.
- Discourage coughing and throat clearing when biopsies have been done.
- Collect sputum specimens as ordered and according to protocols.
- Anti-angiogenesis drugs, e.g., vascular endothelial growth factor and epidermal growth factor receptor inhibitors, have recently been approved in the treatment of non-small-cell lung cancer.

> ### CLINICAL ALERT
>
> - Rarely, deaths have occurred from excessive premedication or topical anesthesia, respiratory arrest, hemorrhage, or spasms.
> - Watch for signs and symptoms of bleeding, shock, cardiac arrhythmias, allergic reaction, hypoxemia or hypoxia, or respiratory failure.
> - If fever, tachycardia, and hypotension develop, this may indicate onset of gram-negative sepsis. Blood cultures and aggressive antibiotic therapies, together with other supportive therapies, usually are instituted.
> - Laryngospasm or bronchospasm (indicated by respiratory stridor, dyspnea, or wheezing) is an emergency situation.
> - Decreased or absent breath sounds, cyanosis, dyspnea, and sharp pain may indicate pneumothorax and must be treated as an emergency.

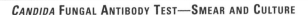

Candida Fungal Antibody Test—Smear and Culture

Blood, Urine, Sputum, Tissue, Skin, Infected Nails, Cerebrospinal fluid (CSF)

This test detects the presence of antibody to *Candida albicans* and is helpful in the diagnosis of systemic *Candida* infection, which occurs in immunocompromised individuals with depressed T-cell levels and can be life threatening.

Indications
- Evaluate *Candida* infection when the diagnosis of systemic infection cannot be shown by culture or tissue sample.
- Evaluate *Candida* infection when positive culture results are obtained from specimens with high potential for contamination, such as that from the urinary tract.

Reference Values

Normal
- Negative for *Candida* antibodies or presence of candidal infection in smears and cultures.

Clinical Implications
- A titer greater than 1:8 using latex agglutination indicates systemic infection.
- A fourfold rise in titer of paired blood samples 10 to 14 days apart indicates acute infection.
- Patients on long-term intravenous therapy treated with broad-spectrum antibiotics and persons with diabetes commonly have disseminated infections caused by *C. albicans.* The disease also occurs in bottle-fed newborns and in the urinary bladder of catheterized patients.
- Vulvovaginal candidiasis, common in late pregnancy, can transmit candidiasis to the infant in the birth canal.

Interfering Factors
- Cross-reaction can occur in cryptococcoses and tuberculosis.
- False-positive results can occur in superficial mucocutaneous candidiasis or severe vaginitis.

• Immunocompromised patients frequently have false-negative results because of their impaired ability to produce antibody.

Procedure
• Serum (7 mL) is obtained by venipuncture, using a red-top Vacutainer.
• Smears and cultures may also be obtained.
• Observe standard precautions and place specimen in a biohazard bag for transport.

Nursing Interventions
▸*Pretest*
• Assess the patient's knowledge about the test and symptom history. Symptoms include pain, burning, discharge, swelling, erythema, and dysuria.
• Explain the *Candida* test purpose and blood-draw procedure. No fasting is required.

▸*Posttest*
• Evaluate the outcome and counsel the patient appropriately about infection and possible treatment (eg, medications). Check venipuncture sites for signs of infection.

C-REACTIVE PROTEIN (CRP) AND HIGH-SENSITIVITY C-REACTIVE PROTEIN (HS-CRP)

Blood

C-reactive protein (CRP) is an acute-phase plasma protein produced in the liver in response to infection or injury virtually absent from the blood of healthy persons. CRP has been associated with atherothrombosis and has been used as a predictor of cardiovascular events (e.g., myocardial infarction and stroke), and hypertension.

Indications
• Monitor acute inflammation, bacterial infection, and acute tissue destruction.
• Evaluate progress of rheumatic fever under treatment and postoperative recovery.
• Predict cardiovascular disease risk.
• Monitor healing process in cases of burns and organ transplantation.

- Identify patients at higher risk of stenosis before percutaneous coronary intervention (PCI), such as coronary stenting.

Reference Values

Normal
- CRP: <0.8 mg/dL or <8 mg/L, determined by rate nephelometry
- hs-CRP: <0.1 mg/dL or <1 mg/L, determined by immunoturbidimetric assay

Clinical Implications
- Positive reaction indicates the presence of an active inflammatory process: rheumatic fever, rheumatoid arthritis, myocardial infarction, or active, widespread malignancy.
- Failure of CRP to decrease during the postoperative period suggests postoperative infection or tissue necrosis.

Interfering Factors
- Oral contraceptives and estrogens may affect CRP levels.
- Smoking and exercise increase CRP levels.

Procedure
- A 7-mL serum sample is obtained by venipuncture, using a red-top tube.
- Observe standard precautions and transport the specimen to the laboratory in a biohazard bag.

Nursing Interventions
▸Pretest
- Assess the patient's knowledge about the test and the signs and symptoms of systemic infection.
- Explain the blood test purpose and procedure. A fasting sample is preferred.
- Determine whether the patient is taking oral contraceptives.

▸Posttest
- Evaluate the outcome and monitor the patient for inflammatory processes.
- Advise the patient that repeat testing is often done during the postoperative period or during the treatment of autoimmune disease.
- A positive test result indicates active inflammation but not its cause.

C3 AND C4 COMPLEMENT COMPONENTS

Blood

Testing for the C3 and C4 components of complement is performed when the total complement (CH_{50}) level is decreased. C3 is synthesized in the liver, macrophages, fibroblasts, lymphoid cells, and skin. C4 is synthesized in bone and lung tissue.

Indications
- C3 and C4

  Investigate an abnormally decreased total complement (CH_{50}) level. Assess connective tissue and autoimmune diseases (eg, SLE).
- C3—Investigate a history of repeated infections; assess degree of nephritis severity.
- C4—Confirm hereditary angioedema.

Reference Values

Normal

Adult normal values: C3 = 75–175 mg/dL (0.75–1.75 g/L) by rate nephelometry; C4 = 14–40 mg/dL (140–400 mg/L) by rate nephelometry; CH_{50} = 95–185 U/mL (95–185 kU/L)

Clinical Implications
- Decreased C3 levels are associated with most active diseases with immune complex formation, such as severe recurrent bacterial infections caused by C3 homozygous deficiency, active SLE, acute poststreptococcal glomerulonephritis (APSGN), membranoproliferative glomerulonephritis (MPGN), end-stage liver disease, and absence of C3b inactivator factor.
- Increased levels of C3 are found in numerous inflammatory states.
- Decreased C4 levels are associated with acute SLE, early glomerulonephritis, cryoglobulinemia, hereditary angioneurotic edema, in-born C4 deficiency, and immune complex diseases.
- Increased levels of C4 are associated with malignancies.

Interfering Factors
- Analysis requires that specimen for C3 or C4 be separated from a clot and immediately frozen.

Procedure
- A 7-mL serum sample for both C3 and C4 is obtained by venipuncture using a red-topped tube.

Nursing Interventions

▶*Pretest*

- Explain that C3 and C4 are used for determining whether a patient has an immune complex disease, such as SLE or rheumatoid arthritis; C3 is further used for assessing renal involvement.

▶*Posttest*

- Evaluate the results, counsel the patient appropriately about repeat testing, and monitor for inflammations and malignancies.

CARDIAC CATHETERIZATION AND ANGIOGRAPHY, HEART CATHETERIZATION, ANGIOCARDIOGRAPHY, CORONARY ARTERIOGRAPHY

Special Heart Interventional Study, X-ray Imaging with Contrast

These procedures are performed to detect abnormalities in the cardiac chambers, valves, and vasculature by means of invasive arterial and venous catheters that carry contrast agents to measure hemodynamics in the right and left sides of the heart. Injected contrast agents provide a visual definition of cardiac structures. Often, interventions such as angioplasty (transluminal balloon and laser angioplasty), stent placement, and septostomy (for infants with congenital heart defects) are performed in conjunction with diagnostic catheterization.

Indications

- Diagnose heart disease type and severity, extent of damage, congenital abnormalities, blood flow, and identify cardiac structure and function before surgery and response to therapy.
- Evaluate abnormal stress tests.
- Measure pressure gradients, cardiac output, ejection fractions, and cardiac blood samples for O_2 content and saturation.
- Evaluate angina, other types of chest pain, syncope, abnormal resting or exercise ECGs, symptoms after revascularization, coronary insufficiency, ventricular aneurysm, and cardiac neurosis.
- Evaluate vessel stenosis during an acute myocardial infarction episode (the patient can be sent to surgery immediately after the procedure).
- Perform therapeutic interventions, such as pacemaker insertion, aortic balloon pump, vena cava filter, or others.

Reference Values

Normal

- Normal heart valves, chamber size, and patent coronary arteries
- Normal wall and valve motion
- Normal cardiac output (CO): 4–8 L/min
- Normal percentage of oxygen content (15–22 vol %) and oxygen saturation (95%–100% or 0.95–1.00)

Normal Cardiac Volumes

End-diastolic volume (EDV): 50–90 mL/m^2 (body surface area)
End-systolic volume (ESV): 25 mL/m^2
Stroke volume (SV): 45 ± 12 mL/m^2
Ejection fraction (EF): 0.67 ± 0.07

Clinical Implications

- Abnormal pressures in the heart, in great vessels, and between chambers indicate valvular stenosis or insufficiency, ventricular failure, idiopathic hypertrophic subaortic stenosis (IHSS), septal defects, and cardiovascular shunts.
- Abnormal blood gas studies indicate circulatory shunting (congenital or acquired), septal defects, leaks, or abnormal sequence of blood circulation.
- Other deviations include aneurysm or enlargement, stenosis, altered contractility, tumors, and constriction.
- Pericarditis: bacterial, restrictive post–myocardial infarction (MI).

CLINICAL ALERT

- The benefits of the procedure usually outweigh the risks to the patient. Some possible contraindications include severe heart failure, hypotension, allergy to contrast, severe renal disease, recent myocardial infarction, digitalis toxicity, recent subacute bacterial endocarditis, uncontrolled dysrhythmias, bundle branch block, fever, or marked obesity.

Procedure

- Moderate sedation/analgesia usually is administered via IV access before the procedure.
- The patient lies on an x-ray table, with an imaging camera nearby. It is tilted at various angles during the procedure to permit better visualization.

- The catheter insertion site is injected with local anesthetic before catheter insertion.
- For right heart catheterization, the medial cubital, brachial, or femoral vein may be used. The catheter is threaded through the superior vena cava to the right atrium and through the tricuspid valve and right ventricle to the pulmonary artery.
- For left heart catheterization, the catheter is threaded through the femoral or brachial artery and through the aortic valve to the left ventricle.
- After the catheter is removed, direct pressure is applied to the arterial site, and vascular closure devices are used to close the access site (eg, hemostasis-promoting pads or patches, and inserts).
- The catheterized extremity may be immobilized to reduce movement.

Nursing Interventions
▸*Pretest*
- Explain the test purpose and procedure.
- Describe the sensations the patient may feel (eg, "pressure" with catheter insertion, transient hot flashes with the injection of contrast medium, nausea, vomiting, headache, cough).
- Explain that sedation and analgesia are used.
- Emphasize that chest pain needs to be reported promptly so that medication to relieve pain may be administered.

CLINICAL ALERT

- Assess allergies and anticoagulant status. NPO status is required for 6 to 12 hours before procedure unless otherwise ordered.

▸*Intratest*
- Provide ordered sedation as necessary and orient the patient for fluoroscopy.
- Reassure the patient frequently.

▸*Posttest*
- Bed rest is usually maintained for 6 to 12 hours after the test, based on the nature of the procedure, the physician's protocols, and the patient's status.
- Check vital signs frequently according to institutional protocols. At the same time, check the catheter insertion site for hematomas, swelling, bleeding, or bruits. Neurovascular checks should be done

along with assessment of vital signs in bilateral extremities and results should be compared. Report significant changes immediately.
- Administer prophylactic antibiotics, if needed.
- Encourage fluid intake unless contraindicated.
- Interpret test results and monitor the patient appropriately for cardiac, circulatory, neurovascular, and pulmonary problems.

CLINICAL ALERT

- Complications include the following:
  Dysrhythmias
  Allergic reactions to contrast agent, evidenced by urticaria, pruritus, conjunctivitis, or anaphylaxis
  Thrombophlebitis
  Insertion site infection
  Pneumothorax
  Hemopericardium
  Embolism
  Liver lacerations, especially in infants and children
- Notify attending physician immediately about increased bleeding, hematoma, dramatic fall or elevation in BP, or decreased peripheral circulation and abnormal or changed neurovascular findings. Rapid treatment may prevent more severe complications.

CARDIAC ENZYMES, CARDIAC INJURY STUDIES, CARDIAC MARKERS

Blood, Serum, Plasma

Creatine Kinase (CK), CK Isoenzymes (CK-1/CK-BB, CK-2/CK-MB, CK-3/CK-MM), Myoglobin, Cardiac Troponin T and I; Atrial Natriuretic Factor (ANF) or Atrial Natriuretic Hormone (ANH), and Brain Natriuretic Peptide (BNP)

Cardiac markers are intracellular proteins, enzymes, or neurohormones released from dead or damaged cells. The markers differ in their location within the myocyte, release kinetics after damage, and clearance from the peripheral circulation. For example, ANF is released by the atria in response to an increase in blood pressure, whereas BNP is released by the ventricles in response to volume expansion, that is, a decrease in the ejection fraction. The markers are usually used for the differential diagnosis of cardiac disease. Cardiac troponins are considered to be the gold standard for identifying myocardial infarctions (MIs) and cardiac injury and have replaced CK-MB as the marker for MIs.

Indications

- Diagnose acute MI and the severity of disease.
- Differential diagnosis of other cardiac diseases, eg, congestive heart failure, myocardial infarct, unstable angina pectoris, and myocarditis.
- Troponins T and I are cardiac specific, rise above the upper reference limit at 2 to 6 hours, and remain elevated up to 4 to 14 days after an acute MI.
- Evaluate the success of thrombolytic therapy (ie, streptokinase and tPA) and reperfusion.

Reference Values

Normal

CREATINE KINASE

TOTAL CK

Adults
  Males: 38–174 U/L (0.65–2.96 μkat/L)
  Females: 26–140 U/L (0.46–2.38 μkat/L)

Infants: 2–3 times adult levels

CPK ISOENZYMES

CK_3-MM: 97%–100%
CK_2-MB: <3%
CK_1-BB: Trace or absent

MYOGLOBIN

Males: 28–72 ng/mL
Females: 25–58 ng/mL

For consistency with cardiac troponin and CK-MB, the 99th percentile of the reference population should be used as the reference cutoff.

CARDIAC TROPONIN

The joint European Society of Cardiology/American College of Cardiology guidelines redefined myocardial infarction. The preferred biomarker for myocardial damage is a cardiac troponin, with an increased value being defined as a measurement exceeding the 99th percentile of a reference control group in the appropriate clinical setting, using an assay with a CV <10% at this value.

REFERENCE RANGE AT THE 99TH PERCENTILE FOR FDA-APPROVED CARDIAC TROPONIN ASSAYS (μg/L) BY GENDER AND RACE

ASSAY	ALL	MALES	FEMALES	CAUCASIAN	AFRICAN AMERICAN	HISPANIC	ASIAN
Abbottt AxSYM	0.8	0.8	0.7	0.8	0.5	0.5	1.1
Siemens Centaur	0.15	0.17	0.14	0.17	0.17	0.00	0.09
Siemens Dimension	0.06	0.06	0.06	0.04	0.03	0.01	0.09
Siemens Immulite	0.21	0.21	<0.2	0.21	<0.2	<0.2	<0.2
Orthoclinical Diagnostics Vitros	0.10	0.11	0.09	0.11	0.10	0.02	0.07
Roche	<0.01	<0.01	<0.01	<0.01	<0.01	N/A	N/A
Beckman Coulter Access	0.08	0.10	0.04	0.07	0.08	0.02	0.10

NATRIURETIC PEPTIDES

ANF (ANH): 20–77 pg/mL or 6.5–25.0 pmol/L
BNP: <100 pg/mL or <100 ng/L

Clinical Implications: CK

- *CK total levels are elevated* in acute myocardial infarction (MI). Levels rise after an attack (4–6 hours) and reach a peak several times the normal value within 24 hours; they return to normal 48 to 72 hours after infarction unless there is new tissue damage.
- *CK total levels increase* in severe myocarditis, cardioversion (cardiac defibrillation), after open-heart surgery, and in many other noncardiac syndromes.
- *CK_3 (CK-MM) isoenzyme levels* are elevated in most conditions in which total CK is increased. CK-MM is predominant in both heart and skeletal muscle and is found in normal serum.
- *CK_2 (CK-MB) isoenzyme levels* increase in MI (rises in 4–6 hours after MI; not demonstrated after 26–36 hours), myocarditis, myocardial ischemia, Duchenne's muscular dystrophy, extensive rhabdomyolysis, polymyositis, subarachnoid hemorrhage, Reye's syndrome, chronic renal failure, malignant hyperthermia, and Rocky Mountain spotted fever.
- *CK_1 (CK-BB)* is rarely found. CK-BB has been described as a marker for adenocarcinoma of the prostate, breast, ovary, colon,

and gastrointestinal tract and for small-cell anaplastic carcinoma of lung. CK-BB has been reported with severe shock and/or hypothermia, infarction of bowel, brain injury, and stroke, as a genetic marker in some families with malignant pyrexia, and with MB in alcoholic myopathy.

Interfering Factors: CK Isoenzymes

- Strenuous exercise (up to three times normal for MB fraction of CK with exercise) is an interfering factor. Athletes have a higher value due to greater muscle mass.
- Multiple intramuscular injections increase enzyme levels, as do childbirth and hypothermia.
- False-positive results may be caused by drugs, including Decadron (dexamethasone), Lasix (furosemide), morphine, anticoagulants, some anesthetics, ampicillin, aspirin, amphotericin B, clofibrate, and carbenicillin, and alcohol.

Clinical Implications: Myoglobin

- Diagnose skeletal or myocardial muscle injury.
- Myoglobin is generally detectable earlier than is CK or CK-MB increase in patients with acute myocardial infarction.
- Myoglobin is found in 50% of patients with acute coronary insufficiency and is thought to define a population of small infarcts of myocardium. It correlates with size of infarct.
- Diagnose rhabdomyolysis.
- Myoglobin appears with trauma, ischemia, malignant hyperthermia, exertion, dermatomyositis, polymyositis, and muscular dystrophy.

Interfering Factors: Myoglobin

- It has a very short half-life of 10 minutes in blood and is rapidly cleared by the kidneys. As an index of myocardial infarct, myoglobin returns rapidly to baseline levels.
- It is known for its excellent clinical sensitivity early after MI but is not a widely used test due to its lack of tissue specificity.
- Myoglobin levels may be increased after intramuscular injections and have been reported after a high-voltage electrical accident.

CLINICAL ALERT

- Because RBCs and kidney cells contain the same isoenzymes as heart muscle, patients with pernicious anemia or renal infarction may have the same serum isoenzyme patterns as those with myocardial infarctions.

Clinical Implications: Troponins
- Cardiac troponin is released even with very low levels of myocardial damage as early as 2 to 6 hours after injury and remains high for 14 days or longer; however, it has low sensitivity for the early diagnosis of acute MI. Troponin T can identify small infarcts, which have been undetectable by conventional diagnostic methods and previously diagnosed as unstable angina.
- Elevated cardiac troponin levels are indicative of myocardial injury but are not synonymous with MI or an ischemic mechanism of injury. Elevated levels indicate acute MI, other cardiac diseases, unstable angina pectoris, and myocarditis.

Interfering Factors: Troponin
- False-positive results: elevations in acute and chronic renal failure and chronic muscle disease.

Clinical Implications: ANF (ANH)
- Increased levels occur in congestive heart failure.

Clinical Implications: BNP
- Elevated levels are consistent with an increase in the end-diastolic volume, that is, a decrease in the ventricular ejection fraction (left ventricular dysfunction).

Procedure
- Serum (7–10 mL, 1 mL minimum for individual test) obtained by venipuncture, using a red-top tube (prechilled lavender-top tube for ANF).
- Avoid hemolysis.
- Food and fluids are not restricted. (Fasting sample is required for ANF.)
- Most cardiac enzymes must be retested 3 days in succession (eg, 1–2 hours for the first 12 hours and then every 12 hours for 24 hours) to have clinical significance. Cardiac troponin concentrations should be measured on serial blood samples collected at least 6 to 9 hours after the onset of symptoms, before a patient is ruled in or ruled out for MI. If cardiac troponin assays are not available, the best alternative is creatine kinase MB (CK-MB).

Nursing Interventions
▶*Pretest*
- Explain the purpose and procedure of the test and need for serial testing.

▸*Posttest*

- Apply pressure or a pressure dressing to the venipuncture site and monitor for bleeding or infection.
- Report all elevated enzyme levels to the physician immediately so that appropriate medical interventions are not delayed.
- Evaluate outcomes and counsel the patient appropriately (eg, for newly diagnosed MI, consider the need for lifestyle adjustment, rest, activity and diet changes, medications, work, and leisure activity).
- Further testing may be needed to monitor success of thrombolytic therapy for acute MIs.

CARDIAC FLOW STUDIES: FIRST-PASS AND SHUNT IMAGING

Nuclear Medicine Scans, Cardiac Imaging

Cardiac flow studies evaluate blood flow through the great vessels and after vessel surgery and determine the right and left ventricular ejection fractions.

Indications

- Examine heart chamber disorders, especially left-to-right (the gold standard technique) and right-to-left shunts.
- For pediatric patients, evaluate congenital heart disease, transposition of the great vessels, atrial or ventricular septal defects, and quantitative assessment of valvular regurgitation.

Reference Values

Normal

- Normal right and left ventricular function
- Normal wall motion and ejection fraction
- Normal pulmonary transit times and normal sequence of chamber filling
- No cardiac shunting

Clinical Implications

- Abnormal first-pass ejection fraction values are associated with the following:
  Congestive heart failure
  Regurgitation due to valvular disease

Change in ventricular function due to infarction
Ventricular aneurysm formation
Persistent arrhythmias from poor ventricular function
Pulmonary emboli
Lung transplantation
- Abnormal heart shunts reveal the following:
Left-to-right shunt
Tetralogy of Fallot (as seen more often in children)
Right-to-left shunt

Interfering Factors
- Inability to access jugular vein with an intravenous line.

Procedure
- The patient is placed in the supine position, with the head slightly elevated.
- A three-way stopcock with saline flush is used for radionuclide injection in the jugular vein or the antecubital fossa. For a shunt evaluation, the radionuclide is injected in the external jugular vein via a large-bore needle to ensure a compact bolus.
- Immediately after the injection, the camera traces the flow of the radiopharmaceutical in its "first pass" through the heart in multiple rapid images.
- Resting multigated acquisition (MUGA) scan with a shunt study is performed.
- The total procedure time is approximately 20 to 30 minutes; the actual imaging time is only 5 minutes.

Nursing Interventions
▶ Pretest
- Explain the purpose, procedure, benefits, and risks of scans.
- An intravenous line is required.

▶ Intratest
- Reassure the patient.

▶ Posttest
- Interpret test outcomes, monitor injection site, and counsel the patient appropriately about further ordered testing and treatment.

CAT (COMPUTERIZED AXIAL TOMOGRAPHY) SCAN—
CT (COMPUTED TOMOGRAPHY) SCAN, CT OF HEAD,
BODY, ABDOMEN, PELVIS, SPINE, EXTREMITIES

X-ray Imaging with Contrast of Head and Body

CT is a specialized procedure in which a thin beam of x-rays is directed at and moves around some stationary body part, with resultant computer-manipulated pictures that are not obscured by overlying anatomy.

Indications

- CT screening is done to detect the amount of calcium plaque in the coronary arteries and for the presence of lung masses.
- Evaluate head trauma and rule out intracranial lesions, aneurysms, and hydrocephalus.
- Evaluate prolonged, severe headache and changes in mental status.
- Rule out pathologies within the abdomen, pelvis, spine, chest, or extremities.
- Cancer staging and treatment planning.
- Biopsy guidance.

Reference Values

Normal

- No apparent tumor or pathology.
- Normal size, location, and appearance of body structures and organs.

Clinical Implications

- Head CT abnormalities refer to aneurysms, cysts, tumors, abscesses, intracranial hemorrhage, hematomas, hydrocephalus, fractures, and degenerative processes.
- Body CT abnormalities refer to abscesses; neoplasms; metastases; cysts; enlarged lymph nodes; ascites; organ enlargement; aneurysms; diffuse changes as in cirrhosis or fatty liver; cancer of kidneys, spleen, pancreas, uterus, or prostate; collections of blood, fluid, or fat; retroperitoneal lymphadenopathy; or enlarged lymph nodes.
- Skeletal CT abnormalities refer to bone metastasis and fractures.

Interfering Factors

- Patient movement results in suboptimal images.
- Retained barium may obscure organs in upper and lower abdominal regions.

Procedure

Head CT

- The patient lies on a motorized couch with the head supported in appropriate position. The couch is moved into a donut-shaped gantry that encases the x-ray apparatus and detectors.
- Contrast is usually administered by intravenous injection.
- Multiple images are taken while the patient remains motionless. Sedation and analgesics may be ordered if it is difficult for the patient to lie quietly. The total examination time is 10 to 30 minutes.

Body or Abdomen CT

- The procedure is the same as for the head, with the following exceptions. An oral contrast is consumed before the examination if the upper gastrointestinal tract is to be examined. Iodine contrast is usually administered intravenously for other examinations.
- In *CT scans of the spine*, the protocol is similar except that CT of the spine performed to rule out fractures does not require contrast media administration or preparation. CT of spine for cord and paraspinous evaluation usually requires intrathecal contrast administration and may be performed in conjunction with a *myelogram.*
- *CT scans of the extremities* may be ordered. No contrast or preparation is required if being performed to evaluate bony detail. Extremity CT scans performed for the assessment of soft tissue abnormalities may require contrast administration.

Nursing Interventions

▸*Pretest*

- Assess for test contraindications (pregnancy, iodine hypersensitivity), evidence of severe renal impairment (elevated BUN, creatinine), and food or beverage consumed within 4 hours before contrast administration.
- Explain the examination purpose and procedure. Food and fluid restrictions before contrast-enhanced studies are generally indicated.
- Special attention is necessary for diabetic patients. Because of pretest fasting, the administration of insulin or oral hypoglycemic agents may be contraindicated. Check with the x-ray department.

CLINICAL ALERT

- Diabetic patients who take the oral drug metformin (Glucophage) may require preprocedure and postprocedure modifications. There is a potential for renal failure with lactic acidosis when iodinated contrast is administered in combination with metformin. Consult with the x-ray department to determine whether medications must be discontinued the day of and several days after the test.

♦Intratest
- Observe for evidence of reactions such as nausea, rashes, and hives. Administer antihistamines to reduce the more severe symptoms. Document and inform the physician.

♦Posttest
- Evaluate the outcome, provide the patient with support and counseling, and explain possible further testing, such as biopsy.

Cerebrospinal Fluid Analysis, Lumbar Puncture, Spinal Tap

Spinal Fluid, Lumbar Puncture

Appearance, Volume, Pressure, Chloride, Sodium, Potassium, Glucose, Protein, Total Cell Count, Syphilis Test, Culture

Cerebrospinal fluid (CSF), a clear, colorless fluid found within the lateral ventricles of the brain, provides nutrients for the brain covering (meninges), serves as a shock absorber to prevent brain injury, regulates intracranial pressure, and removes waste products.

The lumbar sac, located at L4 to L5, is the usual site used for puncture to obtain CSF specimens, because damage to the nervous system is less likely to occur in this area.

Certain observations are made each time a lumbar puncture is performed:

- CSF pressure is measured.
- General appearance, consistency, and tendency of the CSF to clot are noted.
- CSF cell count is performed to distinguish types of cells present; this must be done within 2 hours of obtaining the CSF sample.

- CSF protein and glucose concentrations are determined.
- Other blood serologic and bacteriologic tests are done when the patient's condition warrants attention (eg, cultures for aerobes and anaerobes or tuberculosis).
- Tumor markers may be present in CSF; these tests are useful as supplements to CSF cytology analysis.

CLINICAL ALERT

- Before lumbar puncture, check eyegrounds for evidence of papilledema, because its presence may signal potential problems or complications of lumbar puncture.
- A mass lesion should be confirmed by CT scan before lumbar puncture, because this can lead to brain stem herniation.

Indications

- Diagnose spinal cord and brain diseases such as meningitis, intracranial hemorrhage, CNS malignancy, and demyelinating diseases and determination of the cause of seizure disorders and confused states.
- Measure the level of pressure to determine impairment of CSF flow.
- Determine extent of stroke or CVA.
- Lower intracranial pressure by removal of a volume of fluid.
- Check protein in all cases as a nonspecific indicator of damage to the blood-brain barrier.
- Introduce anesthetics, drugs, or contrast agents into the spinal cord.

Reference Values

Normal

Appearance: Crystal clear, colorless
Volume: 90–150 mL; children: 60–100 mL
Pressure: 90–180 mm H_2O; children: 10–100 mm H_2O
Chloride: 115–130 mEq/L (mmol/L)
Sodium: 135–160 mEq/L (mmol/L)
Potassium: 2.6–3.0 mEq/L (mmol/L)
Total blood cell count: 0–5 white blood cells (WBCs), no RBCs, 40%–80% (0.40–0.80) lymphocytes
Glucose: 40–70 mg/dL (2.2–3.9 mmol/L)
Lumbar protein: neonates: 15–100 mg/dL (150–1000 mg/L); adults: 15–45 mg/dL (150–450 mg/L); elderly (>60 years): 15–60 mg/dL (150–600 mg/L)

Syphilis: Venereal Disease Research Laboratory (VDRL) negative
Culture: Negative; no bacteria or viruses are detected

Critical Values

Total protein: none or >45 mg/dL (>450 mg/L)
Glucose: <20 mg/dL (<1.1 mmol/L)
WBCs: >20 segmented neutrophils

Clinical Implications

- *Increased pressure* occurs with intracranial tumors or abscesses, meningitis, inflammatory processes, subarachnoid hemorrhage, cerebral edema, and thrombosis of venous sinuses.
- *Decreased pressure* occurs with leaking of spinal fluid, subarachnoid block, circulatory collapse, and severe dehydration and hyperosmolality.
- *Change in color or appearance* occurs in inflammatory diseases, hemorrhage, and tumors that bring about an elevated cell count. *Blood evenly mixed in all three tubes* occurs in subarachnoid and cerebral hemorrhage. *Xanthochromia* (pale pink to dark yellow, grading is 1 to 4+) is associated with bilirubin, oxyhemoglobin, methemoglobin, increased CSF protein, carotene, and melanoma.
- *Chloride decreases* are associated with tubercular and bacterial meningitis.
- *Glucose level is decreased* with bacterial activity and acute bacterial meningitis. All types of organisms consume glucose (ie, pyogenic, tubercular, amebic, and fungal meningitis).
- *Glucose level is increased* with diabetes and diabetic coma.
- *Protein level is increased* with increased permeability of CSF barriers in infections, hemorrhage, endocrine disorders, and metabolic conditions. Increased levels are associated with obstructions of CSF circulation in tumors and abscesses and with meningitis, Guillain-Barré syndrome, multiple sclerosis, and neurosyphilis.
- *Protein level is decreased* with CSF leakage and volume removal, intracranial hypertension, and hyperthyroidism.
- *WBC levels are increased* (ie, pleocytosis) in inflammation, bacterial infections, hemorrhage, neoplasms, and trauma. Increased levels are also associated with repeated lumbar puncture, pneumoencephalogram, injection of contrast medium anticancer drugs, lumbar puncture contaminated by detergent, and malignant cells found with metastatic brain tumors. Increased plasma cell levels are associated with lymphocytic reactions.

Interfering Factors
- *Pressure:* Anxiety, breath holding, and abnormal venous compression.
- *Appearance:* Traumatic tap and skin disinfectant cause abnormal color.
- *Chloride:* Concurrent intravenous chloride and traumatic tap invalidate results.
- *Glucose:* Decreased levels result from cellular and bacterial metabolism if the test sample is not processed immediately.
- *Protein:* Traumatic tap invalidates the protein test results.

Procedure
- A local anesthetic is injected slowly into the dermis after the skin is cleaned with an antiseptic solution. A spinal needle with a stylet is inserted in the midline between the spines of the lumbar sac (between L4 and L5) or lower (subarachnoid space). A sterile manometer is attached to the needle and the opening CSF pressure is measured and documented. Four sterile collection tubes are filled with 2 to 3 mL of CSF.
- A specimen consisting of up to 20 mL of CSF is removed. Up to four samples of 2 to 3 mL each are taken, placed in separate sterile vials, and labeled sequentially. Vial no. 1 is used for chemistry and serology; vial no. 2 for microbiology studies; vial no. 3 for hematology cell counts; and vial no. 4 for special studies such as cryptococcal antigens, syphilis testing (Venereal Disease Research Laboratory [VDRL]), protein electrophoresis, and other immunologic studies. A closing pressure reading may be taken before the needle is withdrawn. In cases of increased intracranial pressure (ICP), no more than 2 mL of CSF is withdrawn because of the risk that the brain stem may shift.
- A small, sterile dressing is applied to the puncture site.
- Record the procedure start and completion times, the patient's status, CSF appearance, and CSF pressure readings.

Nursing Interventions
▶*Pretest*
- Assess for contraindications to the procedure, such as soft tissue or other skin conditions and skin infection at the puncture site. Infectious processes often increase the intracranial pressure. Severe degenerative vertebral joint disease, severe psychiatric problems, and chronic back pain need to be considered.
- Perform a baseline neurologic assessment, including strength, sensation, and movement of the legs and vital signs.

- Explain the test purpose and procedure. No fasting is necessary. Explain the equipment used and the sensations patient may feel (ie, "pop" of the needle through the dura mater), even though an anesthetic is used with the procedure.
- Instruct the patient to empty the bladder and bowels before the procedure.
- Explain that it is important to lie very still throughout the procedure to avoid traumatic injury. Instruct the patient how to relax by taking deep breaths slowly, inhaling through the nose and exhaling through the mouth.

▶*Intratest*

- Assist the patient throughout the test to maintain side-lying position with the head flexed onto the chest and the knees drawn up but not compressing the abdomen (ie, fetal position or lateral decubitus).
- Label tubes with the patient's name, date, room number, and tube number. Take the specimens to the laboratory immediately (never refrigerate) for analysis.
- Note any leakage of the fluid after the test is completed.
- Apply a bandage dressing to the puncture site.
- Record the time of the procedure, condition and reaction of the patient, appearance of CSF, pressure readings, time the specimen was sent to the laboratory, and tests requested in the patient's record.

CLINICAL ALERT

- If the initial pressure is near 200 mm H_2O, only 1 to 2 mL of the fluid should be removed to avoid spinal cord compression or cerebellar herniation. If the initial pressure is normal, the Queckenstedt test (ie, application of pressure on both jugular veins to produce increased CSF pressure) may be performed. This test is not done if a central nervous system tumor is suspected.

▶*Posttest*

- Instruct the patient to lie prone (flat or horizontal) for at least 2 hours. Turning from side to side is permitted.
- Headaches are common because of spinal fluid leakage from the site of lumbar puncture. Administer ordered analgesics for these and encourage a longer period of bed rest.
- Encourage fluids to help replace lost CSF, thereby aiding in the prevention or relief of headache.

- Assess for neurologic status and changes such as increased temperature, increased BP, change in the level of conscious state, irritability, change in pupil reaction, and numbness and tingling sensations in extremities.
- Check puncture site frequently for fluid leakage and report immediately to the physician.
- Counsel the patient and the family regarding the posttest outcomes and explain or reinforce the outcomes as discussed by the physician.

CHEMISTRY OR METABOLIC PROFILES

Blood, 24-Hour Urine

These serum studies are a collection of commonly ordered tests (12 to >48) that can be done at one time. They are commonly called SMAC (sequential multiple analysis by computer), CMP (comprehensive metabolic panel), MSSP, etc. (based on the commercial automation devices used). These tests vary widely among laboratories, and the battery of tests may include many different configurations.

Indications
- Provide baseline results on admission panel.
- Differentiate MI from other diagnoses.
- Survey multiple organs.
- Evaluate patients with possible diagnostic problems, alcoholism, and toxic states.
- Use in preoperative patients and after surgery.

COMMONLY MEASURED VALUES

Albumin
Alkaline phosphatase
Anion gap
AST (SGOT)
Bicarbonate
Bilirubin, total
Blood urea nitrogen (BUN)
Calcium
Carbon dioxide (CO_2)
Chloride
Cholesterol
Creatinine, creatinine clearance
Electrolytes

Globulin
Glucose
Lactate dehydrogenase (LDH)
Magnesium
Osmolality
pH
Phosphorous
Potassium
Protein, total
Sodium
Uric acid

Procedure

- Collect a venous blood specimen for serum analysis or a 24-hour urine sample. (See Chapter 2 for collection guidelines.)

CHEST RADIOGRAPHY (CHEST X-RAY)

X-ray of Chest and Bony Thorax

The chest x-ray is a common procedure used to demonstrate the appearance of lungs, mediastinum, bony thorax, diaphragm, chest wall, cardiac silhouette, and thyroid gland.

Indications

- Evaluate suspected pulmonary or cardiac disease and trauma to chest.
- Determine the location of chest tubes, feeding tubes, or subclavian catheters.
- Follow the progress of disease, such as TB.
- Check for pneumothorax after bronchoscopy and following biopsy.

Reference Values

Normal

- Normal appearing and normally positioned chest, bony thorax, soft tissues, mediastinum, lungs, pleura, heart, and aortic arch.

Interfering Factors

- Optimal chest x-ray films require the patient to be in an upright position to reveal fluid levels. Inability to hold the breath and take a deep inspiration may affect image quality.

• Obesity, pain, congestive heart failure, and scarring of lung tissues may affect breathing and should be considered when evaluating x-rays.

Procedure

• Clothing is removed to the waist. X-rays can penetrate through a hospital gown that does not contain any buttons, pins, metal snaps, or jewelry.
• Generally, two views of the chest are taken with the patient in an upright position. Sustained full inspiration is required during the x-ray procedure. The procedure takes only a few minutes.

Nursing Interventions
▶*Pretest*

• Explain the purpose and procedure of obtaining a chest x-ray and assure the patient that the test is painless.
• No preparation is necessary but make certain that jewelry and metallic objects are removed from the chest area.
• Screen for pregnancy status and, if positive, advise the radiology department.

▶*Posttest*

• Evaluate the outcome, monitor pulmonary and chest disorders, and provide the patient with support and counseling.
• Explain the need for repeat chest x-ray films (if necessary) and follow-up tests (eg, bronchoscopy).

CHOLESTEROL (C) TEST OR LIPOPROTEIN PROFILE TESTS, LIPID TESTS/LIPOPROTEIN TESTS

Blood, Fasting, Lipids, Nonfasting Palm Skin Test

Cholesterol (C), Triglycerides and Lipoproteins, High-Density Lipoprotein Cholesterol (HDL-C), Low-Density Lipoprotein Cholesterol (LDL-C), and Very Low-Density Lipoprotein (VLDL)

These tests are performed to evaluate the risk for myocardial or coronary artery occlusion and coronary heart disease and to determine total cholesterol, the "bad" cholesterol (LDL-C), the "good" cholesterol (HDL-C), and triglyceride levels.

Indications

- Cholesterol screens for coronary heart disease risk factors, part of a lipid profile.
- Assess other diseases, such as liver, biliary, thyroid, and renal diseases, and diabetes mellitus.
- Monitor the effectiveness of diet, medication, lifestyle changes (eg, exercise), and stress management on test outcomes and lowered risk.

Reference Values

Normal

CHOLESTEROL (C) FASTING

Normal values vary with age, diet, and geographic location. The desirable values are given in the following ranges:

Adults:
Desirable level: 140–199 mg/dL or 3.63–5.15 mmol/L
Borderline high: 200–239 mg/dL or 5.18–6.19 mmol/L
High: >240 mg/dL or >6.20 mmol/L

Children and adolescents (12–18 years):
Desirable level: <170 mg/dL or <4.39 mmol/L
Borderline high: 170–199 mg/dL or 4.40–5.16 mmol/L
High: >200 mg/dL or >5.18 mmol/L

TRIGLYCERIDES FASTING

Values are related to age, sex, and diet:
Normal <150 mg/dL or <1.70 mmol/L
Borderline: 150–199 mg/dL or 1.70–2.25 mmol/L
High: 200–499 mg/dL or 2.26–5.64 mmol/L
Very high: ≥500 mg/dL or ≥5.65 mmol/L

HIGH-DENSITY LIPOPROTEIN CHOLESTEROL (HDL-C) FASTING

Adults:
Males: 35–65 mg/dL or 0.91–1.68 mmol/L
Females: 35–80 mg/dL or 0/91–2.07 mmol/L

LOW-DENSITY LIPOPROTEIN CHOLESTEROL (LDL-C)

Optimal: <100 mg/dL or <2.85 mmol/L
Near optimal: <130 mg/dL or <3.37 mmol/L
Borderline high: 130–159 mg/dL or 3.37–4.12 mmol/L
High: 160–189 mg/dL or 4.14–4.90 mmol/L
Very high: ≥190 mg/dL or ≥4.92 mmol/L

Very Low-Density Lipoproteins (VLDLs)

Normal: 25%–50% of total triglyceride levels

Clinical Implications: Cholesterol (C)

• *Elevated cholesterol levels* (hypercholesteremia) occur in cardio-vascular disease and atherosclerosis, type II familial hypercholes-terolemia, hyperlipoproteinemia, hepatocellular disease, biliary cirrhosis, hypothyroidism, von Gierke's disease, pancreatic and prostate neoplasms, Werner's syndrome, poorly controlled diabetes mellitus, chronic nephritis, glomerulosclerosis, obesity, and dietary "affluence."

• *Decreased cholesterol levels* (hypocholesteremia) occur in malab-sorption, starvation, severe liver disease, hyperthyroidism, chronic obstructive lung disease, mesoblastic, sideroblastic, chronic ane-mias, Tangier disease, severe burns, acute illness, chronic obstruc-tive lung disease, and mental retardation.

Interfering Factors: Cholesterol (C)

• Cholesterol normally has slight seasonal variations: Levels are higher in the fall and winter and lower in the spring and summer; pregnancy increases levels; positional variations.

• Drugs that cause decreased levels include thyroxine, estrogens, androgens, aspirin, antibiotics (tetracycline and neomycin), nico-tinic acid, heparin, colchicine, MAO inhibitors, allopurinol, and bile salts.

• Drugs that may cause increased levels include oral contraceptives, epinephrine, phenothiazines, vitamins A and D, phenytoin, ACTH, anabolic steroids, beta-adrenergic blocking agents, sulfonamide, and thiazide diuretics.

Clinical Implications: Triglycerides

• *Increased levels* of triglycerides occur in types I, IIb, III, IV, and V hyperlipoproteinemias; liver disease; alcoholism; nephrotic syndrome; renal disease; hypothyroidism; poorly controlled dia-betes mellitus; pancreatitis; gout; glycogen storage disease; myocardial infarction (increases may last 1 year); hypothyroidism; von Gierke's disease (ie, glycogen storage disease); MI (elevated levels for several months); anorexia nervosa; and Down's syndrome.

• *Decreased levels* occur with malnutrition, malabsorption syndrome, hyperthyroidism, hyperparathyroidism, congenital alpha-beta lipoproteinemia, brain infarction, and chronic obstructive lung disease.

CLINICAL ALERT

A triglyceride level of >5000 mg/dL (>56.5 mmol/L) is associated with eruptive xanthoma, corneal arcus, lipemia retinalis, and an enlarged liver and spleen.

Interfering Factors: Triglycerides
- Ingestion of a fatty meal or alcohol increases levels.
- Pregnancy may increase levels.
- Drugs that may *decrease levels* include ascorbic acid, clofibrate, phenformin, metformin, asparaginase, and colestipol.
- Drugs that may *increase levels* include estrogen, oral contraceptives, and cholestyramine.
- *Levels are increased* in acute illness, colds, and flu.

Clinical Implications: HDL-C (Good Cholesterol)
- *Increased levels* (>60 mg/dL or 1.55 mmol/L) help lower the risk for heart disease and are also associated with chronic liver disease or chronic alcoholism, long-term aerobic exercise, and vigorous exercise.
- *Decreased levels* (<40 mg/dL or <1.03 mmol/L) indicate an increased risk for coronary heart disease, familial hypo-alpha-lipoproteinemia (ie, Tangier disease) and hypertriglyceridemia, hepatocellular disease, Apo CIII disease, uncontrolled diabetes mellitus, obesity, chronic renal failure, uremia, and Niemann-Pick disease.

Interfering Factors: HDL-C
- Moderate alcohol intake *increases* HDL-C levels.
- Smoking *decreases* HDL-C levels.
- Iodine contrast substances interfere with test results; recent weight gain or loss interferes with test results.
- Exercise raises HDL-C levels; drugs such as aspirin, estrogen, and steroids and insulin therapy may increase levels or cause false-positive results. Other drugs may cause false-negative results.

Clinical Implications: LDL-C and VLDL Levels
- *Increased LDL-C levels* occur with familial type 2 hyperlipidemia, familial hypercholesteremia, and secondary causes such as a diet high in cholesterol and saturated fat, nephrotic syndrome, chronic renal failure, pregnancy, porphyria, diabetes mellitus, multiple myeloma, steroids, progestins, and androgens.

- *Increased VLDL levels* occur with familial hyperlipidemia and secondary causes such as alcoholism, obesity, diabetes mellitus, chronic renal disease, pancreatitis, pregnancy, estrogen, birth-control pills, and progestins.
- *Decreased LDL-C and VLDL levels* occur with malnutrition and malabsorption.

Procedure

- Blood (5–10 mL) is obtained by venipuncture, using a red-top Vacutainer tube.
- A foam pad with a liquid enzyme (Prevu Skin Sterol Test) is placed on the palm. A change in liquid color is compared against a color chart that correlates with the amount of cholesterol.

Nursing Interventions
▶ Pretest

- Explain the purpose and procedure of cholesterol tests and stress the importance of fasting (no food or fluids for 12–16 hours before drawing blood) before the test to avoid false outcomes.
- Withhold medications according to physician's directives and as related to each specific test; for example, hold oral contraceptives, estrogen, and salicylates before lipoprotein testing.
- Note if the patient has had any drastic weight change last few weeks before HDL testing.

CLINICAL ALERT

- Stress and illness affect HDL (eg, after MI) and testing should not be done until 3 months after an illness.

▶ Posttest

- Monitor the venipuncture site for bleeding or infection and allow the patient to resume the pretest diet and medications.
- Evaluate outcomes and counsel the patient appropriately (eg, for high cholesterol levels instruct on the importance of decreased animal fat, replacement of saturated fats with polyunsaturated fats, a consistent exercise program, maintenance of an appropriate body weight, and stress reduction).

CHORIONIC VILLUS SAMPLING (CVS)

Special Tissue (Fetal Origin) Study and Biopsy

Chorionic villus sampling (CVS) can provide very early diagnosis of fetal genetic or biochemical disorders. CVS involves extraction of a small amount of tissue from the villi of the chorion frondosum. This tissue is composed of rapidly proliferating trophoblastic cells that ultimately form the placenta. Although not part of the fetus, these villi cells are genetically identical to the fetus and are considered fetal rather than maternal in nature.

Indications
- Abnormal ultrasound test.
- Fetus at risk for detectable Mendelian disorders: Tay-Sachs disease, hemoglobinopathies, cystic fibrosis, muscular dystrophy.
- Birth of previous child with evidence of chromosome abnormality.
- Parent with known structural chromosomal rearrangement.
- Diagnosis of fetal infection.

Reference Values

Normal
- Normal chromosomal arrangement; negative for DNA abnormalities.
- No fetal metabolic enzyme or blood disorders.

Clinical Implications
- *Abnormal* CVS results indicate chromosomal abnormalities, abnormal fetal tissue, fetal metabolic blood disorders, and fetal infection.

Procedure
- Patient is positioned on her back to permit ultrasound documentation of fetal viability, the number of fetuses in utero, and the localization of trophoblastic tissue. A bimanual pelvic examination is often performed concurrently with this preliminary ultrasound examination. The patient then assumes a lithotomy position. A sterile speculum is inserted after the vagina is cleansed with an iodine-based antiseptic.
- A sterile flexible catheter (visually tracked by ultrasound) with a stainless steel obturator is introduced into the vaginal canal, through the cervical canal, and into the trophoblastic tissue.

• After the catheter is in place, approximately 5 mL of tissue is extracted and immediately examined under a low-power microscope to determine if the quantity and quality are acceptable. After sufficient tissue has been gathered, ultrasound is again used to monitor fetal viability.

CLINICAL ALERT

• CVS risks include loss of amniotic fluid, bleeding, severe limb deformities, intrauterine infection, spontaneous abortion, Rh isoimmunization, and fetal death (5%).

Nursing Interventions

▸ Pretest
• Involve both parents in genetic counseling that include all risks of a genetic defect and the decision-making process regarding a positive result.
• Explain the test procedure and assess for contraindications.
• Obtain baseline maternal vital signs and fetal heart rate (FHR).
• Explain to the patient the possibility of nausea, vertigo, and cramps during the procedure.
• Instruct the patient to drink four 8-oz glasses of water before the procedure and not to void.

▸ Intratest
• Provide reassurance and support for nausea, vertigo, cramps, and anxiety.

▸ Posttest
• A left side-lying position is necessary.
• Assess maternal BP, pulse, respirations, and fetal heart rate for the first half hour after the test.
• Assess for uterine activity and use a fetal monitor every 15 minutes for the first hour after test completion.
• Instruct the patient to notify the clinician about amniotic fluid leakage, signs of labor, abnormal discharge, pain, bleeding, fever, chills, and a lack of fetal movement.
• Rh-negative women should receive a RhoGAM injection to prevent sensitization.
• Counsel the patient regarding test results in collaboration with the physician.

CISTERNOGRAM

Nuclear Medicine Scan, CSF Imaging, Lumbar Puncture

This study, in which a radiopharmaceutical (usually ^{111}In-DTPA) is injected intrathecally during a lumbar puncture, is a sensitive indicator of altered flow and reabsorption of CSF and is ordered to evaluate congenital hydrocephalus.

Indications
- Aid in the selection of the type of shunt and pathway, monitor shunting, and treatment of hydrocephalus.
- Determine the prognosis of both shunting and hydrocephalus.
- Determine blockages in the CSF pathway.
- Evaluate CSF leakage into the nasal cavity.

Reference Values

Normal
- Unobstructed CSF flow and normal reabsorption.

Clinical Implications

Abnormal filling patterns reveal the following:

Cause of hydrocephalus (eg, trauma, inflammation, bleeding, intracranial tumors)
Parencephalic and subarachnoid cysts
Communicating versus noncommunicating hydrocephalus
Subdural hematoma
Spinal mass lesions
Shunt patency or rhinorrhea and otorrhea
Posterior fossa cysts
CSF leakage due to tumor or infection

Procedure
- A sterile lumbar puncture is performed after the patient has been positioned and prepared. At this time, the radionuclide is injected through the subarachnoid space into the cerebrospinal circulation.
- The patient must lie flat after the puncture; the length of time depends on the physician's order.

- Imaging is done between 2 and 6 hours after the injection, again at 24 hours and at 48 hours, and at 72 hours if the physician so directs.
- The examining time is 1 hour for each imaging.

Nursing Interventions
▸*Pretest*
- Explain the purposes, procedures, benefits, and risks for lumbar puncture and cisternography.
- Advise the patient that it may take as long as 1 hour for each imaging session.

▸*Posttest*
- See Posttest instructions under Cerebrospinal Fluid Analysis, Lumbar Puncture.

CLINICAL ALERT

- Be alert to complications of lumbar puncture, such as meningitis, allergic reaction to the anesthetic, bleeding into the spinal canal, herniation of brain tissue, and mild to severe headaches.

COAGULATION STUDIES

Blood, Bleeding and Coagulation Times

Prothrombin Time or Protime (PT), International Normalized Ratio (INR), Activated Partial Thromboplastin Time (APTT), Thrombin Time (TT) or Thrombin Clotting Time (TCT), Platelet Function Assay (PFA), and Activated Coagulation Time (ACT)

These series of tests measure the clotting mechanisms of the body and identify the type and extent of suspected coagulation disorders.

The template bleeding time (Ivy bleeding time) has been replaced by most hospitals with the platelet function assay on the PFA-100® analyzer. The PFA test is a new laboratory screening test of platelet function that measures both platelet adhesion and aggregation (primary hemostasis). The PFA-100® analyzer uses two cartridges: the primary cartridge is the Collagen/Epinephrine (COL/EPI) test to detect platelet dysfunction induced by intrinsic platelet defects, von

Willebrand's disease, or exposure to platelet inhibiting agents, whereas the Collagen/ADP (COL/ADP) test cartridge is used to indicate if an abnormal COL/EPI result may have been caused by the effect of acetyl salicylic acid (ASA) or other medications containing ASA.

Indications

- Conduct a PT screen for prothrombin deficiency and evaluate heparin and Coumadin effects, liver failure, and vitamin K deficiency.
- Investigate symptoms of easy bruising, petechiae, gastrointestinal bleeding, nosebleeds, and heavy menstrual flow.
- Evaluate disseminated intravascular coagulation (DIC).
- Adjust dosage of anticoagulants and monitor streptokinase therapy (plasminogen activators).
- Perform a PFA to aid in the detection of platelet dysfunction (acquired, inherited, or induced).
- Conduct ACT test to titrate a heparin infusion, reverse with protamine, and during dialysis, coronary bypass, arteriograms, and coronary arteriography.
- Conduct TT test to detect a decrease in fibrinogen levels and presence of fibrin and fibrin degradation products (FDPs)

Reference Values

Normal

PT: 11–13 seconds (can vary by laboratory; INR is now used exclusively). Standard and SI unit values are the same.

The INR was devised to standardize PT results because of differences between different batches and manufacturers of tissue factor. The INR is the ratio of a patient's PT to a normal (control) sample PT, raised to the power of the ISI value for the control sample used. Each manufacturer gives an ISI (International Sensitivity Index) for any tissue factor it makes. The ISI value indicates how the particular batch of tissue factor compares with an internationally standardized sample. The ISI is usually between 1.0 and 1.4.

Normal INR: 0.8–1.2

Therapeutic INR range for monitoring patients on warfarin: 2.0–3.0

Therapeutic INR range for patients with mechanical heart valves: 3.0–4.0

TT/TCT: 17–23 seconds, but highly variable depending on the reagent/instrument used.

PFA:

COL/EPI Cartridge: Closure time ≤185 seconds
COL/ADP Cartridge: Closure time ≤120 seconds

APTT (PTT): 21.0–35.0 seconds; therapeutic range for heparin is 2.0–2.5 times the normal limit (56–86 seconds)

ACT: 90–120 seconds; therapeutic range for heparin is 2 times the normal limit (180–240 seconds)

Critical Values

APTT: none or >78 seconds
INR: >5
PT: >30 seconds

Clinical Implications

Conditions that cause *increased PT* include the following:

- Deficiency of factors II (prothrombin), V, VII, or X
- Vitamin K deficiency; newborns of mothers with vitamin K deficiency
- Hemorrhagic disease of the newborn
- Liver disease (eg, alcoholic hepatitis), liver damage
- Current anticoagulant therapy with warfarin (Coumadin)
- Biliary obstruction
- Poor fat absorption (eg, sprue, celiac disease, chronic diarrhea)
- Current anticoagulant therapy with heparin
- Disseminated intravascular coagulation (DIC)
- Zollinger-Ellison syndrome
- Hypofibrinogenemia (factor I deficiency), dysfibrinogenemia
- (Circulating anticoagulants); lupus anticoagulant
- Premature newborns

Conditions that *do not affect the PT* include the following:

- Polycythemia vera
- Tannin disease
- Christmas disease (factor IX deficiency)
- Hemophilia A (factor VIII deficiency)
- von Willebrand's disease
- Platelet disorders (idiopathic thrombocytopenic purpura)

CLINICAL ALERT

- PT of >30 seconds or INR of >6.0 is associated with spontaneous bleeding.

Interfering Factors: PT

- Many drugs lengthen or shorten the PT:

Increases with corticosteroids, EDTA, oral contraceptives, anticoagulants, asparaginase, bishydroxycoumarin, clofibrate, erythromycin, heparin, ethanol, and tetracycline

Decreases with vitamin K, dehydration, and high hematocrit (Hct)

- Careful venipuncture is required; otherwise, the PT can be shortened because of trauma, tissue fluid contamination, hemolysis, or improper filling of tube.

Clinical Implications: PFA

- Normal COL/EPI closure time indicates no evident platelet dysfunction.
- Prolonged COL/EPI closure time with a normal COL/ADP closure time indicates drug-induced platelet dysfunction commonly seen after aspirin ingestion.
- Prolonged COL/EPI and COL/ADP closure times indicate platelet dysfunction or low platelet counts. Platelet dysfunction is most commonly seen in patients with von Willebrand's disease or congenital platelet defects.

Interfering Factors: PFA

The closure time may be prolonged by hematocrit levels <35% or platelet counts <150,000/mL.

Clinical Implications: APTT

- APTT is *prolonged* in hemophilia A and B; congenital deficiency of Fitzgerald factor; Fletcher factor (prekallikrein); use of heparin, streptokinase and urokinase, and warfarin (Coumadin)-like therapy; vitamin K deficiency; hypofibrinogenemia; liver disease; DIC (chronic or acute); and FDPs.
- APTT is *decreased or shortened* in extensive cancer, except when the liver is involved, in very early DIC, and immediately after acute hemorrhage.

CLINICAL ALERT

- APTT of more than 78 seconds indicates spontaneous bleeding.

Procedure

Procedures for PT, TCT, PTT, and APTT

- For these procedures, obtain 7 mL of venous blood, using a light blue-top Vacutainer tube (sodium citrate as anticoagulant) and mixing gently.

- Do not draw from a heparin lock or heparinized catheter.
- Deliver the tube to the laboratory immediately.

Procedure for PFA
- Collect blood in three light blue–top Vacutainer tubes (sodium cit-rate as anticoagulant) and mix gently.
- Do *not* refrigerate the tubes.
- Do *not* centrifuge the tubes.
- Do *not* transport the tubes in a pneumatic tube system.

Procedure for ACT
- A 0.4-mL whole blood sample (no anticoagulant) is drawn and put in special test tubes containing celite.
- The ACT test is difficult to standardize. No controls are available; therefore, this test is used with caution, mainly in cardiac surgery.

Nursing Interventions
▶*Pretest*
- Obtain a careful drug history and family history of bleeding and thrombosis for persons examined through coagulation studies.
- Explain the test purpose and procedure. No aspirin or aspirin-containing drugs are allowed for at least 7 days before the bleed-ing time test.
- For APTT tests and heparin therapy, explain that testing is done to monitor heparin anticoagulant dosage at baseline before therapy is started, 1 hour before the scheduled dose, and when there are signs of bleeding during therapy.
- For the PT test and Coumadin therapy, explain that testing is done to monitor Coumadin anticoagulant dosage.
- Counsel the patient regarding self-medication. Many prescriptions and over-the-counter drugs increase or decrease the effect of anti-coagulants and affect test outcomes.

▶*Intratest*
- Observe and record the appearance of petechiae after applying tourniquet for venipuncture; this provides an indication of the patient's bleeding tendency.

▶*Posttest*
- Evaluate outcomes and counsel the patient appropriately about the treatment (adjustment of dosage).
- Assess for bleeding when the times are prolonged or increased.
- Examine skin for bruises on extremities and on parts of the body the patient cannot easily see. Record bleeding from the venipunc-ture and injection sites, nose, or groin.

Cold Agglutinins (Acute and Convalescent Studies)

Blood, Infection

This test measures IgM autoantibodies that cause the agglutination of the patient's own red blood cells (RBCs). Cold agglutinins are formed in response to infections and cause RBCs to clump together at low temperatures (0°C–10°C).

Indications
- Assess atypical viral pneumonia with *Mycoplasma pneumoniae* in patients having a respiratory infection or fever of unknown origin (FUO).
- Diagnose certain hemolytic anemias.

Reference Values

Normal
- Normal titer: <1:16 by agglutination of the patient's own RBCs at 4°C

Clinical Implications
- A titer greater than 1:32 suggests infection with *Mycoplasma pneumoniae*. A fourfold risk in titer during the course of illness is more important than a single high titer.
- Normal individuals may have low levels of cold agglutinins.

Interfering Factors
- A high titer of cold agglutinins interferes with the blood type and crossmatch procedure.
- High titers sometimes occur spontaneously in older persons and persist for years.
- Antibiotic therapy may interfere with the development of cold agglutinins.
- Improper transport and processing of specimen may cause false-negative results.

Procedure
- Obtain serum (7 mL, using a red-top Vacutainer) by venipuncture and transport it to the laboratory at 37°C.
- The specimen should be prewarmed at 37°C for 30 minutes before the separation of serum from RBCs to allow the cold agglutinins to "elute" from the membranes of RBCs. Failure to perform this step produces a false-negative result.

Nursing Interventions

▸Pretest

- Assess the patient's knowledge about the test and related clinical history.
- Explain the purpose and blood test procedure. Explain that culture of suspected organisms is difficult and that this test is an important aid in the diagnosis of *M. pneumoniae* infection.

▸Posttest

- Evaluate outcomes and counsel the patient appropriately about the treatment.
- Repeat testing later (2–3 weeks) in the course of the illness to confirm the diagnosis.

COLONOSCOPY, VIRTUAL COLONOSCOPY (VC)

Endoscopic GI Imaging Optical Colonoscopy

Colonoscopy is the visual examination of the large intestine from the anus to the ileocecal valve by means of a flexible fiber-optic or video colonoscope, which can also produce photographs of the area. This technique can differentiate inflammatory disease from neoplastic disease and can evaluate polypoid lesions that are beyond the reach of the sigmoidoscope.

Virtual colonoscopy transforms the computed tomographic data into a form that mimics visualization of the colon from within during optical colonoscopy.

Indications

- Evaluate chronic constipation, diarrhea, persistent bleeding, or lower abdominal pain in the absence of definitive findings from proctosigmoidoscopy and barium enema. Locate source of lower GI bleeding.
- Periodic follow-up for recurrent disease or pathology (eg, polyps, colon cancer) and monitoring effectiveness of treatment.
- Biopsies, removal of foreign bodies and polyps, and other interventional procedures.
- Recommended as primary diagnostic tool for first-degree relatives of colon cancer patients.

Reference Values

Normal
- Normal large intestine mucosa from the anus to the cecum.

Clinical Implications
- Benign or malignant tumors, polyps, ulcerations, inflammatory processes, bleeding sites, colitis, diverticulitis or diverticulosis, strictures, or presence of foreign bodies.

Procedure
- Traditional bowel cleansing precedes the procedure, as well as the administration of moderate sedation/analgesia.
- The patient is positioned on the left side or Sims' position and draped properly.
- A well-lubricated colonoscope is inserted about 12 cm into the bowel. The patient should take deep, slow breaths through the mouth during this time. Air is introduced into the bowel through a special port on the colonoscope to aid in visualization. As the scope is advanced, the patient may need to be repositioned several times to aid in proper visualization of the colon. Better visualization occurs as scope is withdrawn.
- For virtual (optical) colonoscopy, the patient is instructed to perform a Fleet enema the day before the test and the morning of the procedure. A small rectal catheter with a balloon tip is inserted into the rectum. The patient uses a "squeeze bulb" to self-administer air via the catheter into the balloon tip. This helps control the overdistention of the colon.
- Once adequately inflated, the colon is scanned.
- Examination time is 30 to 60 minutes.

Nursing Interventions
◆Pretest
- Explain the purpose and test procedure and indicate that the examination can be fairly lengthy.
- Aspirin (ASA) and aspirin-containing products should be discontinued 1 week before the examination because of potential for bleeding or hemorrhage.
- Iron preparations should be discontinued 3 to 4 days before the test because iron residues produce inky, black, sticky stool that may interfere with visualization, and the stool can be viscous and difficult to clear.

- Instruct the patient regarding a clear liquid diet for up to 72 hours before the examination (according to physician's orders). The patient must fast for 8 hours before the procedure, except for medications (check with the physician).
- Laxatives need to be taken to thoroughly clean the bowel.

▶Intratest

- Administer intravenous analgesics, anticholinergics, or glucagon as ordered. Monitor for respiratory depression, hypotension, diaphoresis, bradycardia, or changes in mental status.
- Coach the patient to breathe deeply and relax.
- Take vital signs according to protocols. Use a pulse oximeter. Properly preserve specimens and transport them to the laboratory immediately.

▶Posttest

- Check vital signs frequently after the procedure according to protocols. Inform the patient that he or she may expel large amounts of flatus.
- Observe for complications of bowel perforation, hemorrhage, abdominal pain, hypotension, and cardiac or respiratory arrest (can be caused by oversedation or vagal stimulation from the instrumentation).
- Observe for visible blood in the stool.
- The most frequent adverse reactions to oral purgatives include nausea, vomiting, bloating, rectal irritation, chills, and feelings of weakness.
- Interpret test outcomes and counsel the patient appropriately.

CLINICAL ALERT

- Patients with congestive heart failure or renal failure are at greater risk for fluid volume overload when prepared with oral washout solutions.
- Washout preparations are contraindicated for patients with ulcer disease, gastric outlet obstruction, toxic colitis, or megacolon and for those with less than 20 kg of body weight.
- Signs of bowel perforation indicate malaise, rectal bleeding, abdominal pain, distention, and fever.
- Antibiotics may be ordered for patients with known valvular or other heart diseases.
- Diabetic persons are usually advised not to take insulin before the procedure, but they should bring insulin with them to the clinic or testing area.

COLPOSCOPY, CERVICOGRAPHY

Endoscopic Vaginal, Cervical, and Genital Imaging

Colposcopy permits examination of the vagina and cervix by means of a colposcope, a special instrument with a magnifying lens. It is also used to evaluate males and females for genital lesions from sexually transmitted diseases, such as syphilitic ulcers, chancroid, condylomata, and human papillomavirus (HPV).

Indications
- Evaluate persistent abnormal Papanicolaou (Pap) smears, cervicitis, benign, precarcinoma, carcinomatous lesions of the cervix or vagina, and other abnormal-appearing genital and vulvovaginal wall tissues.
- Study possible invasive carcinoma and glandular lesions.
- Assess women with a history of diethylstilbestrol.

Reference Values

Normal
- Normal-appearing vagina, cervix, vulva, and genital area.
- Normal pink squamous epithelium and capillaries.
- Normal color, tone, and surface contours.

Clinical Implications
- Abnormal lesions or unusual epithelial patterns, including leukoplakia; abnormal vasculature; slight, moderate, or marked dysplasia; and abnormal-appearing tissue classified by punctuation, mosaic pattern, or hyperkeratosis.
- Extent of abnormal epithelium (with acetic acid) and extent of nonstaining with iodine.
- Clinical cervical cancer; cervical exfetation pain.
- Acute inflammation with human papillomavirus or bacterial infections (e.g., chlamydial infection), bacterial vaginosis, and gonorrhea.

Interfering Factors
- Colposcopy cannot accurately detect endocervical lesions.
- Cervical scarring may prevent satisfactory visualization.

Procedure
- The patient is placed in a modified lithotomy position and the cervix is exposed using a bivalve speculum.

- The cervix, vagina, or male genital areas are swabbed with 3% acetic acid (ie, improves visibility of epithelial tissue). Mucus must be completely removed. Use of cottonwool swabs is discouraged because fibers left on cervix interfere with proper visualization.
- The colposcope does not enter the vagina. Examination begins with a field of white light and decreased magnification and is then switched to a green filter to better see vascular changes. Suspicious lesions are diagrammed, photographed, and biopsied (not done if cone biopsy is to be performed at a later date; done if there is suspicion of invasion).
- Cervicography (for early detection of cervical neoplasia and cancer) may be performed in conjunction with colposcopy in women. This method allows photographic images of entire cervix to be taken. The cervix is cleaned and 5% acetic acid is swabbed onto the area before taking photographs. A second set of photographs are taken after aqueous iodine is applied to the cervix.
- An endocervical smear is transferred onto a slide to be evaluated later.

Nursing Interventions
▶*Pretest*
- Assess the patient's level of knowledge about the colposcopy examination process and procedure and explain the purpose and procedure.
- Obtain a pertinent gynecologic history.
- Obtain a urine specimen.
- Administer ibuprofen for cramps.

▶*Intratest*
- Offer reassurance in a sensitive and understanding manner. Explain that some discomfort may be felt if biopsies are taken. If a patient experiences a vasovagal response, watch for bradycardia and hypotension.
- Assist with a paracervical block if used within the procedure.
- Place specimens in the proper preservative, label accurately, and route to the appropriate department in a timely fashion.

▶*Posttest*
- Monitor for complications (eg, pelvic inflammatory disease). Instruct the patient to watch for infection, bleeding, and pain and advise her regarding physician contact.
- Provide sterile saline or water for perineal cleaning; acetic acid may produce a burning sensation. Explain that a small amount of

vaginal bleeding or cramping for a few hours is normal; provide vaginal pads for the patient's use.

- If cervicography has been done, tell the patient that a brown vaginal discharge (from Schiller's iodine) may persist for a few days. Excessive bleeding, pain, fever, or purulent, abnormal vaginal discharge should be reported to the physician immediately.

- Evaluate and document outcomes and counsel the patient about follow-up treatments and tests, such as cone biopsy radiation, surgery, or loop electrocautery excision procedure (LEEP).

COMPLETE BLOOD COUNT (CBC) WITH DIFFERENTIAL (DIFF), HEMOGRAM (CBC WITHOUT DIFF)

Blood, Cells

Red Blood Cell (RBC) Count, Hematocrit (Hct), Hemoglobin (Hgb) Concentration, Mean Corpuscular Volume (MCV), Mean Corpuscular Hemoglobin (MCH), Mean Corpuscular Hemoglobin Concentration (MCHC), White Blood Cell (WBC) Count, Differential (Diff) Count, Platelets, Bands, Segmented Neutrophils, Eosinophils, Basophils, Monocytes, Lymphocytes, Reticulocytes

The CBC (with the platelet and differential counts) and the hemogram (CBC without the differential count) are basic screening tests and the most frequently ordered laboratory procedures.

The CBC and hemogram findings give valuable diagnostic information about the hematologic and other body systems, prognosis, response to treatment, and recovery. The CBC consists of a series of tests that determine the number, variety, percentage, concentrations, and quality of blood cells.

Indications
- Use WBCs as a guide to indicate the severity of the disease process.
- Use RBCs, hematocrit (Hct), and hemoglobin (Hgb) in the evaluation of anemia and polycythemia.
- Use reticulocyte count to recognize occult disease and chronic hemorrhage.
- Screen in physical examinations and in preoperative and postoperative evaluations.

- Diagnose anemia, inflammatory conditions, polycythemia, leukemia, and myeloproliferative disorders.
- Evaluate prognosis, response to treatment, recovery from anemia, polycythemia, bleeding disorders, and bone marrow failure.

Reference Values

Normal

Normal WBCs, RBCs, Hct, Hgb, MCV, MCH, and platelet counts.

WBCs

4500–10,500 cells/mm^3 or (4.5–10.5) $\times$ 10^9 cells/L

RBCs

Men: (4.2–5.4) $\times$ 10^6/mm^3 or (4.3–5.9) $\times$10^{12} cells/L
Women: (3.6–5.0) $\times$ 10^6/mm^3 or (3.6–5.0) $\times$ 10^{12} cells/L

HCT

Men: 42%–52% or 0.42–0.52
Women: 36%–48% or 0.36–0.48

HGB

Men: 14–17 g/dL or 140–170 g/L
Women: 12–16 g/dL or 120–160 g/L

MCV

82–98 mm^3 or 82–98 fL (femtoliters)

MCH

26–34 pg/cell or 0.40–0.53 fmol/cell (femtomoles)

MCHC

32–36 g/dL or 320–360 g/L

RETICULOCYTE COUNT

0.5%–1.5% of total RBCs or 0.005–0.015

PLATELET COUNT

(140–400) $\times$ 10^3/mm^3 or (140–400) $\times$ 10^9/L

MEAN PLATELET VOLUME

7.4–10.4 mm^3 or 7.4–10.4 fL

Critical Values

WBC: <2000 cells/mm^3 (<2.0 $\times$ 10^9 cells/L) or >30,000/mm^3 (>30 $\times$ 10^9 cells/L)

Hct: <20% (<0.20) or >60% (>0.60)
Hgb: <7.0 g/dL (<70 g/L) or >20.0 g/dL (>200 g/L)

Clinical Implications: RBCs/Erythrocytes

- The RBC count *decreases* in anemias, Hodgkin's disease, multiple myeloma, acute and chronic hemorrhage, leukemia, SLE, Addison's disease, rheumatic fever, subacute endocarditis, and chronic infection.
- The RBC count *increases* in primary and secondary polycythemias, as in erythropoietin-secreting tumors and renal disorders.
- The relative RBC count *increases* with decreased plasma volume, as in severe burns, shock, persistent vomiting, and untreated intestinal obstruction.

Interfering Factors: RBCs

- Many physiologic variants affect outcomes: posture, exercise, age, altitude, pregnancy, and many drugs.

Clinical Implications: Hematocrit

- Hct or packed cell volume (PCV) *decreases* are an indication of anemia. An Hct of 30% or less means that the patient is moderately to severely anemic.
- Hct is *decreased* in leukemia, lymphomas, Hodgkin's disease, adrenal insufficiency, hemolytic reaction, and chronic disease.

> **CLINICAL ALERT**
>
> - Hct of less than 20% can lead to cardiac failure and death.
> - An Hct greater than 60% is associated with spontaneous clotting of blood.

Interfering Factors: Hematocrit

- Physiologic variants affect Hct outcomes: age, sex, and physiologic hydremia of pregnancy.

Clinical Implications: Hemoglobin

- Hgb *decreases* in anemia, hyperthyroidism, liver and kidney diseases, cancer, various hemolytic reactions, and systemic diseases such as SLE, Hodgkin's disease, leukemia, and lymphoma.
- Hgb *increases* with hemoconcentration, burns, polycythemia, chronic obstructive pulmonary disease, and congestive heart failure (not all inclusive).

CLINICAL ALERT

- A hemoglobin value of less than 5.0 g/dL (<50 g/L) leads to heart failure and death.
- An Hgb value of greater than 20.0 g/dL (>200 g/L) results in hemoconcentration and clogging of capillaries.

Interfering Factors: Hemoglobin

- Physiologic variations affect test outcomes: high altitude, excessive fluid intake, age, pregnancy, and many drugs.

Clinical Implications: MCV, MCHC, MCH

- *Mean corpuscular volume* (MCV) changes in certain conditions. Microcytic RBCs and an MCV less than 80 mm^3 (<80 fL) occur with iron deficiency, excessive iron requirements, pyridoxine-response anemia, thalassemia, lead poisoning, and chronic inflammation. Normocytic RBCs and an MCV of 82 to 98 mm^3 (82–98 fL) occur after hemorrhage, hemolytic anemia, and anemias due to inadequate blood formation. Macrocytic RBCs, with a MCV of more than 98 mm^3 (>98 fL), occur in some anemias: vitamin B$_{12}$ deficiency, pernicious anemia, folic acid deficiency in pregnancy and inflammation, fish and tapeworm infestation, liver disease, alcohol intoxication, after total gastrectomy, and strict vegetarianism.
- *Mean corpuscular hemoglobin concentration* (MCHC) *decreases* signify that RBCs contain less hemoglobin than normal, as in iron deficiency microcytic anemias, chronic blood loss anemia, pyridoxine-responsive anemia, and thalassemia.
- *MCHC increases* indicate spherocytosis.
- *Mean corpuscular hemoglobin* (MCH) *decreases* in microcytic anemia.

Interfering Factors: MCHC

- High values may occur in newborns and infants.
- Presence of leukemia or cold agglutinins may increase levels. MCHC is falsely elevated with a high blood concentration of heparin.

Interfering Factors: MCH

- Hyperlipidemia and high heparin concentrations falsely elevate MCH values.
- WBC counts greater than 50,000/mm^3 falsely elevate Hgb and MCH values.

Clinical Implications: WBC Count

- *WBC count increases* (ie, leukocytosis) above $10 \times 10^3/mm^3$ ($>10 \times 10^9/L$), usually because of an increase in only one type of WBC (increase is given the name of the type of cell that shows the main increase, such as neutrophilia or lymphocytosis), and can occur with acute infection in which the degree of increase in WBCs depends on the severity of infection, age, resistance, and presence of leukemia, trauma, tissue necrosis or inflammation, and hemorrhage.
- *WBC count decreases* (ie, leukopenia) below $4.0 \times 10^3/mm^3$ ($<4 \times 10^9/L$) because of viral infections, hypersplenism, bone marrow depression due to drugs, irradiation, heavy metal intoxication, and primary bone marrow disorders.

> **CLINICAL ALERT**
>
> - A WBC count below $2.0 \times 10^3/mm^3$ ($<2.0 \times 10^9/L$) represents a critical value. A WBC count below $0.5 \times 10^3/mm^3$ ($<0.5 \times 10^9/L$) is extremely dangerous and is often fatal.

Interfering Factors: WBC Count

- Hourly variation, age, exercise, pain, temperature, and anesthesia affect test results.

Clinical Implications: Differential Count—Segs, Bands, Eos, Basos, Lymphs, Monos

- *Seg count increases* (ie, neutrophilia) in acute, localized, and general bacterial infections; gout and uremia; poisoning by chemicals and drugs; acute hemorrhage and hemolysis of RBCs; myelogenous leukemia; and tissue necrosis.
- *Seg count decreases* (ie, neutropenia) in acute bacterial infection (poor prognosis); viral infections; rickettsial disease; some parasitic, blood, aplastic, and pernicious anemias; aleukemic leukemia; hormonal conditions; anaphylactic shock; and severe renal disease.
- *Band neutrophils* (ie, more immature form of segmented neutrophils) increase in appendicitis, neonatal sepsis, and pharyngitis, and they provide an early indication of sepsis.
- *Abnormal ratio of segmented neutrophils to band neutrophils* may occur. Normally, 1% to 3% of neutrophils are band (stab) or immature forms that multiply quickly in acute infection. A *degenerative* shift to the left means that, in some overwhelming infections, there

is an increase in band forms with no leukocytosis (ie, leukopenia), a condition that has a poor prognosis. A *regenerative* shift to the left refers to an increase in band forms with leukocytosis, which has a good prognosis in cases of bacterial infection.

- *Eosinophil increases* (ie, eosinophilia) are caused by allergies, hay fever, asthma, parasitic diseases (especially with tissue invasion), Addison's disease, hypopituitarism, Hodgkin's disease, lymphoma, myeloproliferative disorders, polycythemia, chronic skin infection, immunodeficiency disorders, and some infectious and collagen diseases.
- *Eosinophil decreases* (ie, eosinopenia) result from increased adrenal steroid production that accompanies most conditions of bodily stress as in acute infections, congestive heart failure, infectious with neutrophilia, and disorders with neutropenia.

Interfering Factors: Neutrophils and Eosinophils

- Physiologic conditions such as stress, excitement, exercise, and obstetric labor increase neutrophil levels.
- The eosinophil count is lowest in the morning and then rises from noon until after midnight. Do repeat tests at the same time every day. Stressful states such as burns, postoperative states, and obstetric labor decrease the count. Drugs such as steroids, epinephrine, and thyroxine affect eosinophil levels.

Clinical Implications: Basophils, Monocytes, and Lymphocytes

- *Basophil count increases* (ie, basophilia) with granulocytic and basophilic leukemia, myeloid metaplasia, and Hodgkin's disease. It also increases with allergy, sinusitis, inflammation, and infection, with a positive correlation between high basophil counts and high concentrations of blood histamines.
- *Basophil count decreases* (ie, basopenia) in the acute phase of infection, in hyperthyroidism, after prolonged steroid therapy, and in hereditary basopenia. The presence of mast cells (tissue basophils), normally absent in peripheral blood, is associated with rheumatoid arthritis, asthma, anaphylactic shock, hypoadrenalism, lymphoma, mast cell leukemia, and macroglobulinemia.
- *Monocyte or monomorphonuclear monocyte count increases* (ie, monocytosis) in monocytic and other leukemias, myeloproliferative disorders, Hodgkin's disease and other lymphomas, recovering state of acute infections, lipid storage disease, some parasitic and rickettsial diseases, certain bacterial disorders as tuberculosis and subacute endocarditis, sarcoidosis, collagen disease, and chronic ulcerative colitis and sprue. Phagocytic

monocytes (ie, macrophages) are found in small numbers in many conditions.

- *Monocyte count decreases* (ie, monocytopenia) are not usually identified with specific diseases but are found in cases of HIV infection, hairy cell leukemia, prednisone treatment, and overwhelming infection.
- *Lymphocyte or monomorphonuclear lymphocyte count increases* (ie, lymphocytosis) in lymphocytic leukemia, lymphoma, infectious lymphocytosis (mainly in children), infectious mononucleosis, other viral disorders, and some bacterial diseases. The count also increases with serum sickness, drug hypersensitivity, Crohn's disease, ulcerative colitis, and hypoadrenalism.
- *Lymphocyte count decreases* (ie, lymphopenia) with chemotherapy, radiation treatment, and steroid administration. There is increased lymphocyte loss through the gastrointestinal tract and in aplastic anemia, Hodgkin's disease, other malignancies, AIDS, immune system dysfunction, and severe or debilitating diseases of any kind.

Clinical Implications: Platelets

- *Platelet count increases* (ie, thrombocytosis) in thrombocythemia ($>1000 \times 10^3/mm^3$ or $>1000 \times 10^9/L$), malignancies, polycythemia vera, primary thrombocytosis, rheumatoid arthritis, acute infections, and inflammatory disease. The count also increases with iron deficiency, posthemorrhagic anemia, heart disease, and recovery from bone marrow suppression.
- *Platelets and thrombocytes decrease* (ie, thrombocytopenia) with the toxic effects of many drugs; bone marrow lesions; during chemotherapy or irradiation, in allergic conditions; in idiopathic thrombocytopenia purpura (ITP), in pernicious, aplastic, and hemolytic anemias; with the dilution effect of blood transfusion; and in viral infections.

Interfering Factors: Platelets

- Physiologic factors include high altitudes, strenuous exercise, excitement, and premenstrual and postpartum effects.
- A partially clotted blood specimen affects the test outcome.

CLINICAL ALERT

- A critical decrease of less than $20 \times 10^3/mm^3$ ($<20 \times 10^9/L$) in platelet values is associated with a tendency to spontaneous bleeding, prolonged bleeding time, petechiae, and ecchymosis.

Procedure
- Venous plasma (5–7 mL) with EDTA additive is obtained by venipuncture, using a purple-top Vacutainer tube. The blood cannot have any clots present for the CBC to be valid.

Nursing Interventions
▸*Pretest*
- Explain the blood count purpose and procedure.
- Explain that fasting is not required.

▸*Posttest*
- Monitor venipuncture sites for signs of bleeding or infection.
- Evaluate the outcome and counsel the patient appropriately about anemia, polycythemia, risk of infection, and related blood disorders.
- Monitor patients with serious platelet defects for signs and symptoms of gastrointestinal bleeding, hemolysis, hematuria, petechiae, vaginal bleeding, epistaxis, and bleeding from gums.
- Monitor patients with prolonged, severely decreased WBC counts for signs and symptoms of infections. Often, such patients have only fever. In cases of severe granulocytopenia, give no fresh fruits or vegetables, use a minimal-bacteria or commercially sterile diet, and administer no intramuscular injections, no rectal temperatures, no rectal suppositories, and no aspirin or NSAIDs.
- Treatment for anemia can include transfusion or erythropoieses-stimulating agents, e.g., erythropoietin and darbepoetin.

Coombs' Antiglobulin Test (Direct and Indirect), Antihemoglobulin (AHG), Direct Antibody Test (DAT), Direct IgG Test

Blood

The Coombs' test shows the presence of antigen-antibody complexes. The *direct Coombs' test* detects antigen-antibody complexes on the RBC membrane and RBC sensitization. The *indirect Coombs' test* detects serum antibodies, reveals maternal anti-Rh antibodies during pregnancy, and can detect incompatibilities not found by other methods.

Indications
- Diagnose hemolytic disease of the newborn when the RBCs of the infant are sensitized.
- Diagnose acquired hemolytic anemia in adults (ie, autosensitization in vivo).

- Investigate transfusion reaction when the patient may have received incompatible blood that sensitized his or her own red blood cells.
- Detect drug-induced hemolytic anemia.

Reference Values

Normal
- *Direct Coombs' test:* No agglutination
- *Indirect Coombs' test:* No agglutination

Clinical Implications
- Direct Coombs' test is positive (1+ to 4+) in the presence of transfusion reactions; autoimmune hemolytic anemia (most cases); cephalothin therapy (75% of cases); drugs such as alpha-methyldopa (Aldomet), penicillin and insulin therapy; hemolytic disease of newborn; paroxysmal cold hemoglobinuria (PCH); and cold agglutinin syndrome.
- Direct Coombs' test is negative in nonautoimmune hemolytic anemias.
- Indirect Coombs' test is positive (1+ to 4+) in the presence of specific antibodies, usually from a previous transfusion or pregnancy, and nonspecific antibodies, as in cold agglutinants.

CLINICAL ALERT
- Antibody identification is performed when the antibody screen or direct antiglobulin tests are positive and when unexpected blood group antibodies need to be classified.
- Antibody identification tests are an important part of pretransfusion testing so that the appropriate antigen-negative blood can be transfused.

Procedure
- A 7-mL venous blood sample with added EDTA and 20 mL of clotted blood are studied.
- Notify the laboratory about the diagnosis, history of recent and past transfusions, pregnancy, and any drug therapy.

Nursing Interventions
▶*Pretest*
- Explain the purpose and procedure of the Coombs' test.

▶*Posttest*

• Interpret the test outcome and counsel the patient appropriately. Hemolytic disease of newborn can occur when mother is Rh negative and the fetus is Rh positive. The diagnosis is derived from the following information: The mother is Rh negative, the newborn is Rh positive, and the direct Coombs' test is positive (+). Newborn jaundice results from Rh incompatibility. More often, the jaundice results from an ABO incompatibility.

CREATININE, CREATININE CLEARANCE

Timed Urine with Blood

This renal function test is used to estimate the glomerular filtration rate (GFR), which measures the rate at which creatinine is cleared from the blood by the kidney, is co-ordered with virtually every quantitative urine test, and is measured along with other urinary constituents.

Indications

• Assess kidney function, primarily glomerular function.
• Follow progression of renal disease.
• Evaluate diseases associated with muscle destruction.

Reference Values

Normal

Urine creatinine: men: 14–26 mg/kg/24 hours or 124–230 μmol/kg/day; women: 11–20 mg/kg/24 hours or 97–177 μmol/kg/day

Blood creatinine: 0.8–1.2 mg/dL or 71–106 μmol/L

Creatinine clearance is measured in units of mL/min/1.73 m² or mL/s/m².

The National Kidney Disease Education Program (NKDEP) recommends that clinical laboratories report an estimated glomerular filtration rate (eGFR) when reporting serum creatinine.

$$\text{eGFR (mL/min/1.73 m}^2) = 186 \times (S_{cr})^{-1.154} \times (\text{age})^{-0.203}$$
$$\times (0.742 \text{ if female}) \times (1.210 \text{ if African American})$$

Females: 72–110 mL/min/1.73 m² or 0.69–1.06 mL/s/m²
Males: 94–140 mL/min/1.73 m² or 0.91–1.35 mL/s/m²

Clinical Implications: Creatinine Clearance
- *Decreased clearance* occurs in any condition that decreases renal blood flow and with impaired kidney function, intrinsic renal disease, nephrotic syndromes, amyloidosis, shock, hemorrhage, and congestive heart failure.
- *Increased clearance* occurs with high cardiac output, burns, and carbon monoxide poisoning.

Clinical Implications: Urine Creatinine
- *Decreased levels* occur with hyperthyroidism, amyotrophic lateral sclerosis (ALS), progressive muscular dystrophy, anemia, leukemia, and advanced renal disease.
- *Increased levels* occur with acromegaly, gigantism, hypothyroidism, and diabetes mellitus.

Interfering Factors
- Pregnancy substantially increases creatinine clearance.
- Drugs that cause increased levels include antibiotics (eg, cephalosporins, Garamycin [gentamicin], aminoglycosides), L-dopa, alpha-methyldopa (Aldomet), ascorbic acid, steroids, lithium carbonate, and cefoxitin, among others.
- Drugs that cause decreased levels include phenacetin, steroids, and thiazides, among others.
- Strenuous exercise causes increased creatinine clearance.

Procedure
- Collect urine for 24 hours in a clean container. Refrigeration is required.
- A venous blood sample (7 mL) for serum creatinine testing is obtained the morning of the day that the 24-hour collection will be completed. Use a red-top Vacutainer tube.
- Record the patient's height and weight on the urine container. This is needed to calculate the body surface area on which the creatinine clearance values are based.
- See Chapter 2 for standards of timed urine collection.

Nursing Interventions
‣Pretest
- If possible, medications (especially cephalosporins) should be stopped before the test is begun.
- Assess the patient's ability to comply and knowledge base before explaining the test purpose and procedure. Instruct the patient not to eat meat or consume tea or coffee 6 hours before the test.

- Record the patient's height and weight to determine the body surface area of the patient.

▸*Intratest*

- Encourage water intake for good hydration and tell the patient to avoid strenuous exercise.
- Accurate test results depend on proper collection, preservation, and labeling. Be sure to include the test start and completion times.

▸*Posttest*

- Instruct the patient to resume normal activity and intake of food and fluids.
- Evaluate the outcome and provide the patient with counseling, monitoring as appropriate for kidney, heart, and thyroid diseases, and possible medical treatment.

CROSSMATCH (MAJOR COMPATIBILITY TEST), TYPE AND CROSSMATCH

Blood Pretransfusion Tests

Pretransfusion

The primary purpose of the major crossmatch, or compatibility test, is to prevent a possible transfusion reaction by testing the recipient serum directly against the donor RBCs. The major crossmatch detects clinically significant antibodies in the recipient's serum that may damage or destroy the cells of the proposed donor blood. The type and screen determine the ABO and Rh (D) type (under alphabetical listing), as well as the presence or absence of unexpected antibodies from the recipient.

Indications

- Prevent transfusion reaction when transfusion may be required.

Reference Values

Normal

- *Major compatibility* between the recipient serum and donor RBCs, no cell clumping or hemolysis, and absence of agglutination when serum and cells are appropriately mixed and incubated.

The major crossmatch shows compatibility between the recipient's blood serum and the donor's blood cells; the minor crossmatch shows compatibility between the recipient's cells and the donor's serum.

- *Type and crossmatch:* Recipient ABO and Rh (D) type and compatibility, as described under alphabetical listing.

Clinical Implications
- *Incompatibility* implies that the recipient cannot receive the incompatible unit of blood because antibodies are present.

CLINICAL ALERT

- Patients receiving a series of transfusions are at risk for forming RBC antibodies.
- The probable benefits of each blood transfusion must be weighed against the risks; these include hemolytic transfusion reactions due to the infusion of incompatible blood (can be fatal), febrile or allergic reactions, transmission of infectious disease (eg, hepatitis), and stimulation of antibody production, which could complicate later transfusions or childbearing.
- The most common cause of hemolytic transfusion reaction is the administration of incompatible blood to the recipient because of faulty matching in the laboratory, improper patient identification, or incorrect labeling of donor blood.

Procedure
- Obtain a 10-mL venous blood sample using a red-top tube.

Nursing Interventions
▶Pretest
- Explain the purpose and procedure of crossmatching (to prevent a transfusion reaction).

▶Posttest
- Interpret the test outcome and counsel the patient regarding actual or potential transfusion reactions.
- See DISPLAY 3.5 for types of transfusion reactions.
- Document transfusion reaction signs and symptoms; notify the blood bank of a transfusion reaction; and carry out follow-up interventions.

DISPLAY 3.5 Types of Transfusion Reactions

Acute Hemolytic Transfusion Reaction (HTR)
- HTR is triggered by an antigen-antibody reaction and activates the complement and coagulation systems. These reactions are usually caused by ABO incompatibility because of misidentification that results in the patient receiving incompatible blood. Symptoms include fever, chills, backache, vague uneasiness, and red urine. HTR reactions are potentially fatal.

Bacterial Contamination
- Bacteria may enter the blood during phlebotomy. These microbes multiply faster in components stored at room temperature than in refrigerated components. Although rare, bacteria in blood or its components can cause a septic transfusion reaction. Symptoms include high fever, shock, hemoglobinuria, disseminated intravascular coagulation, and renal failure. Such reactions can be fatal.

Cutaneous Hypersensitivity Reactions
- Urticarial reactions are common, second in frequency only to febrile nonhemolytic reactions, and are usually characterized by erythema, hives, and itching. Allergy to some soluble substance in donor plasma is suspected.

Noncardiogenic Pulmonary Reactions (NPR)
- Transfusion-related acute lung injury (TRALI) should be considered whenever a transfusion recipient experiences acute respiratory insufficiency or x-ray films show findings consistent with pulmonary edema without evidence of cardiac failure. These are possibly reactions between the donor's leukocyte antibodies and the recipient's leukocytes. TRALI produces white blood cell aggregates that become trapped in the pulmonary microcirculation. The findings on chest x-ray films are typical of acute pulmonary edema. If subsequent transfusions are needed, leukocyte-reduced red blood cells may prevent NPR reactions.

Febrile Nonhemolytic Reaction (FNH)
- FNH reactions are defined as a temperature increase of 1°C or more. They are seldom dangerous and may be caused by an antibody-antigen reaction.

Anaphylactic Reactions
- Anaphylactic reactions occur after infusion of as little as a few milliliters of blood or plasma.
- Anaphylaxis is characterized by coughing, bronchospasm, respiratory distress, vascular instability, nausea, abdominal cramps, vomiting, diarrhea, shock, and loss of consciousness.

(display continues on page 227)

DISPLAY 3.5 (continued)

- Some reactions occur in IgA-deficient patients who have developed anti-IgA antibodies after immunization through a previous transfusion or pregnancy.
- These reactions can be prevented by giving IgA-deficient blood components.

Circulatory Overload

Rapid increases in blood volume are not tolerated well by patients with compromised cardiac or pulmonary function. Symptoms of circulatory overload include coughing, cyanosis, orthopnea, difficulty in breathing, and a rapid increase in systolic blood pressure.

CYSTOSCOPY, CYSTOURETHROSCOPY

Endoscopic Imaging, Genitourinary System

These examinations are used to view, diagnose, and treat disorders of the lower urinary tract, interior bladder, urethra, male prostatic urethra, and ureteral orifices by means of cystoscopes or cystourethroscopes. Urethroscopy is an important part of this examination because it allows visualization of the male prostate gland. Cystoscopy is the most common of all urologic diagnostic procedures.

Indications

- Evaluate unexplained hematuria (ie, gross or microscopic), infections (ie, chronic, recurrent, and resistant to treatment), and other unexplained urinary symptoms such as dysuria, frequency, urgency, incontinence, retention, hesitancy, intermittency, straining, or enuresis.
- Investigate benign and malignant bladder tumors.
- Cystoscopy may be used to perform meatotomy and to crush and retrieve small stones; other foreign bodies from the urethra, ureter, and bladder; and stents placed during previous surgeries.
- Bladder tumors can be fulgurated and strictures can be dilated through the cystoscope.

Reference Values

Normal

- Normal structure and function of the interior bladder, urethra, ureteral orifices, and male prostatic urethra.

Clinical Implications
- Abnormal findings indicate prostatic hyperplasia, prostatitis, hypertrophy, polyps, cancer of the bladder, bladder stones, urethral strictures or abnormalities, vesical neck stenosis, urinary fistulas, ureterocele, diverticula, abnormally small or large bladder capacity, or ureteral reflux (as shown on a cystogram).

Procedure

- The external genitalia are prepped with an antiseptic solution such as povidone-iodine after the patient is placed in the lithotomy position, with his or her legs in stirrups. The patient is properly gowned, padded, and draped.
- A local anesthetic jelly is instilled into the urethra 5 to 10 minutes before passage of the scope. For males, the anesthesia is retained in the urethra by a clamp applied to the end of the penis. The scope is connected to an irrigation system.
- The time frame is 25 to 50 minutes, depending on the treatment procedures: tissue biopsy, bladder stone crushing, bladder tumor fulguration, and stricture dilatation.
- The scope is connected to an irrigation system and fluid is infused into the bladder throughout the procedure. This solution also distends the bladder to allow better visualization. The infusion is stopped and the bladder is drained when it becomes filled with 300 to 500 mL of fluid. If blood or other matter is in the bladder, the fiber-optic urethroscope cannot provide as clear a view as a rigid cystoscope because it is more difficult to flush.

Nursing Interventions

▶ Pretest
- Explain the test purpose and procedure.
- Liquids may be encouraged until the time of the examination to promote urine formation if the procedure is a simple cystoscopy performed under local anesthesia. Fasting guidelines are followed when spinal or general anesthesia is planned.
- Bowel preparation and other laboratory and diagnostic tests may be necessary if extensive procedures are planned.

▶ Intratest
- An intravenous line may be started for the administration of moderate sedation/analgesia according to protocols.
- Instruct the patient to relax the abdominal muscles to lessen discomfort.
- Monitor for side effects.

▶*Posttest*
- Monitor vital signs frequently in the immediate postexamination period. The intake of fluid should be encouraged to prevent infection.
- Administer medications as ordered (ie, antibiotics and rectal opium suppositories).
- Monitor the patient's (or instruct to self-monitor) voiding patterns and bladder emptying. Evaluate and instruct the patient to watch for edema.
- Provide routine or prescribed catheter care if a retention or ureteral catheter is placed.
- Interpret test outcomes and counsel the patient appropriately.
- Administer pain medications (younger men may experience more discomfort than do older men) for bladder spasms. Instruct the patient to rest.

CLINICAL ALERT

- Report heavy bleeding or difficult urination to physician promptly. Sometimes, clots form and cause difficulty in voiding. This may occur several days after the procedure.
- Assess urinary frequency, dysuria, pink to light red-wine–colored urine, and urethral burning, which are common events after cystoscopy.
- Monitor for signs of complications. Observe for and promptly report gram-negative shock, heavy bleeding, chills, fever, increasing tachycardia, hypotension, back pain, and edema to the physician.

CYTOKINES

Blood, Urine, Feces, Amniotic Fluid, CSF, Synovial Fluid, Bronchial Secretion

Cytokines, a diverse group of proteins and peptides secreted by many cells (eg, lymphocytes, T cells, monocytes, B cells, eosinophils), respond to an immunologic challenge. Cytokines have been implicated in a number of diseases, such as asthma, interstitial cystitis, rheumatoid arthritis, septic shock, transplant rejection, pre-eclampsia, cirrhosis, and multiple sclerosis.

Indications
- Evaluate allergy, skin hypersensitivity, and asthma.
- Assess immune function and rheumatic diseases.

- Evaluate fever, inflammation, and healing.
- Use as tumor marker and marker for pre-eclampsia and abnormal placenta.

Reference Values

Normal

- Physiologic levels are normally low.
- Values depend on the cytokine being measured (eg, interleukins, interferons, or chemokines).

Clinical Implications

- Pathophysiologic levels may indicate inflammation or cancer. Increases are associated with the severity of disease.
- Elevated levels in synovial fluid, CSF, amniotic fluid, and bronchoalveolar fluid may indicate immune disorders, SLE, and other pathological or degenerative conditions.

Procedure

- Collect a venous blood sample in a tube with endotoxin-free heparin for serum analysis.
- Examine the specimen within 5 hours. Avoid a freezing-thawing cycle in storage.

Nursing Interventions

▶*Pretest*

- Explain the cytokine testing purpose and procedure and the complexities involved.

▶*Posttest*

- Interpret laboratory test outcomes.
- Explain the need for further testing for identification of the cause of chronic disease and possible treatment.

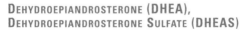

DEHYDROEPIANDROSTERONE (DHEA), DEHYDROEPIANDROSTERONE SULFATE (DHEAS)

Blood, 24-Hour Urine

Dehydroepiandrosterone (DHEA) is an adrenal androgen product and is secreted together with cortisol under the control of corticotropin (ACTH) and prolactin.

Indications

- Differential diagnosis of virilization.
- Work up for infertility, amenorrhea, or hirsutism to identify the source of excessive androgen.
- Evaluate adrenal carcinomas, which frequently secrete large amounts of DHEA.
- Monitor treatment effectiveness of congenital disease.

Reference Values

Normal

SERUM

Males: <6.0 μg/mL or <16.4 μmol/L
Females: <3.0 μg/mL or <8.2 μmol/L

URINE

Male: 0.0–3.1 mg/24 hours or 0–10.7 μmol/day
Female: 0–1.5 mg/24 hours or 0–5.2 μmol/day

Clinical Implications

- DHEAS levels are *increased* in females with hirsutism, acne, congenital adrenal hyperplasia, adrenal cortex tumors, Cushing's disease, and polycystic ovary disease.
- DHEAS levels are *decreased* in persons with adrenal insufficiency, Addison's disease, and adrenal hypoplasia.

Interfering Factors

- Recently administered radioisotopes
- Drugs such as dexamethasone, prednisone, and other cortisones decrease levels.

Procedure

- Serum (5 mL) is obtained by venipuncture, using a red-top Vacutainer tube.
- Obtain a 24-hour urine specimen, using a special container.

Nursing Interventions

▸Pretest

- Assess the patient's compliance and knowledge base before explaining the test purpose and procedure.
- Drugs that could interfere with test should not be taken for 48 hours before the test; check with the physician.

▶*Posttest*
- Resume prescribed medications.
- Evaluate the outcome and provide the patient with counseling and support as appropriate for endocrine dysfunction.

DIABETES TESTING

Whole Blood, Serum, or Plasma

Criteria for Diagnosing Diabetes Mellitus Type 1 and Type 2, Prediabetes, Glucose Tolerance Testing (GTT), Gestational Diabetes Mellitus (GDM), Long-Term Glucose Control, Related Tests that Influence Glucose Metabolism (Hormones and Antibodies that Are Not Part of Criteria)

Fasting Blood

The American Association of Clinical Endocrinologists (AACE) diagnostic criteria for diabetes mellitus (DM) include the following: (1) symptoms of DM (polyuria, polydipsia, unexplained weight loss) plus random plasma glucose concentration >200 mg/dL (>11.1 mmol/L), or (2) fasting plasma glucose concentration ≥126 mg/dL (≥7 mmol/L), or (3) a 2-hour postchallenge glucose concentration ≥200 mg/dL (≥11.1 mmol/L) during a 75-g oral glucose tolerance test. One of these three criteria listed is sufficient to establish the diagnosis of DM after being confirmed by repeat testing on a subsequent day in the absence of unequivocal hyperglycemia. (*Note:* The 2007 diagnosis and classification criteria of DM by the American Diabetes Association parallels the criteria of the AACE. Adapted from American Diabetes Association. (2008). Diagnosis and classification of diabetes mellitus. *Diabetes Care, 31*, S55–S60.)

Fasting Versus Random Plasma Glucose

Fasting Plasma Glucose (FPG), Casual or Random Plasma Glucose (PG)

Fasting (no caloric intake for at least 8 hours) blood plasma glucose is a vital component of diabetes management. The term "random/casual" is defined as any time of day without regard to time since the last meal.

Indications

- Diagnose prediabetes, also known as impaired glucose tolerance or impaired fasting glucose.
- Diagnose diabetes mellitus.

Normal

PG or FPG

- Fasting adults/children: 65–99 mg/dL or 3.6–5.5 mmol/L
- Impaired fasting glucose/prediabetes mellitus: 100–125 mg/dL or 5.6–6.9 mmol/L
- Diabetes mellitus: $\geq$126 mg/dL or $\geq$7.0 mmol/L
- Fasting neonates: 30–60 mg/dL or 1.7–3.3 mmol/L

Clinical Implications

- Elevated blood glucose levels (hyperglycemia) occur in diabetes mellitus (a fasting glucose level >126 mg/dL [>7.0 mmol/L]) or a 2-hour postprandial load (75-g) plasma glucose >200 mg/dL (>11.1 mmol/L) during an oral GTT.
- Other conditions that produce elevated blood plasma glucose levels include Cushing's disease; acute emotional or physical stress situations; pheochromocytoma, acromegaly, and gigantism; pituitary adenoma; hemochromatosis; pancreatitis, neoplasms of the pancreas; glucagonoma; advanced liver disease; chronic renal disease; vitamin B deficiency, Wernicke's encephalopathy; and pregnancy (may signal potential for onset of diabetes later in life).
- Decreased blood plasma glucose (hypoglycemia) occurs in pancreatic islet cell carcinoma (insulinomas); extrapancreatic stomach tumors (carcinoma); Addison's disease; carcinoma of the adrenal gland; hypopituitarism, hypothyroidism, adrenocorticotropic hormone (ACTH) deficiency; starvation, malabsorption; liver damage; premature infant or infant delivered to a mother with diabetes; enzyme-deficiency disease (eg, galactosemia, inherited maple syrup urine disease, von Gierke's disease); insulin overdose; reactive hypoglycemia, including alimentary hyperinsulinism, prediabetes, and endocrine deficiency; and postprandial hypoglycemia occurring after GI surgery. Such hypoglycemia is described with hereditary fructose intolerance, galactosemia, and leucine sensitivity.

Interfering Factors

- Elevate glucose: steroids, diuretics, and other drugs; pregnancy (a slight blood glucose elevation normally occurs); surgical procedures and anesthesia; obesity or sedentary lifestyle; parenteral glucose administration (eg, from total parenteral nutrition); IV glucose (recent or current); and heavy smoking.

- Decrease glucose: hematocrit >55%; prolonged contact with red blood cells, intense exercise; toxic doses of aspirin, salicylates, and acetaminophen; and other drugs, including ethanol, quinine, and haloperidol.

Procedure

- Obtain serum (1.0 mL) by venipuncture, using a SST or red-top tube. A gray-topped tube, which contains sodium fluoride, is acceptable for 24 hours without separation.
- Place in a biohazard bag and transport to clinical laboratory for analysis.

Nursing Interventions

▸*Pretest*

- Explain the test purpose and blood-drawing procedure.
- Tell the patient that the test requires at least an overnight fast (8–10 hours); water is permitted. Instruct the patient to defer insulin or oral hypoglycemic agents until after blood is drawn, unless specifically instructed to do otherwise.

▸*Posttest*

- Tell the patient that he or she may eat and drink after the blood is drawn.
- Interpret test results and monitor appropriately for hyperglycemia and hypoglycemia. Counsel regarding necessary lifestyle changes (eg, diet, exercise, glucose monitoring, medication).
- Advise the patient to make sure the doctor inspects his or her feet as part of every visit.
- Inform the patient of benefits of using a team approach to help make decisions about care. The team may include a doctor, a nurse diabetes educator, a dietician, a pharmacist, and the patient's family.
- Advise the patient of other healthcare professionals who may assist with care, including an eye specialist (ophthalmologist or optometrist), an exercise physiologist, a podiatrist, and a psychologist.
- Counsel the patient to follow the most healthful lifestyle possible.
- Place persons with glucose levels >200 mg/dL (>11.1 mmol/L) on a strict intake and output program.

CLINICAL ALERT

- If a person with known or suspected diabetes experiences headaches, irritability, dizziness, weakness, fainting, or impaired cognition, a blood glucose test or fingerstick test must be done before giving insulin. If a blood glucose level cannot be obtained and one is uncertain regarding the situation, glucose may be given in the form of orange juice, sugar-containing soda, or candy (eg, Life Savers or jelly beans). Make certain the person is sufficiently conscious to manage eating or swallowing. In the acute care setting, IV glucose may be administered in the event of severe hypoglycemia. A glucose gel is also commercially available and may be rubbed on the inside of the mouth by another person if the person with diabetes is unable to swallow or to respond properly. Instruct persons prone to hypoglycemia to carry sugar-type items with them and to wear a necklace or bracelet that identifies the person as diabetic.

- When blood glucose values are >300 mg/dL (>16.6 mmol/L), urine output increases, as does the risk for dehydration.

- Panic/critical values for fasting blood glucose: <40 mg/dL (<2.22 mmol/L) may cause brain damage; >450 mg/dL (>25 mmol/L) may cause coma.

- Diabetes is a "disease of the moment." Persons living with diabetes are continually affected by fluctuations in blood glucose levels and must learn to manage and adapt their lifestyles within this framework. For some, adaptation is relatively straightforward; for others, especially those identified as being "brittle," lifestyle changes and management are more complicated and these patients require constant vigilance, attention, encouragement, and support. Each person with diabetes may experience certain symptoms in his or her own unique way and in a unique pattern.

- Infants with tremors, convulsions, or respiratory distress should have glucose testing done STAT, particularly in the presence of maternal diabetes or with hemolytic disease of the newborn.

- Newborns who are too small or too large for gestational age should have glucose levels measured on the first day of life.

- Diseases related to neonatal hypoglycemia include glycogen storage diseases, galactosemia, hereditary fructose intolerance, ketogenic hypoglycemia of infancy, and carnitine deficiency (Reye's syndrome).

Fasting Blood

Use of Hormones and Antibodies

These tests are performed only when specially ordered and in research and complex diagnostic situations.

Insulin Indications
• Evaluation of fasting hypoglycemia.
• Assessment of pancreatic beta-cell activity.
• Investigation of insulin resistance.

Reference Values

Normal: Adult fasting: <29 μIU/mL or <202 pmol/L
Abnormal: Increase in insulinoma and obesity

C-Peptide Indications
• Evaluation of pancreatic beta-cell activity, insulin-secreting neoplasms versus factitious hypoglycemia
• Monitor postpancreatectomy and islet cell transplants
• Perform test in conjunction with FPG, FBG, or GTT

Reference Values

Normal: Fasting: 0.9–4.3 ng/mL or 297–1419 pmol/L
Abnormal: Insulin is increased in insulin-secreting neoplasms; decrease reflects pancreatic loss

Glucagon Indications
• Diagnosis of pancreatic alpha-2 cell tumors

Reference Values

Normal: Adults: 40–130 pg/mL or ng/L
Abnormal: Increased glucagonomas (pancreatic alpha-2 cell tumors) >900 pg/mL or ng/L

Insulin Antibodies Indications
• Evaluation of type 1 diabetes, which is characterized by circulating autoantibodies against a variety of islet cell antigens, including glutamic acid decarboxylase (GAD), tyrosine phosphatase (IA_2), and insulin.

- The autoimmune destruction of the insulin-producing pancreatic beta cells is thought to be the primary cause of type 1 diabetes.
- The presence of these autoantibodies provides early evidence of autoimmune disease activity, and their measurement can be useful in assisting the physician with the prediction, diagnosis, and management of patients with diabetes.
- Identify state of insulin resistance and determine most appropriate treatment of certain diabetic patients.

Reference Values

Normal: Negative, <3% binding of labeled human, beef, or pork insulin by patient's serum

Abnormal: Increase in insulin resistance and allergies to insulin.

Blood Timed

Glucose Tolerance Test (GTT); Oral Glucose Tolerance Test (OGTT)

This is a timed test for glucose tolerance. In a healthy individual, the insulin response to a large oral glucose dose is almost immediate. It peaks in 30 to 60 minutes and returns to normal levels within 3 hours when sufficient insulin is present to metabolize the glucose ingested at the beginning of the test. The test should be performed according to World Health Organization (WHO) guidelines, using a glucose load containing the equivalent of 75 g of anhydrous glucose dissolved in water or another solution.

Indications

- If fasting and postload glucose tests give borderline results for diabetes, the GTT can support or rule out a diagnosis of diabetes mellitus.
- The GTT/OGTT test should be ordered when there is sugar in the urine or when the fasting blood sugar level is significantly elevated. The GTT/OGTT should *not* be used as a screening test for children or nonpregnant women.

Reference Values

Normal

(All blood values must be within normal limits to be considered normal.)

- *Fasting plasma glucose (PG):*
  Adults: Normal: 65–99 mg/dL or 3.6–5.5 mmol/L
- *120-minute (2-hour) PG after 75-g glucose load:*
  Adults: Normal: <140 mg/dL or <7.8 mmol/L
  > Impaired glucose tolerance/prediabetes mellitus: 140–199 mg/dL
  > or 7.8–11.0 mmol/L
  > Diabetes mellitus: >200 mg/dL or >11.1 mmol/L

Interfering Factors

- Smoking increases glucose levels.
- Weight reduction before testing can diminish carbohydrate tolerance and suggest "false diabetes."
- Glucose levels normally tend to increase with aging.
- Prolonged oral contraceptive use causes significantly higher glucose levels in the second hour or in later blood specimens.
- Infectious diseases, illnesses, and operative procedures affect glucose tolerance. Two weeks of recovery should be allowed before performing the test.
- Certain drugs impair glucose tolerance levels, including, but not limited to, the following: insulin; oral hypoglycemic agents, large doses of salicylates or anti-inflammatories, thiazide diuretics, oral contraceptives, corticosteroids, estrogens, heparin, nicotinic acid, phenothiazines, lithium, and metyrapone (Metopirone [metyrapone]). If possible, these drugs should be discontinued for at least 3 days before testing. Check with the clinician for specific orders. Prolonged bed rest influences glucose tolerance results. If possible, the patient should be ambulatory. A GTT in a hospitalized patient has limited value.

Procedure

This is a timed test for glucose tolerance. Blood plasma glucose is tested after a glucose load (75 g). There is a peak at 30 to 60 minutes and a return to normal at 3 hours.

- Have the patient eat a diet of >150 g of carbohydrates for 3 days before the test.
- If ordered, discontinue the following drugs 3 days before the test because these may influence test results: hormones, oral contraceptives and steroids, salicylates, anti-inflammatory drugs, diuretic agents, hypoglycemic agents, antihypertensive drugs, and anticonvulsants.
- Insulin and oral hypoglycemic agents should be withheld until the test is completed.

- The patient's weight should be recorded. Pediatric doses of glucose are based on body weight, calculated as 1.75 g/kg, and are not to exceed a total of 75 g.
- Pregnant women receive 75 or 100 g of glucose (AACE criteria based on 75-g OGTT).
- Nonpregnant adults receive 75 g of glucose.
- A 5-mL fasting (12–16 hours) sample of venous blood is drawn. Gray-topped tubes are used. After the blood is drawn, the patient drinks all of a specially formulated glucose solution within a 5-minute time frame.
- Blood samples are obtained at 1 hour and 2 hours following 75-g glucose administration, and at 1, 2, and 3 hours after 100-g glucose ingestion. Specimens taken 4 hours after ingestion may be significant for detecting hypoglycemia.
- Tolerance tests can also be performed for pentose, lactose, galactose, and D-xylose.
- The GTT is not indicated in the following situations: persistent fasting hyperglycemia >126 mg/dL or >7.0 mmol/L, persistent fasting normal plasma glucose, overt diabetes mellitus, and persistent 2-hour plasma glucose >200 mg/dL or >11.1 mmol/L.

Clinical Implications

- The presence of abnormal GTT values (decreased tolerance to glucose) is based on the International Classification for Diabetes Mellitus and the following glucose intolerance categories: at least two GTT values must be abnormal for a diagnosis of diabetes mellitus to be validated; in cases of overt diabetes, no insulin is secreted and abnormally high glucose levels persist throughout the test; and glucose values that are above normal values but fall below the diagnostic criteria for diabetes or impaired glucose tolerance (IGT) should be considered nondiagnostic.
- See TABLE 3.2 for an interpretation of oral glucose tolerance levels.
- Decreased glucose tolerance occurs with high glucose values in the following conditions: diabetes mellitus; postgastrectomy; hyperthyroidism; excess glucose ingestion; hyperlipidemia types II, IV, and V; hemochromatosis; Cushing's disease (steroid effect); CNS lesions; pheochromocytoma.
- Decreased glucose tolerance with hypoglycemia can be found in persons with von Gierke's disease, severe liver damage, or increased epinephrine levels.
- Increased glucose tolerance with a flat curve (ie, glucose level does not increase, but it may decrease to hypoglycemic levels)

TABLE 3.2 ORAL GLUCOSE TOLERANCE TEST LEVELS

2-HOUR OGTT (75-g LOAD)	DIAGNOSIS
<140 mg/dL (7.8 mmol/L)	Normal
140–199 mg/dL (7.8–11 mmol/L)	Prediabetes (impaired glucose tolerance)
≥200 mg/dL (≥11.1 mmol/L)	Diabetes

DIAGNOSTIC CRITERIA FOR GESTATIONAL DIABETES	
2-HOUR OGTT (75-g LOAD)	
STATE AT PLASMA GLUCOSE MEASUREMENT	PLASMA GLUCOSE CONCENTRATION*
Fasting	>95 mg/dL (>5.3 mmol/L)
1-Hour post–glucose administration	>180 mg/dL (>10 mmol/L)
2-Hour post–glucose adminstration	>155 mg/dL (>8.6 mmol/L)
3-HOUR OGTT (100-g LOAD)	
STATE AT PLASMA GLUCOSE MEASUREMENT	PLASMA GLUCOSE CONCENTRATION*
Fasting	>95 mg/dL (>5.3 mmol/L)
1-Hour post–glucose administration	>180 mg/dL (>10 mmol/L)
2-Hour post–glucose adminstration	>155 mg/dL (>8.6 mmol/L)
3-Hour post–glucose adminstration	>140 mg/dL (>7.8 mmol/L)

*Two or more of these criteria must be met or exceeded for positive diagnosis.

occurs in the following conditions: pancreatic islet cell hyperplasia or tumor; poor intestinal absorption caused by diseases such as sprue, celiac disease, or Whipple's disease; hypoparathyroidism; Addison's disease; liver disease; hypopituitarism; and hypothyroidism.

Nursing Interventions
▸Pretest
- Explain the test purpose and procedure. A written reminder may be helpful.
- Instruct the patient to eat a diet high in carbohydrates (150 g) for 3 days preceding the test and to abstain from alcohol.
- Instruct the patient to fast for at least 12 hours but not more than 16 hours before the test. Only water may be ingested during fasting time and test time.
- Encourage patients to rest or walk quietly during the test period. They may feel weak, faint, or nauseated during the test. Vigorous exercise alters glucose values and should be avoided during testing.
- Collect blood specimens at prescribed times and record exact times of collection. Urine glucose testing is no longer recommended.

◆*Posttest*
- Have the patient resume a normal diet and activities at the end of the test. Encourage complex carbohydrates and protein, if permitted.
- Administer prescribed insulin or oral hypoglycemic agents when the test is done. Arrange for the patient to eat within a short time (30 minutes) after these medications are taken.
- Interpret test results and counsel the patient appropriately.

Blood

Gestational Diabetes Mellitus (GDM); O'Sullivan Test (1-Hour Gestational Diabetes Mellitus Screen)

Glucose intolerance *during* pregnancy (gestational diabetes mellitus [GDM]) is associated with an increase in perinatal morbidity and mortality, especially in women who are older than 25 years, overweight, or hypertensive. Additionally, more than one half of all pregnant women with an abnormal GTT do not have any of the same risk factors. It is therefore recommended that all pregnant women be screened for gestational diabetes.

Indications
- The O'Sullivan test, based on an OGTT, is performed to detect gestational diabetes and screen nonsymptomatic pregnant women. During pregnancy, abnormal carbohydrate metabolism is evaluated by screening all pregnant women at their first prenatal visit and then again at 24 to 28 weeks' gestation.
- Women with a family history of diabetes or previous gestational diabetes should undergo the O'Sullivan test at 15 to 19 weeks' gestation and again at 24 to 28 weeks' gestation.

Reference Values

O'Sullivan (Gestational Diabetes Screen):

1 hour after 50-g glucose load:
Normal: <140 mg/dL (<7.8 mmol/L)
Abnormal: ≥140 mg/dL (≥7.8 mmol/L)
Note: Abnormal O'Sullivan test (Gestational Diabetes Screen) should be followed with a 3-hour OGTT (100-g dose) or a 2-hour OGTT (75-g dose; AACE guidelines)
Refer to TABLE 3.2 for diagnostic criteria for gestational diabetes mellitus.

Clinical Implications

- Abnormal GDM test result after 75-g glucose load and 100-g glucose load reveal glucose intolerance.
- A positive result in a pregnant woman means she is at much greater risk (7 times) for having GDM.
- GDM is any degree of glucose intolerance with onset during pregnancy or first recognized during pregnancy.
- A diagnosis of GDM is based on the following blood glucose results (more than two tests must be met and exceeded): fasting, >95 mg/dL (>5.3 mmol/L); 1 hour, >180 mg/dL (>10.0 mmol/L); 2 hours, >155 mg/dL (>8.6 mmol/L); and 3 hours, >140 mg/dL (>7.8 mmol/L).
- All pregnant women should be tested for gestational diabetes with a 50-g dose of glucose at 24 to 28 weeks' gestation. Pregnant women with abnormal GTT are at risk for pre-eclampsia, eclampsia, and delivery of a large infant.
- If abnormal results occur during pregnancy, repeat GTT at the first postpartum visit.
- During labor, maintain maternal glucose levels at 80 to 100 mg/dL (4.4–5.5 mmol/L); beware of markedly increased insulin sensitivity in the immediate postpartum period.

Procedure

- Draw a 5-mL venous blood sample (sodium fluoride [NaF]) after an 8- to 14-hour fast, at least 3 days of unrestricted diet and activity, and again after glucose load.
- An oral glucose load is administered and blood is examined after 1 hour for glucose levels.
- Measure plasma or serum glucose 2 and 3 hours after GTT (glucose challenge).

Nursing Interventions
▸Pretest

- Explain the test's purpose (to evaluate abnormal carbohydrate metabolism and predict diabetes in later life) and procedure. Fasting may be required. Obtain a pertinent history of diabetes and record any signs or symptoms of diabetes.
- Instruct the woman about obtaining a urine sample for glucose testing to check before drinking the glucose load. Positive urine glucose level should be checked with the physician before administering the glucose load. Those with glycosuria >250 mg/dL (>13.8 mmol/L) must have a blood glucose test before O'Sullivan or GDM testing.
- Give the patient 75–100 g of glucose beverage (150 mL dissolved in water, or Trutol or Orange DEX).

- Explain to the patient that no eating, drinking, smoking, or gum chewing is allowed during the test. The patient should not leave the office. The patient may void if necessary.
- After 1 hour, draw one NaF tube (5-mL venous blood), using standard venipuncture technique. If a 75-g glucose load is given, collect a 2-hour specimen. If a 100-g glucose load is given, obtain 2- and 3-hour specimens.

▸*Posttest*
- Normal activities, eating, and drinking may be resumed.
- Test results are interpreted.
- Six weeks after delivery, the patient should be retested and reclassified. In most cases, glucose will return to normal levels.

Blood

Glycosylated Hemoglobin (HbA$_{1c}$); Glycohemoglobin (G-Hb); Glycated Hemoglobin (GhB); Diabetic Control Index; Glycated Serum Protein (GSP), Fructosamine

Glycohemoglobin is blood glucose bound to hemoglobin. In the presence of hyperglycemia, an increase in glycohemoglobin causes an increase in HbA$_{1c}$. If the glucose concentration increases because of insulin deficiency, then glycosylation is irreversible. Glycosylated hemoglobin values reflect average blood sugar levels for the 2- to 3-month period before the test.

Reference Values

Normal
- G-Hb: 4.0%–7.0% of total hemoglobin or 0.04–0.07
- HbA$_{1c}$: 4.0%–6.7% of total hemoglobin or 0.04–0.067
- HbA$_1$ always 2.0%–4.0% higher than HbA$_{1c}$ or 0.02–0.04

Values vary slightly by method and laboratory. Be certain of the specific test used.
Note: The following equation can be used to calculate an estimated average glucose (eAG) for an HbA1c level:

$$eAG = 28.7 \times HbA1c - 46.7$$

Critical Values
- G-Hb: >8.6% or >0.086
- HbA$_{1c}$: >8.1% or >0.081 (corresponds with glucose >200 mg/dL or >11.1 mmol/L)

Clinical Implications
- Values are frequently increased in persons with poorly controlled or newly diagnosed diabetes.
- With optimal control, the HbA_{1c} moves toward normal levels.

Procedure
- Obtain a 5-mL venous blood sample with EDTA purple-topped anticoagulant additive. Serum may not be used. A blood sample may be drawn at any time.

Nursing Interventions

▶*Pretest*
- Explain purpose and procedure.
- Fasting is not required.

▶*Posttest*
- Interpret test outcome, stressing a target value of <7% for HbA_{1c}.
- Counsel patient as necessary.

D-DIMER
D-Dimers are produced by the action of plasmin on cross-linked fibrin. This test is used when there is a suspicion of hypercoagulability.

Indications
- Diagnose disseminated intravascular coagulation (DIC).
- Analyze the spinal fluid to differentiate cases of subarachnoid hemorrhage (SAH) from a traumatic tap.
- Screen for deep vein thrombosis (DVT).
- Investigate the suspicion of pulmonary embolism (PE).

Reference Values

Normal
- Quantitative: <250 μg/L or <1.37 nmol/L
- Qualitative: no D-dimer fragments present

Procedure
- Collect a 5-mL venous blood sample into a tube containing sodium citrate and aprotinin.
- Place the specimen in a biohazard bag and take to lab immediately.

Clinical Implications

- *Increased* D-Dimer values are associated with DIC, DVT, PE, pre-eclampsia, myocardial infarction, malignancy, inflammation, and severe infection.
- The presence of D-dimer confirms that both thrombin generation and plasmin generation have occurred.

Interfering Factors

- False-positive tests are obtained with high titers of rheumatoid factor, inflammation, and liver disease.
- False-positive D-dimer levels increase as the tumor marker CA-125 for ovarian cancer increases.
- The D-dimer test is positive in patients after surgery or trauma.
- False-positive results found in estrogen therapy, normal pregnancy.

Nursing Interventions

◗Pretest

- Explain test purpose and procedure.
- See Chapter 1 guidelines for safe, effective, informed *pretest* care.

◗Posttest

- Interpret test outcome and monitor appropriately for DIC or thrombin.

DNA TESTING AND FINGERPRINTING

Tissue, Blood, Body Fluids (Urine, Amniotic, Seminal), Plucked Hair, Fingernail Scrapings, Fingerprints from Handled Objects

DNA testing is used during criminal investigations and tracking of parentage by means of laboratory techniques called *restriction fragment length polymorphism* (RFLP) and polymerase chain reaction (PCR). DNA typing and fingerprinting provide the code for individual genetic characteristics through a sequence or "blueprint" that is unique to each person.

CLINICAL ALERT

- The traditional DNA test provides a 99.99% exclusion probability.
- Bones and teeth are the most stable sources of postmortem DNA.

Indications

- Establish identity (ie, military and disaster casualties) by evaluating DNA samples from several sources (shed hair and fingernails contain mitochondrial DNA) to determine matching patterns (similar to comparing codes).
- Determine parentage (eg, infant abduction, possible switch at birth).
- Part of criminal investigation (eg, murder, sexual abuse, rape).
- Use in postconviction cases for the purpose of exoneration.
- Use for confirmation that a urine sample for drug testing is truly from the person who gave the sample.

Reference Values

Normal

- Each person has a unique DNA profile.

Clinical Implications

- Abnormal; no matching patterns.
- In parentage studies, identity is confirmed when there are matching patterns in certain areas of the autoradiographs (ie, autorads).
- In criminal cases, matching DNA characteristics associated with samples from the victim and the suspect may establish presence at the scene of a crime.

Interfering Factors

- Insufficient amounts of DNA (<0.1 g), sample deterioration, and lack of a material database to conduct effective sample comparison.

Procedure

- DNA can be extracted from dried whole blood or from any cellularly dense tissue that contains nucleated cells (eg, skin, saliva, hair shafts, urine, and semen).
- The DNA samples are collected and stored using great care with pristine equipment to prevent contamination and preserve specimens, which may have crucial legal implications.
- Collect venous blood samples in a yellow-top (ACD) tube or lavender-top (EDTA) tube. Prepared blood is stored and shipped at 4°C. Do *not* freeze blood.
- Between 0.1 and 1 g of tissue is obtained and put in a plastic freezing bag. Freeze the tissue sample at −70°C. Keep it frozen until it is shipped to a laboratory. Store tissue at −70°C or in dry ice.
- Samples of DNA can be stored for an indefinite period.

- The DNA samples are processed until DNA fragments can be visually represented on x-ray film. These films are called autorads or autoradiographs; the fragments somewhat resemble bar codes.
- The autorads are compared for matching or nonmatching characteristics among several samples. If a match between two or more different autorads is found, there exists a high probability that the different samples came from the same source or person.

Nursing Interventions

Pretest

- Explain the DNA test purpose and procedure with the concerned individual and family members, being mindful of privacy and confidentiality.
- Check to be sure that transfusions were given 90 days before DNA testing.

CLINICAL ALERT

- Communicate results in confidence.
- DNA specimen collection, identification, packaging, and storage are extremely important. In forensic studies, the issue of chain-of-custody arises.

Posttest

- Counsel appropriate persons about the meaning of test outcomes (eg, no match, low probability that samples did not come from the same person as the DNA source).

DUCTAL LAVAGE, GAIL INDEX OF BREAST CANCER

Breast, Nipple, Milk Ducts

Ductal lavage involves collecting cells from the nipple where most breast cancers begin. If a cytologic study shows abnormal cells, this is an indication of increased risk of breast cancer. A statistical model computes a Gail Index score that indicates risk of developing breast cancer in the next 5 years. The Gail Index score is based on risk factors (eg, age at menarche, age at first live birth, number of previous biopsies, and number of first-degree relatives with breast cancer).

Indications
- Assess breast cancer risk.
- Provide ongoing surveillance

Reference Values

Normal
- No atypical or abnormal cells.
- Gail Index score of <1.7.

Clinical Implications
- Atypical hyperplasia.
- Proliferative breast disease.
- Increased risk of breast cancer.

Procedure
- A local anesthetic cream is applied to the nipple area using a special kit. A suction device draws tiny amounts of fluid droplets from the milk ducts to the nipple surface. These droplets locate the milk ducts' natural opening on the surface of the nipple.
- A very fine (hair-thin) catheter is inserted into the periareolar duct, local anesthetic is administered into the duct, and a saline wash is used to separate the cells.
- The specimen is placed in a special collection vial and sent for examination in a biohazard bag.

Nursing Interventions
▸*Pretest*
- Explain the lavage purpose, procedure, benefits, and risks.
- Describe sensations that might be felt: feelings of fullness, pinching and gentle tugging on the breast, and discomfort but not usually pain.

▸*Posttest*
- Interpret test results and counsel sensitively about follow-up, close monitoring, and preventive drug treatment (eg, tamoxifen and newer antibreast cancer medications).
- Interpret test outcomes in conjunction with mammogram and physical examination findings.

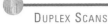

Duplex Scans

Vascular Ultrasound, Doppler Imaging, Segmental Pressures in Extremities

Cerebrovascular, Carotid and Vertebral Artery Scans, Peripheral Scans, Lower Extremity Venous (LEV) Scans, Lower Extremity Arterial (LEA) Scans, Ankle-Brachial Index (ABI), Upper Extremity Venous (UEV), Upper Extremity Arterial (UEA)

These noninvasive Doppler ultrasound procedures provide anatomic and hemodynamic information about the major blood vessels supplying the brain and extremities as indications of blood flow and thromboses. As an adjunct to duplex scans, blood pressures are recorded throughout the extremities. The ankle-brachial index (ABI) is calculated by dividing the ankle pressure (mm Hg) by the brachial pressure (mm Hg).

Indications
- *Carotid:* Evaluate symptoms of transient ischemia, headache, dizziness, hemiparesis, paresthesia, speech and visual disturbances; screen before major cardiovascular surgery and as a follow-up.
- *Extremity:* Evaluate chronic limb swelling, stasis pigmentation, and limb pain (pressures confirm a vascular cause for ischemic rest pain and claudication).
- *Veins:* "Map" veins to be used for grafts (eg, dialysis access).

Reference Values

Normal
- Vascular arterial anatomy of the common carotid artery and internal and external carotids shows no evidence of stenosis or occlusion, triphasic blood flow patterns in these major arteries, no thrombi or occlusive disease, and no plaques.
- Normal venous anatomy is found, demonstrating spontaneous blood flow, phasic flow (ie, flow patterns that respond to the patient's respiratory changes), augmentation (ie, a rush of venous flow superior to compression of the vein), competence of valves, and nonpulsatile flow. Segmental blood pressure is within normal range.
- ABI of more than 1.0 is considered normal when a multiphasic waveform is present.

- No difference between the right and left brachial pressures.
- The gradual pressure drop, as measured from upper thigh or arm to ankle or wrist, does not exceed 20 mm Hg (2.7 kPa) between any two segments.

Clinical Implications

- Evidence of plaques, stenosis, occlusion, dissection, aneurysm, carotid body tumor, and arteritis.
- Venous thrombosis, obstruction, and incompetent valves.
- Asymmetry of more than 10 mm Hg (1.3 kPa) in brachial pressures indicates arterial disease.
- An ABI of less than 1.0 indicates disease. The lower the numeric value for this index, the more severe the disease may be (eg, an ABI of <0.25 is associated with impending tissue loss).
- A difference of 20 mm Hg (2.7 kPa) or more between successive segments on the same extremity and opposite sides may suggest obstructive vascular disease or occlusion.

Interfering Factors

- Cardiac arrhythmias and disease may cause changes in hemodynamic patterns.
- Extreme tortuosity of the blood vessels degrades hemodynamic information.
- Marked obesity may adversely affect examination findings; pressures may be unobtainable.

Procedure

Carotid Examination

- In most cases, the patient is asked to lie on an examination table with the neck slightly extended and the head turned to one side. A coupling agent, usually a gel, is applied to the neck. A handheld transducer is gently moved up and down the neck while images of appropriate blood vessels are made.
- During Doppler evaluation, an audible signal representing blood flow can be heard. The right and left carotid vessels are examined.
- The examination time is approximately 30 to 60 minutes.

Extremity Examination

- The patient is asked to lie on the examination table with the arm or leg turned out slightly and the knee or elbow partially bent. A handheld transducer is moved up and down the limb over blood vessels from the shoulder (upper extremity) or pelvic girdle (lower extremity) to the distal extremity.

- Brief compression of the veins is performed at selected intervals to evaluate vessel pathology.
- Both limbs are examined for comparison.
- The examination time is approximately 30 to 60 minutes.

Obtaining the Brachial-Ankle Index and Pressures

- The patient is asked to lie on a table with the extremity extended.
- Pneumatic cuffs (usually four) are placed at intervals along the extremity.
- A flow-sensing device (often a continuous-wave Doppler device) is placed distal to a cuff. The cuff is inflated (often automatically) to suprasystolic values and slowly deflated until flow resumes. The pressure at which flow resumes is recorded.
- This technique is repeated, distal to each cuff, until the entire extremity has been evaluated. Brachial pressures are measured as well.
- Both extremities are examined. Total examination time (for pressures only) is generally less than 15 minutes.

Nursing Interventions

▶ Pretest

- Explain the examination purpose and procedure.
- Explain that a coupling gel will be applied to skin. Although gel does not stain, advise the patient to avoid wearing nonwashable clothing.
- Advise the patient to remove necklaces and earrings before the examination for safekeeping.
- Instruct the patient to refrain from smoking or consuming caffeine for at least 2 hours before the study.

▶ Posttest

- Remove or instruct the patient to remove any residual gel from the skin.
- Evaluate the outcome and provide the patient with support and counseling about blood flow abnormalities and possible treatment (medical or surgical).

D-XYLOSE ABSORPTION

Timed Urine and Blood

The D-xylose test is used to measure intestinal absorption. D-xylose, a pentose sugar, not normally present in the blood or urine, is easily absorbed by the intestine. When D-xylose is administered orally, blood and urine levels are checked for absorption rates. It is a reliable index of the functional integrity of the jejunum in pediatric patients.

Indications
- Evaluate causes of chronic weight loss.
- Diagnose malabsorption syndrome.

Reference Values

Normal

Blood
- 1-hour absorption of 5-g dose—infants: >15 mg/dL or >1.0 mmol/L
- 1-hour absorption of 5-g dose—children: >20 mg/dL or >1.3 mmol/L
- 2-hour absorption of 5-g dose—adults: >20 mg/dL or >1.3 mmol/L
- 2-hour absorption of 25-g dose—adults: >25 mg/dL or >1.6 mmol/L

Urine Xylose 5-Hour Reference Range for 25-g Dose
- Children: 16%–33% of 5-g dose
- Adults: >16% of 5-g dose or >4.0 g of max (0.5 g/kg to a maximum of 25 g)
- Adults 65 years and older: >14% of dose or >3.5 g of maximum

Procedure
- Have the patient refrain from foods containing pentose for 24 hours before test.
- Do not allow food or liquids by mouth for at least 8 hours before the start of the test. Pediatric patients should fast only 4 hours.
- Have the patient void at the beginning of the test. Discard this urine.
- Administer the oral dose of D-xylose after it has been dissolved in 100 mL of water. Adult dosage is 25 g; for children younger than 12 years, a 5-g oral dose is recommended. For adults, additional water up to 250 mL should be taken at this time and another 250 mL in 1 hour. Record the time of administration. Give no further fluids (except water) or food until the test is completed.
- Draw a 3-mL sample of venous blood at 60 and 120 minutes following D-xylose ingestion.

- Have the patient void 5 hours from the start of the test. Save all urine voided during the test.

Clinical Implications

- Urine D-xylose is *decreased* in intestinal malabsorption (malabsorption syndrome), impaired renal function, small-bowel ischemia, Whipple's disease, viral gastroenteritis, and bacterial overgrowth in small intestine.
- The D-xylose test gives a *normal* result in malabsorption due to pancreatic insufficiency, postgastrectomy, and malnutrition.

Interfering Factors

- Nonfasting state, treatment with hyperalimentation therapy.
- Foods rich in pentose (fruits and preserves).
- Vomiting of the xylose test meal (25-g dose may cause gastrointestinal distress).
- Impaired renal function—use serum test only.

Nursing Interventions

▸Pretest

- Explain purpose and procedure of the test and the urine collection process. The entire 5-hour specimen must be collected.
- The patient must fast at least 8 hours before the start of the test; children younger than 9 years should fast for only 4 hours.
- Water may be taken at any time.
- Weigh the patient to determine the proper dose of D-xylose.

▸Posttest

- Normal food, fluids, and activities can be resumed.
- See Chapter 1 guidelines for safe, effective, informed *posttest* care.

ELECTROCARDIOGRAM (EKG OR ECG), SIGNAL-AVERAGED ELECTROCARDIOGRAM (SAE), VECTORCARDIOGRAM

Special Cardiac Studies

The SAE is an averaged ECG that adds hundreds of an individual's ECGs together to detect small, late potentials that are indicative of arrhythmias. The vectorcardiogram is an ECG that records a three-dimensional display of the heart's electrical activity, whereas the ECG records in a single plane.

Indications
- Identify heart rhythm disturbances and myocardial ischemia.
- Evaluate artificial pacemaker function.
- Use SAE to identify persons at risk for malignant ventricular arrhythmias, especially after myocardial infarction.
- Use a vectorcardiogram to diagnose MI and determine hypertrophy or ventricular dilatation. It is more sensitive than an ECG.

Reference Values

Normal
- Normal sinus rhythm and cardiac cycle are represented by a P wave, QRS complex, and T wave (a U wave may also be observed).
- Normal intervals, segments, junctions, and voltage measurements.
- No late potentials for SAE.
- Normal rate, rhythm, conduction velocities, and position of the heart in the chest.

Clinical Implications
- *ECG abnormalities* fall into five categories: rhythm, rate, axis or position, hypertrophy, and infarct or ischemia.
- *SAE* reveals the cause of syncope and can be positive for the presence of a late potential that may be associated with sustained ventricular tachycardia and sudden death.
- Vectorcardiogram abnormalities appear in MI, hypertrophy, and intraventricular conduction.

Interfering Factors
- *Race:* False-positive findings of abnormalities can be more common in African Americans.
- *Anxiety or hyperventilation* causes motion artifacts or morphology changes to the ECG.
- *Deep respiration* may shift the heart's position.
- *Exercise or movement:* Strenuous exercise before ECG or muscle twitching can affect the waveform.
- *Ascites, excess body weight, and pregnancy* can produce a left shift in QRS axis.
- *Medication or drug overdose* and *electrolyte imbalance.*
- For SAE, the patient's movement and talking affect impulse gathering.

Procedure
- Gelled electrodes are placed on the extremities and the chest and attached to the recorder.

- For SAE, electrodes are applied to the abdomen and the anterior and posterior thoraxes.

Nursing Interventions
▶ *Pretest*
- Explain the purpose and procedure of the test.
- Assess the patient's cardiac history, drug history, and interfering factors.
- Instruct the patient regarding the need to remain quiet, to relax completely, and to refrain from talking during test.

▶ *Posttest*
- Clean the electrode sites and equipment used in test.
- The patient may resume pretest activities.
- Evaluate outcomes and provide emotional support and explanations about possible further testing (eg, electrophysiology tests) to the patient, as needed.

CLINICAL ALERT

- The ECG does not show mechanical valvular function. It measures electrical impulses. It therefore may be normal in the presence of heart disease. An abnormal ECG may not necessarily signify heart disease, just as a normal ECG does not always reflect the absence of disease.
- Pacemaker patients should be identified and documentation on the ECG should include whether a magnet was or was not used during the recording process.
- A finding of late potentials in an SAE may be a predictor of sudden death.

ELECTROENCEPHALOGRAPHY (EEG) AND EPILEPSY/SEIZURE MONITORING
Special Brain Study

Evoked Responses/Potentials, Brain Stem Auditory Evoked Response (BAER), Visual Evoked Response (VER), Somatosensory Evoked Response (SSER)

The EEG measures and records electrical impulses from the cortex of the brain by means of electrodes attached to the patient's scalp. The evoked responses/potentials use conventional EEG recording electrodes with specific site placement to evaluate the electrophysiologic integrity of the auditory, visual, and sensory pathways. Epilepsy monitoring uses simultaneous video recording and EEG of brain activity.

Indications

- Diagnose epilepsy, tumors, abscesses, infarcts, injuries, hematomas, cerebrovascular diseases, narcolepsy, tremors, and Alzheimer's disease.
- Ascertain brain death (ie, cerebral silence).
- Evaluate suspected peripheral hearing loss, cerebellopontine angle lesions, brain stem tumors, infarcts, and comatose states, using BAER.
- Assess lesions involving the optic nerves and tracts, multiple sclerosis, and other disorders, using VER.
- Monitor epilepsy episodes to differentiate seizure type, region of seizure onset, and seizure frequency.
- Identify candidates for vagus nerve stimulation or surgery, using EEG.
- Assess spinal cord lesions, stroke, and numbness and weakness of the extremities, using SSER.

Reference Values

Normal

- Brain waves have normal symmetric patterns, amplitudes, frequencies (measured in cycles per second [Hertz], alpha 8–11), and other characteristics (measured in microvolts [μV]).
- No cross-circulation of the internal carotid arteries.
- Normal BAERs, VERs, and SSERs, indicating integrity of the auditory, visual, and sensory pathways.
- Normal cognitive tests.
- Normal event-related potentials (ERPs).

Clinical Implications

- Seizure activity (eg, grand mal, petit mal), if recorded during the seizure.
- Other types of seizures include psychomotor, infantile, myoclonic, and Jacksonian seizures that may occur with brain abscesses; gliomas; CVS; dementia; late stages of metabolic diseases; tumors; vascular lesions; metabolic disorders; meningitis; encephalitis; and posttraumatic head injury.

- Abnormal BAERs are associated with acoustic neuromas, cerebrovascular accidents, multiple sclerosis, auditory nerve lesions, brain stem lesions, or hearing loss in newborns.
- Abnormal VERs are associated with demyelinating disorders (eg, multiple sclerosis), lesions of the optic nerves and eye (prechiasma defects), and lesions of the optic tract and visual cortex (postchiasma defects).
- Abnormal SSERs are associated with spinal cord lesions, multiple sclerosis, and cervical myelopathy after an accident.

Interfering Factors

- Sedatives, mild hypoglycemia, oily hair, hair spray, and artifact from eye and body movements may affect test outcomes.

Procedure

- Electrode placement for evoked potential studies includes the vertex of the scalp and earlobe (for BAER) and over the median nerve at the wrist or peroneal nerve at the knee (for SSER).
- Multiple (up to 21) gelled electrodes are affixed onto the scalp in a definite pattern.
- The patient may be asked to purposely hyperventilate to produce an alkalosis that results in vasoconstriction. This may activate a seizure pattern. Photic stimulation, which is the use of flashing lights over the face at 1 to 30 times per second, may produce an electrical discharge not normally produced on EEG. Sleep deprivation before the test may be ordered to promote rest during the test. Abnormalities frequently surface during sleep.

Nursing Interventions

▶Pretest

- Explain the test purpose and procedure.
- Sleep deprivation may be ordered. A sleep-deprivation EEG requires that the patient sleep only between midnight and 4:00 AM. Special instructions may apply to children.
- Inform patient that food is permitted. The patient should not skip meals. (Hypoglycemia alters brain waves.) However, coffee, tea, colas, and other caffeine-containing products should be withheld for 8 hours before testing.
- Shampoo hair the evening before the test. Use only shampoo (ie, no conditioners or oils).
- Withhold anticonvulsants, tranquilizers, barbiturates, and other sedatives for 24 to 48 hours before the test unless otherwise ordered. Children and some adults may need sedation if they cannot sleep.

Intratest

- Instruct the patient to relax, remain quiet, and close the eyes. Promote a relaxed, quiet environment.
- Look for unusual recorded eye movements and body activity, because these motions can alter brain wave patterns. Be alert for seizure activity and provide proper interventions if necessary.

Posttest

- Shampoo the hair to remove gel and adhesive. If sedation was given, promote rest. Safety precautions should be observed. Otherwise, resume normal activities.
- Observe seizure precautions if applicable.
- Resume medications unless ordered otherwise (consult with the physician first).
- Provide emotional support and teaching to help the patient adjust to disorders. Explanations of the findings and how they relate to behavior may be helpful. Further testing is usually required (eg, MRIs, combined PET/CT scans).

> ## CLINICAL ALERT
>
> - Hyperventilation may cause transient dizziness or numbness and tingling in hands and feet.
> - If needle electrodes are used, a "prickly" sensation may be felt.
> - Abnormal EEGs findings correlate with impaired consciousness—the more profound the change in consciousness, the more abnormal is the EEG result.
> - Between seizures, the EEG pattern may be normal.

ELECTROLYTE STUDIES

Blood, Fasting, Timed Urine

Calcium (Ca), Chloride (Cl), Phosphate (P), Magnesium (Mg), Potassium (K), Sodium (Na)

This series of tests is performed to evaluate electrolytes (ie, ions, negatively [anion] and positively [cation] charged) and acid-base balance in the body. Levels of these ions can be used in the early detection for the potential or actual imbalances so that corrective treatment can be initiated.

Indications

- Calcium ion (Ca^{2+}) in blood for parathyroid function; calcium metabolism and malignancy activity
- Chloride ion (Cl^-) for inferential value (ie, sodium) and for diagnosis of acid-base disorders and correction of hypokalemic alkalosis
- Phosphate (P) for the relationship to calcium levels and parathyroid hormone levels
- Magnesium ion (Mg^{2+}) as an index of renal function, electrolyte status, and magnesium metabolism
- Potassium ion (K^+) to identify unsuspected and anticipated potassium imbalances, which can be lethal; evaluation of acid-base imbalances; and monitoring of acidosis and diabetic ketoacidosis (eg, renal failure, intestinal obstruction)
- Sodium ion (Na^+) for renal and adrenal disturbances, acid-base balance, changes in water balance, dehydration, and water intoxication

Reference Values

Normal

TOTAL CALCIUM IN BLOOD

AGE	MG/DAY	MMOL/L
0–10 days	7.6–10.4	1.90–2.60
10 days–2 years	9.0–11.0	2.25–2.75
2–12 years	9.9–10.1	2.20–2.70
12–18 years	8.4–10.7	2.10–2.55
Adult	8.4–10.2	2.15–2.50

IONIZED CALCIUM IN BLOOD

Adults: 4.65–5.28 mg/dL or 1.16–1.32 mmol/L
Children (1–18 years): 4.80–5.52 mg/dL or 1.20–1.38 mmol/L
Newborns: 4.40–5.48 mg/dL or 1.10–1.37 mmol/L

CALCIUM IN URINE

Adults: 110–300 mg/24 hours on an average diet or 2.50–7.50 mmol/day
50–150 mg/24 hours on a low-calcium diet or 1.25–3.75 mmol/day

CRITICAL VALUES— TOTAL CALCIUM

<6.0 mg/dL (<1.50 mmol/L)

>13 mg/dL (>3.25 mmol/L)

CHLORIDE IN BLOOD

Adults: 98–106 mEq/L or mmol/L
Newborns: 98–113 mEq/L or mmol/L

PHOSPHATE IN BLOOD

Adults: 2.5–4.5 mg/dL or
  1.0–1.5 mmol/L
Children: 4.5–5.5 mg/dL or
  1.45–1.78 mmol/L
Newborns: 4.5–9.0 mg/dL or
  1.45–2.91 mmol/L

CRITICAL VALUES

<1.2 mg/dL (<0.4 mmol/L) or
>9 mg/dL (>3 mmol/L)

MAGNESIUM IN BLOOD

Adults: 1.8–2.4 mg/dL or
  0.66–1.07 mmol/L
Children: 1.7–2.1 mg/dL or
  0.70–0.86 mmol/L
Newborns: 1.4–2.2 mg/dL or
  0.62–0.91 mmol/L

CRITICAL VALUES

<1.0 mg/dL (<0.4 mmol/L) or
>2.7 mg/dL (>1.0 mmol/L)

POTASSIUM IN BLOOD

Adults: 3.5–5.3 mEq/L
  or mmol/L
Children: 3.4–4.7 mEq/L
  or mmol/L
Newborns: 3.7–5.9 mEq/L
  or mmol/L

CRITICAL VALUES

<2.8 mEq/L (mmol/L) or
>6.7 mEq/L (mmol/L)

POTASSIUM IN URINE

Broad range: 25–125 mEq/24 hours or 25–125 mmol/24 hours
Average range: 40–80 mEq/24 hours or 40–80 mmol/24 hours (diet
  dependent)

SODIUM IN BLOOD

Adults: 135–145 mEq/L
  or mmol/L
Premature infant: 132–
  140 mEq/L or mmol/L
Term infants: 133–142 mEq/L
  or mmol/L
Children (1–16 years): 135–
  145 mEq/L or mmol/L

CRITICAL VALUES

<120 mEq/L (mmol/L) or
>160 mEq/L (mmol/L)

Clinical Implications: Calcium

- *Total calcium is increased* (ie, hypercalcemia [>12 mg/dL or >3 mmol/L]) in hyperparathyroidism, cancers, parathyroid hormone–producing tumors, hyperthyroidism, prolonged immobility, granulomatous disease, renal transplant, Paget's disease, and milk-alkali syndrome.
- *Total calcium is decreased* (ie, hypocalcemia [<4.0 mg/dL or <1.0 mmol/L]) with reduced albumin levels (hypoalbuminemia), hyperphosphatemia, hypoparathyroidism, malabsorption of calcium and vitamin D, alkalosis, acute pancreatitis, and vitamin D deficiency.
- *Ionized calcium is increased* in hypoparathyroidism, ectopic PTH-producing tumors, excess vitamin D intake, and some malignancies. Elevated serum protein levels increase calcium.
- *Ionized calcium is decreased* in hyperventilation, bicarbonate administration, acute pancreatitis, diabetic acidosis, sepsis, hypoparathyroidism, vitamin D and magnesium deficiency, toxic shock, and multiple organ failure. Decreased serum protein levels decrease calcium.

Interfering Factors: Calcium

- Many drugs (eg, thiazide diuretics, dialysis resins) cause increases, as do milk intake and excessive antacids.
- Decreases are caused by diarrhea and an excessive use of laxatives.

Clinical Implications: Chloride

- *Chloride is increased* with dehydration, Cushing's syndrome, metabolic acidosis with prolonged diarrhea, hyperparathyroidism, diabetes insipidus, renal tubular acidosis, dehydration, and hyperventilation that causes respiratory alkalosis.
- *Chloride is decreased* with vomiting, gastric suction, chronic respiratory acidosis, burns, metabolic alkalosis, congestive heart failure, Addison's disease, syndrome of inappropriate antidiuretic hormone (SIADH), and overhydration (ie, water intoxication).

Interfering Factors: Chloride

- Many drugs change chloride levels, and levels increase after excessive saline infusions.

Clinical Implications: Phosphorus

- *Phosphorus is increased* (ie, hyperphosphatemia) in renal insufficiency, severe nephritis, hypoparathyroidism, hypocalcemia, excessive alkali intake, healing fractures, bone tumors, Addison's disease, and acromegaly.

- *Phosphorus is decreased* (ie, hypophosphatemia) in hyperparathyroidism, rickets, diabetic coma, hyperinsulinism, liver disease, renal tubular acidoses, continuous intravenous glucose in nondiabetic persons (ie, phosphorus follows glucose into the cells), vomiting, severe malnutrition, and gram-negative septicemia.

Clinical Implications: Magnesium

- *Magnesium is increased* in renal failure or reduced renal function, diabetic acidosis, hypothyroidism, Addison's disease, after adrenalectomy, with dehydration, and with the use of antacids.
- *Magnesium is decreased* with hemodialysis, blood transfusions, chronic renal diseases, hepatic cirrhosis (eg, alcoholism), chronic pancreatitis, hyperaldosteronism, hypoparathyroidism, malabsorption syndromes, severe burns, long-term hyperalimentation, and excessive loss of any body fluid.

Interfering Factors: Magnesium

- Hemolysis invalidates results.
- Magnesium levels are falsely increased with prolonged salicylate therapy, lithium, magnesium antacids, and laxatives and levels are decreased by a number of drugs (eg, calcium gluconate).

Clinical Implications: Potassium

- *Potassium:* A falling trend time (0.1–0.2 mEq/day or mmol/24 hours) indicates a developing potassium deficiency. The most common potassium deficiency is caused by its GI loss. Potassium depletion occurs in patients receiving intravenous solutions without potassium supplementation.
- *Potassium levels are decreased* (ie, hypokalemia) with excessive renal excretion, diarrhea, vomiting, excessive spitting and drooling of saliva, eating disorders, malabsorption, draining wounds, cystic fibrosis, alcoholism, and respiratory alkalosis.
- *Potassium levels are increased* (ie, hyperkalemia) with renal failure, dehydration, cell damage, metabolic acidosis, diabetic ketoacidosis, interstitial nephritis, tubular disorders, pseudohypoaldosteronism, sickle cell anemia, and SLE.

Interfering Factors: Potassium

- Hemolysis causes up to a 50% increase in potassium levels.
- "Pumping" a fist with tourniquet in place increases potassium levels by 10% to 20%.
- Glucose administration and licorice decrease potassium levels.
- Many drugs interfere with potassium levels. IV potassium penicillin causes hyperkalemia; penicillin sodium causes hypokalemia.

- Leukocytosis (ie, leukemia) and thrombocytopenia (ie, polycythemia vera) interfere with potassium measurements.

Clinical Implications: Sodium

- *Sodium level increases* (ie, hypernatremia) are uncommon but do occur with dehydration, insufficient water intake, tracheobronchitis, coma, primary aldosteronism, Cushing's disease, and diabetes insipidus.
- *Sodium level decreases* (ie, hyponatremia) reflect a relative excess of body water rather than a low total body sodium level. Decreased levels occur with severe burns, diarrhea, vomiting, excessive nonelectrolyte intravenously administered solutions, kidney and liver diseases, edema, large intake of water, Addison's obstruction and malabsorption, diuretics, congestive heart failure, stomach suction, diabetic acidosis, and hypothyroidism.

Interfering Factors: Sodium

- Dietary salt or sodium and many drugs cause increases or decreases.

Procedure

- Obtain blood (5–7 mL) by venipuncture, using a red-top tube.
- Deliver specimens to the laboratory for immediate examination.
- For urine calcium, collect urine for 24 hours in an acid-washed bottle if not ordered with other tests. Urine specimens for calcium, sodium, and potassium may be refrigerated. See the timed specimen collection guidelines in Chapter 2.

Nursing Interventions

◆Pretest

- Assess the patient's compliance and knowledge base before explaining the purpose and procedure of testing for electrolyte disorders.
- No calcium supplements should be ingested 8 to 12 hours before the blood sample is obtained.
- If electrolyte disorders are suspected, record the daily weight and BP; accurate fluid intake and output; and color changes in the skin, tongue, and urine.
- Fasting may be required for calcium, chloride, phosphate, and magnesium tests.

◆Intratest

- Accurate test results depend on proper collection, preservation, and labeling.

▶*Posttest*
• Evaluate the outcome and monitor the patient appropriately for signs or symptoms of excess or deficient electrolytes.

CLINICAL ALERT

• Notify the physician and institute appropriate treatment at once for critical or panic values.

ELECTROMYOGRAPHY (EMG), ELECTRONEUROGRAPHY (ENG), ELECTROMYONEUROGRAPHY (EMNG)

Special Nerve and Muscle Studies

Electromyography (muscles) and electroneurography (nerves) are performed to detect neuromuscular abnormalities and differentiate between neuropathy and myopathy.

Indications
• Define the site and cause of motor neuron disorders at the anterior horn of the spinal cord and of peripheral nerves; also identify site and cause of muscle disorders.

Reference Values

Normal
• Normal nerve conduction and muscle action potentials at rest and during minimum and maximum voluntary muscle contractions.

Clinical Implications
• Abnormal neuromuscular activity, which occurs in diseases or disturbances of striated muscle fibers or membranes in the following conditions: muscle fiber disorders (eg, muscular dystrophy); cell membrane hyperirritability; myotonia and myotic disorders; and myasthenia gravis due to a variety of causes.
• Disorders or diseases of the lower motor neurons, including lesions of the anterior horn of the spinal cord (myelopathy) such as tumors, traumas, syringomyelia, muscular dystrophy, congenital amyotonia, anterior poliomyelitis, ALS, and peroneal muscular atrophy.

- Lesions of nerve root (radiculopathy), such as Guillain-Barré or nerve root entrapment from tumor, trauma, herniated disc, spurs, or stenosis.
- Damage or disease to peripheral or axial nerve, caused by entrapment of nerve, endocrine disorders such as hypothyroidism or diabetes, or effects of toxins and peripheral nerve degeneration and regeneration.
- Early peripheral nerve degeneration and regeneration.

Interfering Factors

- Decreased conduction in the elderly, and in the presence of pain, extraneous electrical activity, edema, hemorrhage, or thick, subcutaneous fat.

Procedure

- A ground electrode surface disk is applied to the wrist or ankle. The patient is instructed to relax or to contract certain muscle groups.
- There are two parts to the test:

   The first part is for *nerve conduction*; electrical current is passed through an electrode placed over a specific site. Sensations may be perceived by patient as discomfort.

   The second part determines *muscle potential*. A needle (long, small gauge) electrode is inserted into a muscle and moved or advanced as needed to detect the muscle's normal electrical responses.

Nursing Interventions

▶*Pretest*

- Explain the purpose and procedure of the test.
- Order sedation or analgesics as needed.
- Explain that the length of the test can be from 45 minutes to 3 hours depending on the suspected clinical problem.

▶*Intratest*

- Explain the procedure as it progresses.
- Alert the patient about possible perceived sensations and about the need to inform the diagnostician of pain, because this may alter results.

▶*Posttest*

- Provide pain relief if necessary.
- Promote rest and relaxation, especially if the test was lengthy.

ELECTRO-OCULOGRAPHY (EOG)

Eye

This test is used for evaluating retinal function.

Indications
- Evaluate hereditary and acquired degeneration of the retina.
- Assess the functional state of the retinal pigment epithelium.
- Monitor for retinopathy.

Reference Values

Normal

≥1.85 ratio (Arden ratio: maximum height of the retinal potential in light divided by the minimum height of the potential in the dark)

Clinical Implications
- An Arden ratio of 1.60–1.84 is probably abnormal; a ratio of 1.20–1.59 is definitely abnormal; and a ratio <1.20 is flat. The outcome is usually reported as normal or abnormal.
- The EOG ratio decreases in most retinal degeneration (eg, retinitis pigmentosa); this sometimes parallels the decrease on the electroretinography (ERG) examination.
- In Best's disease (congenital macular degeneration), the EOG is abnormal; however, the ERG is normal.
- In retinopathy, because of toxins such as antimalarial drugs, the EOG may show abnormalities earlier than the ERG.
- Supernormal EOGs have been noted in albinism and aniridia (loss of all or part of the iris) in which the common factor seems to be chronic excessive light exposure resulting in retinal damage.

Procedure
- The patient sits in the examining chair.
- Skin surface electrodes are placed in the inner and outer canthi of the eye. The electrical potentials are recorded on a polygraph unit.
- Two recordings are made: (1) recordings are made for 15 minutes with the patient in total darkness to measure eye movement through a known angle and (2) the patient is asked again to move his or her

eyes through the same angle, this time with the integrating sphere lighted.
- Total examination time is 40–45 minutes.

CLINICAL ALERT

If both fluorescein angiography (FA) and EOG are ordered, the EOG must be performed first because the eyes are dilated for the FA test but not for the EOG test. However, when an ERG and an FA are performed on the same day, the FA should be performed first to avoid corneal edema caused by the corneal electrode used in the ERG procedure. The waiting time between FA and ERG should be at least 2 hours.

Nursing Interventions
▶*Pretest*
- Explain the purpose and procedure of the test. The patient will experience little to no discomfort.

▶*Posttest*
- Interpret test results and monitor the patient appropriately.

ELECTROPHYSIOLOGY STUDY (EPS), HIS BUNDLE PROCEDURE

Special Cardiac Study

An electrophysiology study (EPS) is an invasive procedure (similar to a cardiac catheterization) performed to diagnose and treat supraventricular and ventricular arrhythmias. This is done by measuring the cardiac conduction system through solid electrodes and catheters that are advanced through the veins to the heart using fluoroscopy and x-ray to guide and track the catheter location.

Indications
- Diagnose conduction system defects and differentiation of impulse disorders (supraventricular from ventricular rhythms).
- Establish the mechanisms of impulse disorders or evaluate complaints of syncope or sick sinus syndrome.
- Evaluate antiarrhythmic drug effectiveness and pace the heart to induce certain dysrhythmias during these studies.

Reference Values

Normal

- Normal EP/His bundle procedure
- Normal conduction intervals, refractory periods, and recovery times
- Controlled, induced arrhythmias

Clinical Implications

- Longer or shorter conduction intervals, longer refractory periods, prolonged recovery times, and induced dysrhythmias
- Long atrial His (AH) bundle intervals, indicating atrioventricular (AV) node disease in the absence of vagal and sympathetic influences
- Long ventricular His (VH) bundle intervals, indicating His-Purkinje system disease
- Prolonged sinus node recovery time, indicating sinus mode dysfunction
- Sinoatrial conduction times, indicating sinus exit block
- Recurrent supraventricular and ventricular tachycardia that are inducible and confirm the diagnosis

Procedure

- Local anesthetic is administered.
- IV saline is used to support BP and a 12-lead ECG is performed.
- An antecubital or groin insertion site is chosen (depends on the location of catheter placement in the heart and condition of the patient's veins). Baseline values (eg, time for conduction, response to pacing) are recorded. To measure sinus node recovery times, it may be necessary to perform atrial pacing until the sinus node becomes fatigued and then measure the time to recover.
- Sustained arrhythmias that are symptomatic may require cardioversion or defibrillation.
- Sterile pressure dressings are applied to catheter insertion sites after the procedure.
- The procedure may take several hours, especially with the complex arrhythmias.

Nursing Interventions

▶ Pretest

- Explain the purpose and procedure of the EPS. Procedural or moderate sedation and analgesia may be administered. Describe sensations that may be felt, such as a "racing" heart, lightheadedness, or dizziness. Sensations may include feeling as if a bug is crawling on the arm or neck as the catheter is advanced.

- Evaluate the patient's neurologic status for deficits.
- Patient needs to be NPO for at least 3 hours before the procedure and should void immediately before the study, if possible. Record baseline vital signs.

Intratest

- Explain the procedure and expected sensations as the procedure progresses. A continuous, quiet conversation is held to assess the level of consciousness.
- Record vital signs according to protocols.

Posttest

- Ensure that the patient takes mandatory 4 to 8 hours bed rest lying flat, with no bending or flexing of extremities used for catheter introduction.
- Check vital signs, catheter sites (eg, swelling, bleeding, hematoma, bruit), and neurovascular status (eg, color, motion such as wiggling toes, sensation, warmth, capillary refill times, pulses) according to protocols. Monitor the ECG.
- Interpret test results and stress the importance of compliance with prescribed treatments and medications.

> ### CLINICAL ALERT
>
> - Drug side effects must be considered and anticipated (eg, hypotension, cramping, venous pain, euphoria).
> - Be alert to possibility of hematoma or bleeding at catheter sites, thromboembolism, phlebitis, and hemopericardium.
> - Notify the physician if bleeding, hypotension, altered neurovascular status, decreased distal perfusion, or life-threatening arrhythmias occur. Institute prompt treatment.

ELECTRORETINOGRAPHY (ERG)

Eye

Electroretinography (ERG) is indicated when surgery is considered in cases of questionable retinal viability.

Indications
- Evaluation of color blindness or night blindness
- Assessment for retinal detachment
- Preoperative evaluation for retinal viability

Reference Values

Normal
- Intact retina
- Normal A (photoreceptor cells) and B (Müller cells) waves

Clinical Implications
- Changes in the ERG are associated with the following:
  - Diminished response in ischemic vascular diseases (eg, arteriosclerosis, giant cell arteritis) and siderosis (poisoning of the retina when copper is embedded intraocularly [not associated with stainless steel foreign bodies]).
  - Certain drugs that produce retinal damage (eg, chloroquine, quinine).
  - Retinal detachment.
  - Opacities of ocular media.
  - Decreased response (eg, in vitamin A deficiency or mucopolysaccharidosis).
- Diseases of the macula do not affect the standard ERG. Macular disorder can be detected by a focal ERG.

Procedure
- The patient may be sitting up or lying down, with eyes held open.
- Topical anesthetic eyedrops are instilled.
- Bipolar cotton-wick electrodes, saturated with normal saline, are placed on the cornea.
- Two states of light adaptation are used to detect rod and cone disorders, along with different wavelengths of light to separate rod and cone function. Normally, the more intense the light, the greater the electrical response.
  a. Room (ambient) light
  b. Room darkened for 20 minutes and then a flash of white light
  c. Bright flash
- In infants and small children, who are being tested for a congenital abnormality, chloral hydrate or a general anesthesia may be used.
- Total examining time is about 1 hour.

Nursing Interventions

▶Pretest
- Explain the purpose and procedure of the test.
- For the most part, the patient will experience little to no discomfort. The electrode may feel like an eyelash in the eye.

 CLINICAL ALERT

- The patient should be cautioned not to rub his or her eyes for at least 1 hour after testing to prevent accidental corneal abrasion.

▶Posttest
- Interpret test results and monitor the patient appropriately.

 ENDOSCOPIC RETROGRADE CHOLANGIOPANCREATOGRAPHY (ERCP) AND MANOMETRY

Endoscopic and X-ray Imaging with Contrast, Interventional

This examination of the hepatobiliary system is done through a side-viewing, flexible fiber-optic endoscope, using an x-ray and instillation of a contrast agent into the duodenal papilla or ampulla of Vater. ERCP manometry can be performed to obtain pressure readings in the bile duct, pancreatic duct, and sphincter of Oddi at the papilla.

Indications
- Evaluate jaundice, pancreatitis, persistent abdominal pain, malformations, stenosis, pancreatic tumors, common bile duct stones, extrahepatic and intrahepatic biliary tract diseases, and strictures.
- Follow-up study for confirmed or suspected cases of pancreatic disease.
- Identify abnormal esophageal muscle function, aphagia (ie, difficulty swallowing), heartburn, regurgitation, vomiting, esophagitis, and chest pain of unknown origin.
- Perform procedures such as biopsies, calculi removal, dilatations, and drain insertions.

Reference Values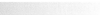

Normal

- Normal appearance and patent pancreatic ducts, hepatic ducts, common bile ducts, duodenal papilla (ampulla of Vater), and gallbladder.
- Manometry: normal pressure readings of the bile and pancreatic ducts and sphincter of Oddi.

Clinical Implications

- Abnormal findings include calculi, papillary stenosis, biliary cirrhosis, fibrosis, primary sclerosing cholangitis, cysts, pseudocysts, pancreatic tumors, chronic pancreatitis, cancer of bile ducts, pancreatic cysts, and cancer of the head of the pancreas.

Procedure

- An intravenous line is started and used for administration of procedural sedation. Intravenous fluids and blood, if needed, are started before the procedure. Pulse oximetry and vital signs are monitored continuously.
- The patient gargles with a topical anesthetic, or the patient's throat is sprayed. The patient assumes the left lateral position with the knees flexed (as endoscope is inserted through a mouthpiece) and changes to prone position, with left arm positioned behind, when instructed to do so.
- Simethicone is instilled to reduce bubbles from bile secretion. Glucagon or anticholinergics may be administered intravenously to relax the duodenum so that the papilla can be cannulated.
- Iodine contrast is instilled to outline pancreatic and common bile ducts after the ampulla of Vater is cannulated. Fluoroscopy and x-ray studies are performed at this time.

CLINICAL ALERT

- Contraindications include acute pancreatitis, cholangitis, acute infections, severe cardiopulmonary disease, recent MI, and coagulopathy.

Nursing Interventions

▸Pretest

- Require fasting for 10–12 hours.
- Explain the purpose and procedure of ERCP.
- Remove the patient's jewelry, contact lenses, and dentures and store these items safely.

- Ascertain how long the patient has been NPO. Check for allergies to medications, iodine, and latex.
- Evaluate the patient's health status relative to complaints of pain, respiratory difficulty, bleeding, or other significant events. Obtain baseline vital signs.

▶ Intratest

- Explain that oral suctioning may be necessary to remove secretions.
- Reposition patient and administer medications as requested by the physician.
- Monitor the patient's respiratory and cardiac status (eg, vital signs, ECG, pulse oximetry) and monitor for side effects and drug allergy reactions (eg, diaphoresis, pallor, restlessness, hypotension, transient flushing, hives, vomiting).

▶ Posttest

- Monitor vital signs, including temperature, and assess for effects of sedation, analgesics, and other medications. Observe respiratory status.
- Withhold fluids and food until the gag reflex returns (about 2 hours). Reassure the patient that a sore throat and abdominal discomfort may persist for several hours.
- Make sure that the patient voids within 8 hours after the procedure.
- Instruct the patient not to perform tasks that require mental alertness or to sign legal documents for 24 hours.
- Gargles, ice chips, oral fluids, or lozenges can soothe a sore throat.
- Explain that some abdominal discomfort may persist for several hours and that drowsiness may last up to 24 hours.

CLINICAL ALERT

- Have resuscitation equipment readily accessible. Flumazenil and naloxone should be available to reverse narcotic and sedation effects, if necessary. Notify the physician of pain with swallowing or neck movement, substernal or epigastric pain worsened with breathing or movement, nausea, vomiting, hypotension, shoulder pain, dyspnea, abdominal or back pain, prolonged cyanosis, fever, chills, or left upper-quadrant pain or tenderness. Potential complications include perforation, cholangitis, pancreatitis, gram-negative septicemia, hemorrhage, and shearing or stripping of gastric mucosa.

Esophagogastroduodenoscopy (EGD), Endoscopic-Gastroscopic Upper Gastrointestinal (UGI) Study, Endoscopy, Gastroscopy

Endoscopic GI Imaging, Interventional

This examination permits visualization of the upper GI tract (ie, mouth to upper jejunum), esophagus, stomach, and duodenum through a fiberoptic scope.

Indications
- Evaluate dysphagia.
- Evaluate ulcers, epigastric or substernal pain, upper GI diseases or injuries, anatomic variations, and dyspepsia.
- Diagnose and control bleeding.
- Remove foreign bodies.
- Obtain biopsies and specimens for laboratory studies.

Reference Values

Normal
- Upper GI tract features are within normal limits.
- Esophagus, stomach, and upper duodenum appear normal (ie, esophagus is yellow-pink, stomach is orange-red, and duodenal bulk is red).

Clinical Implications
- Abnormal findings reveal upper GI bleeding or hemorrhage sites, neoplasms, varices, esophageal rings, stenoses, striations, ulcers (benign or malignant), inflammatory processes, and hiatal hernia.

Interfering Factors
- Chemical ingestion or history of alcohol abuse

Procedure
- A topical anesthetic is applied to the patient's throat, and the patient is placed in a left lateral position with the knees flexed. Procedural sedation is administered.
- The endoscope is gently passed through the opening in the mouthpiece into the esophagus, stomach, and duodenum. Air passed through scope distends the area being examined so that better visualization is achieved.

- Biopsies and brushings are taken for cytologic analysis; photos provide a permanent record of the visual examination.
- A *Campylobacter*-like organism (CLO) test may be done if *Helicobacter pylori* is suspected as the causative agent for active chronic gastritis, duodenal or gastric ulcers, or nonulcer dyspepsia. Gastric mucosal biopsies are taken and immersed into the test gel for rapid analysis of urea-producing organisms.
- A videoendoscopic evaluation of dysphagia (VEED) may be performed as part of the EGD. Pudding and crackers are swallowed and then tracked on video. Views of the nasopharynx, laryngopharynx, and larynx assist in evaluating aspiration associated with dysphagia.

Nursing Interventions
▶ *Pretest*
- Explain the procedure and purpose of the EGD examination, fasting for 8 hours before the test, and the need for sedation and a local anesthetic. Provide written instructions.
- Check for allergies to drugs.
- Perform or assist with oral hygiene.
- The patient must remove dentures, jewelry, hairpieces, glasses, and tight clothing.
- Explain that a full feeling or pressure may be felt with movement of the scope and introduction of air. Have the patient void, if necessary.
- Administer prescribed medications and record baseline vital signs.

▶ *Intratest*
- Advise the patient that sensations of pressure or bloating are normal but that there is usually no pain.
- Assist with positioning the patient's head during the examination. Monitor vital signs as necessary; be alert to adverse medication reactions. Send properly prepared specimens to the laboratory.

▶ *Posttest*
- Allow nothing by mouth (NPO) until the swallowing reflex returns (usually about 2 hours). Record vital signs according to protocols or the patient's status. Keep the sedated patient in a side-lying position. Provide saline gargle for a sore throat after the swallowing reflex is intact.
- Encourage the patient to belch or expel air.

- The following complications, though rare, may occur: perforation, bleeding or hemorrhage, aspiration, infection, complications from drug reaction, complications from unrelated diseases, or death (very rare).
- Signs of perforation include pain with swallowing and neck motion, substernal or epigastric pain, shoulder pain and dyspnea or abdominal pain, back pain, cyanosis, fever, and pleural effusion.

ESTROGEN URINE TOTAL AND FRACTIONS, ESTRADIOL (E₂), ESTRIOL (E₃)

Timed Urine and Blood

These tests are used along with assays of gonadotropins to evaluate fertility problems, menstrual problems, pregnancy, estrogen-producing tumors, and male-feminization characteristics.

Indications

- Evaluate estradiol for menstrual and fertility problems in women and feminization in men.
- Investigate estriol for estrogen-producing tumors and to monitor pregnancy.
- Assess total urine estrogen to determine ovulation time and the optimal time for conception.

Reference Values

Normal

URINE ESTRADIOL (E₂)

Men	0–6 µg/24 hours or 0–22 nmol/day
Women	Follicular phase: 0–3 µg/24 hours or 0–11 nmol/day
	Ovulatory peak: 4–14 µg/24 hours or 15–51 nmol/day
	Luteal phase: 4–10 µg/24 hours or 15–37 nmol/day
	Postmenopausal phase: 0–4 µg/24 hours or 0–15 nmol/day

URINE ESTRIOL (E₃) (WIDE RANGE OF NORMAL)

Men	1–11 µg/24 hours or 4–40 nmol/day
Women	Follicular phase: 0–14 µg/24 hours or 0–51 nmol/day
	Ovulatory phase: 13–54 µg/24 hours or 48–198 nmol/day

Luteal phase: 8–60 μg/24 hours or 29–220 nmol/day
Postmenopausal phase, 0–11 μg/24 hours or
  0–40 nmol/day

Pregnancy   First trimester: 0–800 μg/24 hours or 0–2900 nmol/day
Second trimester: 800–12,000 μg/24 hours or
  2900–44,000 nmol/day
Third trimester: 5000–50,000 μg/24 hours or
  18,000–180,000 nmol/day

URINE TOTAL ESTROGENS

Men   15–40 μg/24 hours or 55–147 nmol/day
Women Menstruating, 15–80 μg/24 hours or 55–294 nmol/day
Postmenopausal phase: <20 μg/24 hours or
  <73 nmol/day
Pregnancy First trimester: 0–800 μg/24 hours or 0–2900 nmol/day
Second trimester: 800–5000 μg/24 hours or
  2900–18,350 nmol/day
Third trimester: 5000–50,000 μg/24 hours or
  18,350–183,000 nmol/day

BLOOD TOTAL ESTROGENS

Men   20–80 pg/mL or 20–80 ng/L
Women 60–400 pg/mL or 60–400 ng/L
Postmenopausal phase: <130 pg/mL or <130 ng/L
Prepuberty: <25 pg/mL or <25 ng/L
Puberty: 30–280 pg/mL or 30–280 ng/mL

Note: Total serum estrogen does not measure estriol (E_3) and should not be used in pregnancy or to assess fetal well-being.

Clinical Implications

- *Increased urine E_2* is found in the following conditions: feminization in children (testicular feminization syndrome), estrogen-producing tumors, precocious puberty related to adrenal tumors, hepatic cirrhosis, hyperthyroidism, and in women during menstruation, before ovulation, and during the 23rd–41st weeks of pregnancy.
- *Decreased urine E_2* occurs in primary and secondary hypogonadism, Kallmann's syndrome, menopause, and hypofunction or dysfunction of the pituitary or adrenal gland.

Interfering Factors

- Drugs that can cause decreases include vitamins and some phenothiazines; tetracycline can increase levels.

- Recently administered radioisotopes and oral contraceptives affect test results.
- Estrogen or progesterone therapy can interfere with test results.

Procedure

- A 10-mL venous serum specimen is obtained using a red-top Vacutainer tube.
- A 24-hour urine sample can be collected using a preservative and refrigeration. See the specimen collection guidelines in Chapter 2.

Nursing Interventions

▶ Pretest

- Assess the patient's compliance and knowledge base before explaining the test purpose and procedure.
- Note any anxiety about testing of sex hormones.

▶ Intratest

- No restriction of food or fluids is required.
- Accurate test results depend on proper collection, preservation, and labeling. Be sure to include the test start and completion times. Note on the laboratory requisition form the phase of patient's menstrual cycle and whether any sex-related hormones are being taken.

▶ Posttest

- Evaluate the outcomes, provide counseling for the patient, and monitor as appropriate for fertility and pregnancy.

ESTROGEN OR ESTRADIOL RECEPTOR (ER), PROGESTERONE RECEPTOR (PR), DNA PLOIDY (TUMOR ANEUPLOIDY)

Tissue and Epithelial Cells

Estrogen and progesterone receptors in the cancerous cells of breast and endometrial tissues are measured to determine whether the cancer is likely to respond to therapy. DNA ploidy measures cell turnover (ie, replication) in specimens identified as cancer and predicts progress, shorter survival, and relapse in some patients with cancer of the bladder, breast, colon, endometrium, prostate, kidney, or thyroid. The predictive value is greater for breast, prostate, and colon cancers.

Indications

- Tests done on cancerous tissues in the laboratory.

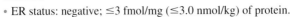

Reference Values

Normal

- ER status: negative; ≤3 fmol/mg (≤3.0 nmol/kg) of protein.
- PR status: negative; ≤5 fmol/mg (≤5.0 nmol/kg) of protein.
- DNA index (DI): 0.9–1.0 u/L (15–17 nkat/L) is normal.
- For DNA ploidy (content) or the diploid state, an interpretive histogram by flow cytometry (Fc) classifies the stained nucleic acid as DNA diploid, DNA tetraploid, DNA uninterpretable, or DNA aneuploid abnormal.

Clinical Implications

- A positive result for ER binding occurs at levels of >10 fmol/mg (>10 nmol/kg) and for PR binding at levels of ≥10 fmol/mg (>10 nmol/kg). Approximately 50% of ER-*positive* tumors respond to antiestrogen therapy, as do 60% to 70% of patients with both ER- and PR-positive tumors.
- ER-*negative* tumors rarely respond to antiestrogen therapy.
- The finding of PR positivity increases the predictive value of selecting patients for hormonal therapy. Some evidence suggests that PR synthesis is estrogen dependent.
- The presence of aneuploid peaks in the replicative activity of neoplastic cells may be prognostically significant, independent of tumor grade and stage.
- The greater the amount of cells in S phase (ie, DNA synthesis) of the cell cycle, the more aggressive is the tumor.
- Positive aneuploidy points to a favorable prognosis in some conditions, such as acute lymphoblastic lymphoma, neuroblastoma, and perhaps transitional cell bladder cancer.

Procedure

- A fresh specimen is obtained by biopsy and is delivered to the histology laboratory.
- A 1-g specimen of quickly frozen tumor is examined for receptor binding, and the result is expressed in a Scatchard plot. The specimen must *not* be placed in formalin. Some laboratories can perform estrogen receptor-to-progesterone receptor ratio (ERA/PRA) studies on paraffin-embedded tissue. Check with your laboratory for specific instructions.
- Specimens for DNA ploidy are examined and classified on the basis of the percentage of epithelial cells that contain diploid (2N) DNA content and nondiploid DNA (aneuploid). DNA content is calculated as the DNA index.

Nursing Interventions

▸*Pretest*

- Explain the purpose and laboratory method for testing.
- Obtain an appropriate clinical history so that this information can be provided with the specimen.

▸*Posttest*

- In conjunction with physician, interpret test results, and counsel the patient appropriately about other tests and possible treatment (eg, antiestrogen therapy).

EYE, EAR, THROAT, AND SINUS CULTURE SWABS OR WASHINGS

Exudate, Drainage

Acute pharyngitis is the most common infection of the upper respiratory tract for which a throat culture is obtained. Eye, ear, and sinus cultures are obtained to isolate pathogenic organisms causing infections (eg, bacterial conjunctivitis, otitis media).

Indications

- Identify the cause of conjunctivitis; symptoms include eye drainage (ie, purulent, mucopurulent, or serosanguineous), eye pain, and redness.
- Identify the cause of throat infection; symptoms may include difficulty swallowing, headache, or fever.
- Identify cause of ear infections; symptoms may include ear pain and itching, tenderness of the tissues around the ear, or drainage of pus.
- Identify cause of acute sinusitis, an infection of one or more of the paranasal sinuses after a common cold, or other viral infections of the upper respiratory tract.

Reference Values

Normal

- Negative for pathogenic organisms or no growth of organisms.

Clinical Implications

- Throat infections are commonly caused by group A-B hemolytic *Streptococcus*, *Corynebacterium diphtheriae*, *Neisseria gonorrhoeae, Bordetella pertussis*, adenovirus, herpes virus, *Mycoplasma*, and *Chlamydia*.

- Ear and eye infections are commonly caused by *Streptococcus pneumoniae, Staphylococcus* sp., *Haemophilus* sp., and *Pseudomonas aeruginosa* (ie, swimmer's ear). Sinusitis is caused by the same organisms and by viruses.

Procedure

- For a throat culture, use a sterile culture kit containing a sterile, polyester-tipped swab with a transport medium. With the patient's head tilted back slightly and the patient instructed to say "ah," the swab is extended between the tonsillary pillars and behind the uvula. A tongue depressor helps prevent touching the tongue. Any purulent exudate in the posterior pharynx should be gently rubbed with the swab. Return the swab to its transport container and expose it to the transport medium.
- Cultures from ear drainage fluid do not reflect the bacterial cause of otitis media unless the tympanic membrane has recently ruptured. The canal must be cleaned and fresh pus must be obtained as it exudes from the tympanic membrane.
- Acute bacterial sinusitis can be determined only by culture of an exudate or rinse of a sinus by direct puncture and aspiration. Culture of nasal pus is unreliable. Sinus puncture should be performed only in cases of intracranial infection or severe immuno-suppression.
- Suppurative material from the conjunctiva of an infected eye should be collected on a sterile swab that is then placed in the transport medium.

Nursing Interventions

▸*Pretest*

- Explain the culture purpose and procedure to the patient or parents.

▸*Intratest*

- Label the specimen with the patient's name, date and time collected, and specific source of the specimen.
- Transport the specimen to the laboratory.

▸*Posttest*

- Counsel the patient regarding positive results, type of treatment (eg, antibiotics), and possible need for further testing to evaluate the effectiveness of therapy.

EYE AND ORBIT SONOGRAMS

Eye

Ultrasound can be used to describe both normal and abnormal tissues of the eye when no alternative visualization is possible because of opacities caused by inflammation or hemorrhage.

Indications
- Management of eyes for keratoprosthesis.
- Detection of orbital lesions.
- Evaluation before vitrectomy or surgery for vitreous hemorrhages.
- Differentiation between inflammatory and congestive causes of exophthalmus.
- Rule out retinal and choroidal detachments.
- Detection and localization of vitreoretinal adhesions and intraocular foreign bodies.

Reference Values

Normal
- Pattern image indicating normal soft tissue of the eye and retrobulbar orbital areas, retina, choroid, and orbital fat.

Clinical Implications
- Abnormal patterns are seen in alkali burns with corneal flattening and loss of anterior chamber, detached retina, keratoprosthesis, extraocular thickening in thyroid eye disease, pupillary membranes, cyclitic membranes, vitreous opacities, orbital mass lesions, inflammatory conditions, vascular malformations, and foreign bodies.
- Abnormal patterns are also seen in tumors of various types on the basis of specific ultrasonic patterns: solid tumors (eg, meningioma, glioma, neurofibroma), cystic tumors (eg, mucocele, dermoid, cavernous hemangioma), angiomatous tumors (eg, diffuse hemangioma), lymphangioma, and infiltrative tumors (eg, metastatic lymphoma, pseudotumor).

Interfering Factors
- If at some time the vitreous humor in a particular patient was replaced by a gas, no result can be obtained.

Procedure

- A small, very high-frequency transducer is placed on the eye directly or is positioned over a water standoff pad placed onto the eye surface. Multiple images and measurements are taken.
- The eye area is anesthetized by instilling eyedrops.
- The patient is asked to fix the gaze and hold very still.
- A probe is gently placed on the corneal surface.
- If a lesion in the eye is detected, as much as 30 minutes may be required to accurately differentiate the pathologic process.
- Orbital examination can be done in 8 to 10 minutes.

Nursing Interventions

 Pretest

- Explain the purpose and procedure of the test.

 Posttest

- Instruct the patient to refrain from rubbing the eyes until the effects of the anesthetic have disappeared. This type of friction could cause corneal abrasions.
- Advise the patient that minor discomfort and blurred vision may be experienced for a short time.

> **CLINICAL ALERT**
>
> - When a ruptured globe is suspected, ophthalmic ultrasound should not be performed. Excessive pressure applied to the globe may cause expulsion of the contents and increase the risk of bacteria introduction.

FETAL BIOPHYSICAL PROFILE (FBP)

Ultrasound Imaging of Fetus/Mother

This prenatal test uses ultrasound to evaluate five noninvasive fetal parameters: muscle tone, fetal movement, fetal breathing, volume of amniotic fluid, and fetal heart acceleration (nonstress test). Each parameter is assessed and assigned a value of 0 to 2; 2 points is optimal. Some centers include placental grading in biophysical profile. Modified FBP includes the nonstress test (NST) and amniotic fluid index (AFI).

Indications
- Monitor later stages of pregnancy to assess fetal well-being.
- Identify the fetus affected by hypoxia.
- Test a high-risk pregnancy beginning by 32 to 34 weeks; severe complications may require testing at 26 to 28 weeks.
- Test a postdated pregnancy with biweekly surveillance of the bio-physical profile.
- Provide information about fetal size, position, and number; placental location; and fetal eye movements and voiding.

Reference Values

Normal
- A maximum score is 10 points for a normal test result and indicates no fetal distress.
- A score of 8 or more indicates fetal well-being based on NST results, movement, breathing, and normal amount of fetal muscle tone and amniotic fluid.

Clinical Implications
- A score lower than 8 points indicates a potential fetal distress or an existing fetal distress.
- Outcomes may be affected by fetal age, fetal behavior states, fetal or maternal infection, hypoglycemia, hyperglycemia, postmaturity, and maternal drug use. Use of magnesium sulfate, alcohol, cocaine, and nicotine can decrease the biophysical profile parameters.

Procedure
- Place the patient on her back as for an obstetric sonogram and apply a gel (coupling agent) on the skin of the lower abdomen.
- Move the ultrasound transducer across the lower abdominal area to visualize the fetus and surrounding structures.
- A contraction stress test (CST) or NST is also done at this time. Examining time varies with fetal age and condition; it is usually 30 minutes.

Nursing Interventions
▶Pretest
- Explain the purpose of the test and how each parameter relates to fetal well-being. If there are no eye movements or evident respirations, the fetus is most likely asleep.
- Obtain the baseline BP, temperature, pulse, respirations, and fetal heart rate (FHR).

▸*Intratest*
• Provide reassurance.

▸*Posttest*
• Interpret the test outcome and counsel the patient in collaboration with the physician. Explain that results may or may not reflect fetal status. Further testing may be needed weekly or two times a week.
• Provide crisis intervention if the test outcome indicates a need for immediate medical attention or delivery.

FETAL WELL-BEING TESTS

Special Studies

Nonstress Test (NST), Contraction Stress Test (CST), Oxytocin Challenge Test (OCT), Breast Stimulation Test (BST)

The nonstress test (NST) for fetal well-being involves the use of an external fetal monitor to observe acceleration of the fetal heart rate (FHR) with fetal movement. Acceleration of the FHR indicates intact central and autonomic nervous systems that are not affected by intrauterine hypoxia. The contraction stress test (CST) involves the use of an external fetal monitor to observe the fetal response to spontaneous or induced uterine contractions by administering oxytocin (OCT) to evaluate placental function.

Indications
• Monitor high-risk pregnancies, including those associated with diabetes, pregnancy-induced hypertension, intrauterine growth retardation, multiple gestation, spontaneous rupture of membranes, postdate pregnancy, and other high-risk situations.
• Assess the FHR in response to uterine contractions by a CST, or assess fetal ability to respond to the fetal environment when not under the stress of labor by performing NST.
• Monitor the FHR reaction to stress when a nonstress test (NST) is nonreactive or CST is positive or unsatisfactory by performing OCT.

CLINICAL ALERT

- CST is contraindicated for third-trimester bleeding, previous cesarean section, and risks of preterm birth such as premature rupture of membranes, incompetent cervix, and multiple gestation.

Reference Values

Normal

- *Negative NST:* Two or more FHR accelerations last at least 15 seconds and accelerate at least 15 beats per minute, with fetal movements in 20-minute segments of a monitor strip.
- *Negative CST:* No late decelerations of FHR occur, with a minimum of three uterine contractions within a 10-minute period.

Clinical Implications

- *Positive NST:* indicates a nonreactive fetus; however, by itself does not mean fetal distress without other supporting tests.
- *Positive CST:* indicates fetoplacental inadequacy.

Procedure

- *NST:* With the patient in the left lateral position, an external fetal monitor records for 20 to 90 minutes to assess FHR accelerations with fetal movement. The patient is instructed to depress a button to mark the monitor strip when she feels fetal movement.
- *CST:* With the patient in a left lateral position, an external fetal monitor records uterine contractions until three contractions occur that last 40 to 60 seconds in 10 minutes. Contractions are achieved by intravenous oxytocin administration or tactile nipple stimulation.
- *OCT:* Oxytocin is infused intravenously to produce three good-quality contractions of at least 40 seconds each in 10 minutes on an external fetal monitor strip.

CLINICAL ALERT

- If uterine contractions are induced by oxytocin or nipple stimulation, there is a risk of hyperstimulation (ie, contractions are closer than every 2 minutes and lasting more than 90 seconds) and late decelerations. There is also risk of inducing preterm labor. Tocolytics can be given for hyperstimulation.

Nursing Interventions
▶ *Pretest*
- Explain the purpose of the test, use of an external fetal monitor, and use of a remote marker for fetal movement.
- Obtain baseline maternal vital signs and the FHR.

▶ *Intratest*
- Provide reassurance.
- If no fetal movement is detected after 30 minutes of NST monitoring, the patient is given orange juice or fruit juice or a light meal to increase blood glucose, or the fetus is manually stimulated.
- In some centers, acoustic or vibroacoustic stimulation of the fetus is used with NST to induce FHR accelerations.
- In CST, if late decelerations occur, oxytocin is discontinued, the patient is placed in a left lateral position, oxygen is given by mask at 6 to 8 L/minute, and the physician is notified.

▶ *Posttest*
- Interpret the test outcome and counsel the patient in collaboration with the physician.
- Provide crisis intervention if the test outcome shows a need for immediate medical attention or immediate delivery of an infant at risk.

FINE-NEEDLE ASPIRATION (FNA), FNA BIOPSY BREAST ASPIRATE

Cells and Tissues of All Body Parts and Fluids

Fine-needle aspiration is a method of obtaining diagnostic material for cytologic (cells) and histologic (tissue) study from all parts of the body—mouth, breast, nipple discharge, liver, genital tracts, respiratory tract and body fluid, urine, cerebrospinal fluid, and effusions—with a minimal amount of trauma to the patient.

Indications
- Identify infectious process.
- Confirm benign conditions (eg, duct papilloma).
- Diagnose primary or metastatic malignancies (eg, intraductal breast cancer).
- Obtain cell and tissue markers to predict cancer development.

Reference Values

Normal

- Cells and tissue are normal.
- No expression of select biomarkers.
- Negative for neoplasia or hyperplasia.

Clinical Implications

- In practice, results of these studies are commonly reported (according to Broders' classification, grade I, II, III, or IV, with grade I being most malignant) as inflammatory, benign, atypical, suspicious for malignancy, or positive for malignancy (in situ vs invasive). A basic method for classifying cancers according to tissue (histologic) or cellular (cytologic) characteristics of the tumor is Broders' classification of malignancy, which identifies differentiated cells and many atypical features. The tumor node metastasis (TNM) system is a method of classifying tumor stages, spread of disease, type of cancer (eg, breast), primary site, extent, and involvement (eg, lymphatic invasion).
- Abnormal findings are indicative of hyperplasia with increased risk of future cancer.
- Expression of certain markers is indicative of risk and malignancy.

Procedure

- Local anesthesia is used in most cases.
- Superficial or palpable lesions may be aspirated without the aid of x-ray films. Nonpalpable lesions are aspirated using x-ray guidance for needle placement.
- After the needle has been properly positioned, the plunger of the syringe is retracted to create negative pressure. The needle is moved up and down and sometimes at different angles to obtain the aspirate. The plunger of the syringe is released and the needle is removed.
- Record the source of the sample and method of collection so that evaluation can be based on complete information.
- Specimens collected from patients in isolation should be clearly labeled on the specimen container and on the requisition form with an appropriate warning sticker. The specimen container is then placed inside two sealed, protective, biohazard bags before transportation.

Nursing Interventions

▶Pretest

- Explain the purpose, procedure, risks (eg, vasovagal response), and benefits of aspiration.
- Allay fears and anxiety.

CLINICAL ALERT

- There are several contraindications (mainly for deep-seated organs): bleeding diathesis (anticoagulant therapy); seriously impaired lung function by advanced emphysema, severe pulmonary hypertension, or severe hypoxemia; highly vascular lesions; suspected hydatid cyst; and uncooperative patient.
- Traumatic complications are rare. Fine-needle aspiration of the lung infrequently results in pneumothorax. Local extension of the malignancy is a consideration, but studies have shown this to be a rare occurrence.
- A negative finding on fine-needle aspiration does not rule out the possibility that a malignancy is present. The cells aspirated may have come from a necrotic area of the tumor or a benign area adjacent to the tumor.

▶*Posttest*

- Monitor for signs of inflammation and care for the site with infection control measures. Treat pain, which may be common in sensitive areas such as the breast, nipple, and scrotum.
- Monitor for specific problems, which vary depending on the site aspirated (eg, hemoptysis after lung aspiration).
- Counsel the patient about further tests (eg, surgical biopsies and treatment of infection [antibiotics] and malignancies [refer to oncologist]).

FLUORESCEIN ANGIOGRAPHY (FA)

Eye

In this test, images of the eye, taken by a special camera, are studied to detect the presence of retinal disorders.

Indications
- Evaluate for vascular disorders of the retina.
- Assess for poor vision.

Reference Values

Normal
- Normal retinal vessels, retina, and circulation.

Clinical Implications
- Abnormal results reveal diabetic retinopathy, aneurysm, macular degeneration, diabetic neovascularization, blocked blood vessels, and leakage of fluid from vessels.

Procedure

- A series of three drops is given to dilate the pupil of the eye. Complete dilatation occurs within 30 minutes of giving the last drop. When dilatation is complete, a series of color photographs of both eyes is taken.
- The patient sits with the head immobilized in a special headrest in front of a fundus camera.
- Fluorescein dye is injected intravenously.
- A series of photographs is taken as the dye flows through the retinal blood vessels over a period of 3–4 minutes.
- A final series of photographs is taken 8–10 minutes after the injection.

CLINICAL ALERT

- Choroidal circulation is not seen with color photographs.
- Some patients may experience nausea for a short period of time following the injection.
- The eyedrops may sting or cause a "burning" sensation.

Nursing Interventions

▶*Pretest*
- Determine whether the patient has any known allergies to medications or contrast agent.
- Instruct the patient about the purpose, procedure, and side effects of the test.

▶*Posttest*
- Advise the patient that he or she may experience color changes in the skin (yellowish) and urine (bright yellow or green) for 36–48 hours after the test.
- Advise the patient to wear dark glasses and not to drive while the pupils remain dilated (4–8 hours).
- Interpret test results and monitor appropriately.

Folic Acid (Folate), Vitamin B$_{12}$

Blood

These B vitamin measurements are usually made together to diagnose macrocytic anemia.

Indications
- Provide differential diagnosis of anemia.
- Diagnose pernicious anemia, leukemia, and other macrocytic anemias.

Reference Values

Normal
- *RBC folate:* 280–791 ng/mL or 634–1791 nmol/L
- *Folic acid:* 5–24 ng/mL or 11.3–54.4 nmol/L
- *Vitamin B$_{12}$:*
  Newborns: 160–1300 pg/mL (118–959 pmol/L)
  Adults: 200–835 pg/mL or 146–616 pmol/L
  Elderly (60–90 years): 110–770 pg/mL or 81–568 pmol/L

Clinical Implications
- *Vitamin B$_{12}$* levels decrease with pernicious anemia, malabsorption, and inflammatory bowel disease; gastrostomy or gastric resection; Zollinger-Ellison syndrome; fish and tapeworm infestation; primary hypothyroidism; and folic acid deficiency.
- *Vitamin B$_{12}$* levels increase with chronic granulocytic leukemia, lymphatic and monocytic leukemia, liver disease, some cancers, chronic renal failure, polycythemia vera, and congestive heart failure.
- *Folic acid levels decrease* with macrocytic (megaloblastic) anemias, insufficient dietary intake, alcoholism, liver disease, hemolytic disorders, malignancies, infantile hyperthyroidism, and adult celiac disease.
- *Folic acid levels increase* with blind loop syndrome, a vegetarian diet, and B$_{12}$ deficiency.

Interfering Factors
- Altered outcomes are seen in persons with recent diagnostic or therapeutic doses of radionuclides, high doses of vitamin C, anticonvulsants, and oral contraceptives. Many drugs affect test outcomes.

- Pregnancy, smoking, age, and a vegetarian diet affect the test outcome.

Procedure
- Vitamin B_{12}: A 10-mL fasting serum sample is obtained in a SST or red-top tube and protected from light. The blood cannot be hemolyzed.
- Folic acid: A 5-mL serum sample is obtained using a SST or red-top tube, and it is protected from light.
- If an RBC folate assay is also ordered, a whole-blood sample is obtained using a purple-top tube.

Nursing Interventions
▶Pretest
- Explain the test purpose and procedures.
- The patient is allowed no food overnight, but water is permitted.

▶Posttest
- Evaluate outcomes, counsel the patient about treatment (for pernicious anemia, monthly vitamin B_{12} injections), and monitor the patient appropriately regarding pernicious and macrocytic anemia and leukemia.
- Advise about foods high in vitamin B_{12} and folic acid.

FOLLICLE-STIMULATING HORMONE (FSH), LUTEINIZING HORMONE (LH)

Blood

The test measures the gonadotropic hormones FSH and LH (produced and stored in the pituitary gland) to determine whether a gonadal insufficiency is primary or caused by insufficient stimulation by the pituitary hormones.

Indications
- Evaluate FSH and primary ovarian or testicular failure.
- Measure FSH and LH in children with endocrine problems related to precocious puberty.
- Support other studies of the cause of hypothyroidism (women) and endocrine dysfunction (men).

Reference Values

Normal

VALUES FOR LUTEINIZING AND FOLLICLE-STIMULATING HORMONES

	LUTEINIZING HORMONE (LH)		FOLLICLE-STIMULATING HORMONE (FSH)	
	(mIU/L) OR (IU/L)		(mIU/L) OR (IU/L)	
Female				
Follicular phase	1.37–9.9	1.37–9.9	1.68–15	1.68–15
Ovulatory peak	6.17–17.2	6.17–17.2	21.9–56.6	21.9–56.6
Luteal phase	1.09–9.2	1.09–9.2	0.61–16.3	0.61–16.3
Post-menopausal phase	19.3–100.6	19.3–100.6	14.2–52.3	14.2–52.3
Male	1.42–15.4	1.42–15.4	1.24–7.8	1.24–7.8

Note: Contact your laboratory for reference values in infants and children. Normal values may vary with method of testing and units used.

Clinical Implications

- *Decreased FSH levels* occur in cases of feminizing and masculinizing ovarian tumors when production is inhibited as a result of increased estrogen, failure of pituitary or hypothalamus, neoplasm of testes or adrenal glands that secrete estrogens or androgens, hemochromatosis, and polycystic ovarian disease.
- *Increased FSH levels* occur in Turner's syndrome (ie, ovarian dysgenesis), hypopituitarism, precocious puberty (idiopathic), Klinefelter's syndrome, Sheehan's syndrome, and castration.
- *Increased FSH and LH levels* occur in hypogonadism, gonadal failure, complete testicular feminization syndrome, absence of testicles (anorchia), and menopause.
- *Inappropriately low FSH and LH levels* occur in pituitary or hypothalamic failure. (FSH and LH are often within the reference range but are inappropriately low for the loss of gonadal steroid negative feedback.)

Interfering Factors

- Certain drugs such as testosterone, estrogens, and oral contraceptives can cause false-negative results for FSH levels.
- Hemolysis of blood sample.
- Pregnancy.

Procedure

- A 5-mL blood serum sample is obtained in a red-top tube.
- For women, the date of the last menstrual period is noted.
- Multiple blood specimens may be needed because of the episodic release of FSH and LH.

Nursing Interventions

▶*Pretest*

- Assess the patient's compliance and knowledge base before explaining the test purpose and procedure.

▶*Intratest*

- Accurate test results depend on proper collection and labeling. Be sure to include the date of the last menstrual period.

▶*Posttest*

- Evaluate the outcome and provide the patient with counseling and support as appropriate for pituitary dysfunction.

Food Poisoning

Stool

These tests are used to detect the underlying pathogen responsible for food poisoning or in some cases contributing factors for neuroparalytic diseases.

Indications

- Identify pathogenic organisms and toxins in GI disturbance (emetic toxin with vomiting and enterotoxin with diarrhea).
- Evaluate cause of infectious diarrhea.
- Assess underlying cause of neuroparalytic diseases (eg, Guillain-Barré syndrome or infant botulism).

Reference Values

Normal

- Negative culture by DNA probe for *Bacillus cereus*, type A *Clostridium perfringens*, *Clostridium botulinum*, *Staphylococcus aureus*, *Campylobacter jejuni*, *Escherichia coli*, and *Salmonella*.

Clinical Implications

- Positive cultures of these pathogens are consistent with food poisoning.
- *C. botulinum* has been implicated as the cause of infant botulism and is associated with the ingestion of soil or honey that may contain *C. botulinum* spores.
- *C. jejuni* has been found to be a contributing factor in Guillain-Barré syndrome.

Procedure

- Collect stool specimens (25–50 g) for culture. (See Chapter 2 for details.)
- Suspected food specimens (eg, contaminated meat, unrefrigerated fried rice with patient symptoms of vomiting, and poultry or mashed potatoes with patient symptoms of diarrhea) may also be tested.
- Refrigerate specimen in clean, sealed, leak-proof containers.
- If a delay of more than 2 hours is anticipated, the specimen should be placed on Cary-Blair transport medium.

Nursing Interventions

⬥ Pretest

- Explain the purpose and procedure for diagnosing food poisoning.
- Take a history of recently ingested, undercooked foods that were not kept hot (eg, foil-wrapped baked potatoes held at room temperature, sautéed onions, or cheese sauce) and were accompanied by symptoms of diarrhea or vomiting.

⬥ Posttest

- Interpret test outcomes.
- Monitor prescribed drug treatment (eg, vancomycin, erythromycin).

CLINICAL ALERT

- Monitor patients diagnosed with botulism for impending respiratory failure. Mechanical ventilation may be needed.
- Administer antitoxin in a timely manner to minimize subsequent nerve damage.

FUNGAL ANTIBODY TESTS

Blood, Infections

Histoplasmosis, Blastomycosis, Coccidioidomycosis (Desert, San Joaquin, or Valley Fever) Cryptococcal Infection

These tests are performed to diagnose fungal infections involving the deep tissues and internal organs caused by *Histoplasma capsulatum*, *Blastomyces*, *Coccidioides immitis*, and *Cryptococcus.*

Indications

- Evaluate fungal infection involving respiratory tract infection in persons with signs (eg, enlargement of lymph nodes) and symptoms (eg, cough and dyspnea) and possible history of inhalation of spores from sources such as contaminated dusts, soil, and bird droppings.
- Assess patients who have symptoms of pulmonary or meningeal infection.
- Evaluate cryptococcal infection in patients with predisposing conditions such as lymphoma, sarcoidosis, steroid therapy, or AIDS.

Reference Values

Normal

- Negative for fungal antibodies; complement-fixation (CF) titer: <1:8.
- Negative for antibodies or antigens to these fungi according to immunodiffusion tests.
- *Cryptococcus* antibodies or antigens: 1:4 titer suggests cryptococcal infection; 1:8 or greater titer indicates active infection.

Clinical Implications

- Antibodies to coccidioidomycosis, blastomycosis, and histoplasmosis appear early in the disease (from first to fourth weeks) and then disappear.

Interfering Factors

- Antibodies against fungi may be found in blood of apparently normal people who live in an area where the fungus is endemic.

- In tests for blastomycosis, there may be cross-reactions with histoplasmosis.
- False-positive results for *Cryptococcus* occur for patients with elevated rheumatoid factor levels.

Procedure
- Serum (7 mL) is obtained by venipuncture, using a red-top or serum separator tube.
- Antibodies to fungi are detected by complement-fixation or immunodiffusion tests.

Nursing Interventions
▸*Pretest*
- Assess the patient's knowledge about the test and travel history to endemic areas.
- Assess for exposure to spores found in dust and soil.
- Explain blood test purpose and procedure. No fasting is required.

▸*Posttest*
- Evaluate the outcome and counsel the patient appropriately. Advise the patient that additional procedures such as skin tests, cultures, and lumbar puncture for CSF may be required to identify the particular fungus involved.

GALLBLADDER, HEPATOBILIARY, AND BILIARY NUCLEAR MEDICINE SCAN

Nuclear Medicine, GI Imaging

This nuclear medicine study uses a radiopharmaceutical and is done to visualize the gallbladder and determine patency of the biliary system.

Indications
- Investigate upper abdominal pain.
- Evaluate cholecystitis and differentiate obstructive from nonobstructive jaundice.
- Evaluate biliary atresia and postsurgical biliary assessment.

Reference Values

Normal
- Normal gallbladder, biliary system, and duodenum.

Clinical Implications
- Abnormal patterns reveal acute and chronic cholecystitis, gallstones, biliary atresia, strictures, and lesions.
- Gallbladder visualization excludes the diagnosis of acute cholecystitis with a high degree of certainty.

Interfering Factors
- Elevated bilirubin level (>10 mg/dL or >171 μmol/L) and some pain medications may affect reliable outcomes.
- Total parenteral nutrition (TPN) and long-term fasting may affect gallbladder visualization.
- Opiates or morphine-based pain medications taken within 6 hours of the test may interfere with transit of the radiopharmaceutical.

Procedure
- A radiopharmaceutical is injected intravenously. Start imaging immediately after injection. A series of images at 5-minute intervals is taken until adequate visualization of the gallbladder and small intestine.
- In the event of biliary obstruction, obtain delayed views.
- In some patients, cholecystokinin (CCK) is administered to differentiate acute from chronic cholecystitis or provide quantification of gallbladder function. Morphine may be given to visualize the gallbladder.

Nursing Interventions
▶*Pretest*
- Explain the test purpose, procedure, risks, and benefits.
- Record accurately the patient's weight.
- Explain that the patient must be NPO for 4 hours (3–4 hours for pediatric patients). In the case of prolonged fasting (>24 hours), notify the nuclear medicine department.
- Reassure the patient regarding the safety of injection of the radiopharmaceutical.

▶*Intratest*
- Provide reassurance and support during the test.

• Evaluate outcomes and counsel the patient appropriately (eg, need for possible treatment).
• Assess the intravenous site for signs of infection or infiltration.

GALLBLADDER (GB) ULTRASOUND, HEPATOBILIARY SONOGRAM, LIVER ULTRASOUND

Ultrasound GI Imaging

These tests are helpful in differentiating hepatic disease from biliary obstruction. Unlike the oral cholecystogram, this procedure allows visualization of the gallbladder and ducts in patients with impaired liver function.

Indications
• Initial study for persons with upper right-quadrant pain.
• Differentiate gallbladder disease from heart disease, detect gallstones or acute chronic cholecystitis, and evaluate nonfunctioning gallbladder that cannot be visualized on x-ray films.
• Guide fine-needle aspiration for biopsy or other interventional procedures.

Reference Values

Normal
• Normal size, position, and configuration of gallbladder and bile ducts.
• No evidence of calculi.
• Normal adjacent liver tissue.

Clinical Implications
• Abnormal patterns, renal size variations, and thickened wall indicative of cholecystic adenomyomatosis or tumor and commonly seen as a manifestation of cholecystopathy in patients with AIDS or other inflammatory processes or neoplasms.
• Presence of inflammation; gallstones in the gallbladder and bile ducts; dilatations, strictures, and obstructions of the biliary tree; and congenital abnormalities (eg, choledochal cysts).
• Benign and malignant lesions such as polyps.
• Liver pathologies such as cirrhosis, cysts, solid lesions, and metastatic tumors.
• If combined with Doppler evaluation, portal hypertension and hepatofugal (portal blood flow away from the liver) flow.

Interfering Factors
• Barium from recent radiographic studies, presence of excessive intestinal gas, and obesity affect visualization.

Procedure
• Ask patient to lie quietly on the examination table in the supine or decubitus position.
• Cover skin with a layer of coupling gel, oil, or lotion.
• Ask the patient to regulate breathing as instructed.
• Examination time is approximately 10–30 minutes.

Nursing Interventions
▶Pretest
• Explain the purpose, benefits, and procedure of the test.
• Instruct the patient to remain NPO at least 8 hours before the examination to fully dilate the gallbladder and to improve anatomic visualization. Some laboratories prefer that the last meal before the study should contain low quantities of fat.
• Assure the patient that there is no pain involved. However, the patient may feel uncomfortable lying quietly for a long period.
• Explain that a liberal coating of coupling agent must be applied to the skin so that there is no air between the skin and the transducer and to allow for easy movement of the transducer over the skin. A sensation of warmth or wetness may be felt. Although the acoustic couplant does not stain, advise the patient not to wear nonwashable clothing for the examination.
• Explain that the patient will be instructed to control breathing patterns while the images are being taken.

▶Posttest
• Patient may resume normal diet and fluid intake.
• Remove the gel, or instruct the patient to clean the remaining gel from the abdomen.
• Evaluate the outcome and counsel appropriately about further treatment or procedures.

GALLIUM (^{67}GA) IMAGING

Nuclear Medicine Scan, Tumor Imaging

This test involves the injection of a radiopharmaceutical to image the entire body for lymph node involvement.

Indications

- Detect the presence, location, and size of lymphomas, infections, and abscesses.
- In patients with fever of unknown origin (FUO).
- In adult and pediatric patients to help stage bronchogenic cancer, Hodgkin's disease, and non-Hodgkin's lymphoma.
- Record tumor regression after radiation or chemotherapy.
- Differentiate malignant from benign lesions and determine the extent of invasion of known malignancies.

Reference Values

Normal

- No evidence of tumor-type activity or infection.
- No abnormal uptake.

Clinical Implications

- Abnormal gallium concentration usually implies the existence of underlying pathology, such as a malignancy, especially in the lung or testes, or a mesothelioma.
- Tumor uptake of ^{67}Ga varies with tumor type, among persons with tumors of the same histologic types, and even within tumor sites of a given patient.
- Tumor uptake of ^{67}Ga may be significantly reduced after effective treatment.

Interfering Factors

- A negative study result does not definitely exclude the presence of disease. (The rate of false-negative results in gallium studies is 40%.)
- It is difficult to detect a single, solitary nodule such as in adenocarcinoma. Lesions <2 cm can be detectable.
- Because gallium does collect in the bowel, there may be an abnormal concentration in the lower abdomen. For this reason, laxatives and enemas may be ordered.
- Degeneration or necrosis of tumor and antineoplastic drugs immediately before imaging can cause false-negative results.

Procedure

- Laxatives, suppositories, and tap water enemas are often ordered before scanning. The patient may eat breakfast the day of imaging.
- The radionuclide is injected 24 to 96 hours before imaging.
- The patient must lie quiet without moving. Anterior and posterior views of the entire body are taken.

- Additional imaging may be done at 24-hour intervals to differentiate normal bowel activity from pathologic concentrations.

Nursing Interventions
▸*Pretest*
- Explain the purpose, procedure, benefits, and risks of the test.
- Some departments request that patient eat a low-residue lunch and clear liquid supper the day before examination.
- Bowel preparation is needed. The usual preparation includes oral laxatives taken the night before the first imaging session and continuing the night before each imaging session. Enemas or suppositories may also be given. These preparations clean normal gallium activity from the bowel.
- Imaging time is 45 to 90 minutes per imaging session.

▸*Intratest*
- Reassure the patient that the follow-up imaging is routine.

▸*Posttest*
- Interpret the outcome and monitor the patient appropriately (eg, injection site for extravasation or infiltration).
- Observe, report, and counsel the patient regarding side effects (ie, rash, hives, and tachycardia) that may occur 1 day after injection.

CLINICAL ALERT
- Breast-feeding should be discontinued for at least 4 weeks after testing.

GASTRIC ANALYSIS (TUBE GASTRIC ANALYSIS)
Gastric Fluid

This test is performed to examine the contents of the stomach for the presence of abnormal substances such as blood, bacteria, and drugs and to measure gastric acidity.

Indications
- Diagnose gastric or duodenal ulcers, pyloric or intestinal obstruction, pernicious anemia, and carcinoma of the stomach.
- Determine the cause of GI bleeding.

- Assess the effectiveness of medical or surgical therapy to treat ulcers.
- Examine gastric washings (tuberculosis studies) to identify mycobacterial infection when previous sputum test results were negative.

Reference Values

Normal

- Fluid: negative for blood, drugs, or bile present in the sample; pH of 1.5–3.5.
- Culture: negative for mycobacterial organisms.
- Fasting specimen total acidity: <2 mEq/L or <2 mmol/L.
- Basal acid output (BAO) without stimulation: 0–5 mEq/hour or 0–5 mmol/hour.
- Maximal acid output (MAO) or normal secretory ability when using a gastric stimulant such as histamine or betazole hydrochloride intramuscularly or pentagastrin subcutaneously: 10–20 mEq/hour or 10–20 mmol/hour.
- BAO/MAO ratio: 1:2.5 to 1:5.

Clinical Implications

- *Decreased levels* of gastric acid (ie, hyposecretion and hypochlorhydria) occur with pernicious anemia, gastric malignancy, atrophic gastritis, adrenal insufficiency, vitiligo, rheumatoid arthritis, thyroid toxicosis, chronic renal failure, and postvagotomy.
- *Increased levels* of gastric acid (ie, hypersecretion and hyperchlorhydria) occur with peptic or duodenal ulcer, Zollinger-Ellison syndrome, hyperplasia and hyperfunction of antral gastric cells, and after massive small intestine resection.

Interfering Factors

- Lubricant or barium from previous studies can affect results.
- Medications such as antacids, histamine blockers, food, and smoking alter gastric acid secretions.
- Insulin treatment of diabetic persons and surgical vagotomy affect test results.
- Problems may be related to passing the nasogastric tube, such as previous nasal surgery, trauma, or a deviated septum.
- Elderly patients have lower levels of gastric hydrochloric acid.

Procedure

- Collect fasting specimens during endoscopy or through a nasogastric (NG) tube inserted for the test.
- Aspirate initial gastric acid through the nasogastric tube with a syringe, test for pH, and discard it. If no acid is present, reposition the nasogastric tube and obtain another specimen.

- Specimens are normally collected via continuous intermittent low suction over 1 to 2 hours at 15-minute intervals, depending on the type of gastric stimulant given. Each specimen is placed in a separate specimen cup and labeled BAO or MAO, along with the patient's name, date, and time collected.
- The nasogastric tube is removed after all specimens are collected.
- Documentation includes date and time, type of procedure, type and size of tubes used, number of specimens collected, appearance, consistency, measured volumes of gastric fluid obtained, the patient's response to the testing, complications, interventions, and other pertinent information.

Nursing Interventions

▶ Pretest

- Assess for contraindications to the procedure, such as carcinoid syndrome, congestive heart failure, or hypertension; histamine for the test may exacerbate these conditions.
- Explain the test purpose and procedure. Instruct the patient to restrict food, fluids, gum chewing, and smoking 8 to 12 hours before the test (usually NPO after midnight). Restrict anticholinergics, cholinergics, adrenergic blockers, antacids, steroids, alcohol, and coffee for at least 24 hours before the test.
- Record baseline vital signs and remove loose dentures before the test.

▶ Intratest

- Explain that panting, mouth breathing, and swallowing can facilitate tube insertion.
- Observe for signs of distress such as coughing or cyanosis when inserting the tube.

CLINICAL ALERT

- If histamine is injected, inform the patient that flushing, dizziness, headache, faintness, and numbness of extremities and abdomen may occur during or immediately after testing. Advise the patient to report changes immediately. Have epinephrine ready for shock treatment if histamine is injected.

▶ Posttest

- Monitor vital signs and observe for possible side effects of stimulants. Observe for respiratory bleeding or distress and gastrointestinal bleeding (may be sign of perforation).

- Counsel the patient in collaboration with the physician about posttest deviations and the need to alter lifestyle, such as stopping smoking, alcohol use, diet changes (ie, caffeine or stimulants), stress reduction, and medication or surgical interventions.

GASTRIC STOMACH EMPTYING IMAGING

Nuclear Medicine Scan, GI Imaging

This study involves administration of an oral radiopharmaceutical in liquid or solid form (mixed with eggs or oatmeal) in adult and pediatric patients to assess gastric motility disorders and in patients with unexplained nausea, vomiting, diarrhea, and abdominal cramping.

Indications

- Assess mechanical and nonmechanical gastric motility disorders. Mechanical disorders include peptic ulcerations, gastric surgery, trauma, and cancer. Nonmechanical disorders include diabetes, uremia, anorexia nervosa, certain drugs (eg, opiates), and neurologic disorders.
- Evaluate stomach emptying.
- Evaluate patients with diabetes and symptoms of nausea, vomiting, and early satiety.
- Monitor response to drug therapy (eg, metoclopramide).

Reference Values

Normal

- Normal half-time clearance ranges are 45 to 110 minutes for solids and 10 to 65 minutes for liquids, depending on the standard normalization of the specific technique and type of imaging equipment used.

Clinical Implications

- Slow or delayed emptying results are usually seen in cases of peptic ulceration, diabetes, or smooth muscle disorders and after radiation therapy.
- Accelerated emptying is often visualized in Zollinger-Ellison syndrome, certain malabsorption syndromes, and after gastric or duodenal surgery.

Interfering Factors
- Administration of certain medications (eg, gastrin, cholecystokinin) interferes with emptying.

Procedure
- This may be a two-phase procedure.
- The fasting patient consumes the solid phase (^{99m}Tc sulfur colloid usually in scrambled eggs or oatmeal), followed (if ordered as dual phase) by the liquid phase (^{111}In-DTPA in 300 mL of water).
- The patient is imaged immediately after ingesting the food.
- Subsequent images are obtained for the next 2 hours.
- The half-time clearance for the liquid and solid phases of gastric emptying time is computed.

Nursing Interventions
▶*Pretest*
- Explain the gastric emptying imaging purpose and the procedure, benefits, and risks.
- Assess for recent medication administration.
- Fasting for 8 hours in adult patients is required for emptying imaging.

▶*Intratest*
- Reassure the patient or parent that the procedure is proceeding normally. Allow the parent to assist with the oral feeding of infants or small children.
- Pregnancy is a contraindication for this procedure.

▶*Posttest*
- Evaluate the outcome and counsel the patient appropriately regarding further tests and possible treatment (eg, medication).

GASTRIC X-RAY; UPPER GASTROINTESTINAL EXAMINATION (UPPER GI [UGI] SERIES); CONTRAST X-RAY OF STOMACH; ESOPHAGUS X-RAY, BARIUM SWALLOW

UGI, Contrast X-ray

Gastric radiography uses fluoroscopic and conventional x-ray techniques to visualize the form, position, mucosal folds, peristaltic activity, and motility of the upper gastrointestinal tract and provide views of the esophagus, stomach, duodenum, and first part of the jejunum. The small-bowel study is generally ordered as a continuation of the upper gastrointestinal (UGI) study to follow and document the filling of the entire small bowel.

Indications

- Exclude gastric ulcers, obstructions, pyloric stenosis, cancer, tumors, hernias, gastric diverticulitis, presence of undigested food, gastritis, congenital anomalies, and stomach polyps.
- Evaluate gastric pain and swallowing difficulties.
- Detect Crohn's disease.
- A video esophagram is typically performed to evaluate swallowing disorders, particularly in stroke patients and after head and neck surgery with plastic surgical repair.

Reference Values

Normal

- Normal position, size, contour, motility, and peristaltic patterns of the esophagus, stomach, and duodenum.
- Normal small intestine position, contour, and filling.

Clinical Implications

- Evidence of congenital abnormalities, gastric ulcers, carcinoma of stomach, masses, foreign bodies, gastric polyps, and diverticula, gastritis and reflux, hiatal hernia, volvulus of the stomach, and Crohn's disease.

Interfering Factors

- Retained food or fluids interfere with optimal film clarity.
- Optimal gastrointestinal studies depend on patient's ability to consume contrast media orally. Inability to do so compromises the examination's quality.
- Severe obesity adversely affects image quality.
- If the patient is debilitated, proper examination may be difficult; it may be impossible to adequately visualize the stomach.

Procedure

- After being NPO for approximately 8 hours before the examination, an oral contrast agent, usually barium, is swallowed to outline the gastrointestinal contents while the patient is positioned in front of the fluoroscopy machine. Follow-up x-ray films are obtained after fluoroscopic examination. Many labs use a "double" or "air" contrast technique. The patient is asked to swallow a "fizzy" agent (effervescent granules) in addition to barium. This material produces gas that improves the visualization of the GI tract. The examination time is 20 to 45 minutes.

- For small-bowel study, the procedure is as previously described, but the examination time is much longer. Because the peristaltic pattern, general activity, and presence of disease influence how quickly contrast moves through the intestinal tract, this study can vary from minutes to several hours.

Nursing Interventions
▶ *Pretest*
- Assess for test contraindications, such as pregnancy or allergies.
- Explain the gastric test purpose and procedure.
- Special attention is necessary for diabetic patients. Because of pretest fasting, the administration of insulin or oral hypoglycemic agents may be contraindicated.
- If the patient is allergic to barium (although rare), this must be communicated to the radiology department so that alternate contrast media can be used.

▶ *Intratest*
- Encourage the patient to follow breathing and positional instructions.

▶ *Posttest*
- Provide plenty of fluids, food, and rest after the study. Administer laxatives and a high-fiber diet, if ordered.
- Observe and record stool color and consistency to determine if all barium has been eliminated.
- Evaluate outcomes, provide support, and counsel the patient that follow-up procedures may be necessary.

GASTROESOPHAGEAL REFLUX IMAGING

Nuclear Medicine Imaging, GI Imaging

This nuclear medicine test involves the oral administration of a radiopharmaceutical to study adult and pediatric patients for esophageal disorders such as regurgitation and helps identify the cause of persistent nausea and vomiting. In infants, the gastroesophageal reflux scan is used to distinguish between vomiting and reflux (for those with more severe symptoms).

Indications
- Verify or exclude gastric reflux before and after imaging, because the symptoms of gastric reflux and cardiac pain are similar.
- Investigate unexplained nausea and vomiting.
- Determine the presence of pulmonary aspiration.

Reference Values

Normal
- Computer-generated curve shows less than 4% gastric reflux across the esophageal sphincter.

Clinical Implications
- Greater than 4% reflux at any pressure level is considered an abnormal finding.
- Evidence of pulmonary aspiration.

Interfering Factors
- Prior upper gastrointestinal x-ray procedures performed may interfere with this test.

Procedure
- After an overnight or 4-hour fast, the radiopharmaceutical (^{99m}Tc sulfur colloid) is administered orally in orange juice, milk, or scrambled eggs. For infants, the test is usually performed at the normal infant feeding time to determine esophageal transit.
- The infant is burped before being given the remainder. Then, some unlabeled milk is given to clear the esophagus of the radioactive material. If a nasogastric tube is required for radiopharmaceutical administration, the tube must be removed before the imaging occurs for reflux because it could cause a false-positive result.
- Images are obtained for 2 hours.
- A computer analysis generates and calculates a time-activity reflux curve.

CLINICAL ALERT
- Patients who have esophageal motor disorders, hiatal hernias, or swallowing difficulties and infants should have an endogastric tube inserted for the procedure.

Nursing Interventions

▸*Pretest*

- Explain the gastrointestinal reflux imaging purpose, procedure, benefits, and risks.
- Ensure overnight fasting or fasting 4 hours before the test.
- Ensure oral intake of the radiopharmaceutical in orange juice, milk, or scrambled eggs.
- Perform imaging with the patient in a supine position.

▸*Intratest*

- Reassure the patient that the test is proceeding normally.
- Allow a parent to assist with oral feeding of infants or small children.
- Pregnancy is a contraindication to this procedure.

▸*Posttest*

- Remove gastric tubes, if placed for the examination, after the procedure.
- Evaluate outcomes and monitor the patient appropriately (eg, injection site).
- Routinely dispose of body fluids and excretions unless the patient is also receiving therapeutic doses of radiopharmaceuticals to treat a disease.
- Document the outcomes accurately and completely. Include patient evidence-based outcomes as appropriate.

GASTROINTESTINAL (GI) BLEEDING IMAGING

Nuclear Medicine Imaging, GI Imaging

This nuclear medicine study, using ^{99m}Tc pertechnetate, detects suspected active bleeding sites distal to the ligament of Treitz.

Indications

- Detect sites of acute, active GI bleeding (patients with bright-red blood per rectum) and the need for transfusion.
- Locate peritoneal and retroperitoneal sites of recent hemorrhage.
- Assess the patient with melena.
- Guide for surgery and assessment for angiography, aggressive treatment, and transfusion.

Reference Values

Normal
- Normal gastrointestinal bleed imaging; no sites of actual bleeding.

Clinical Implications
- Abnormal concentrations of RBCs with areas of radioactivity greater than the background activity are associated with the approximate geographic location of active gastrointestinal bleeding sites (peritoneal and retroperitoneal) of 0.2 to 0.5 mL/min.
- Hepatic hemangioma

Interfering Factors
- Presence of barium in gastrointestinal tract may obscure the site of bleeding because of the high density of barium and the inability of the technetium to penetrate the barium.
- Drugs that interfere with RBCs falsely include contrast agents, digoxin (Lanoxin), doxorubicin (Adriamycin), heparin, hydralazine hydrochloride, prazosin (Minipress), propranolol (Inderal), penicillin, and quinidine.

Procedure
- A venous blood sample is obtained.
- ^{99m}Tc-labeled RBCs are injected intravenously.
- Imaging begins immediately after injection and is continued every few minutes. Images are obtained anteriorly over the abdomen at 5-minute intervals for 60 minutes or until the bleeding is located. If the study is negative at 1 hour, delayed images can be obtained at 2, 6, and sometimes 24 hours later, when necessary, to identify the location of difficult to determine bleeding sites.
- The patient is assessed for signs of active bleeding during the examination period.
- Total examining time varies.

Nursing Interventions
▶Pretest
- Explain the gastrointestinal bleed imaging purpose, procedure, benefits, and risks.
- Determine whether the patient has received barium as a diagnostic agent in the last 24 hours.
- Advise the patient that delayed images may be necessary. If active bleeding is not seen on the initial scans, additional images must be

obtained for up to 24 hours after injection, whenever the patient has clinical signs of active bleeding.

◆Intratest

- Provide support and reassurance during administration of radioactive medications and imaging throughout period.

◆Posttest

- Evaluate outcomes and counsel the patient appropriately about further testing or treatment (eg, blood transfusion).
- The patient may eat and drink normally after completion of the procedure.
- Dispose of body fluids and excretions in routine ways unless the patient is also receiving therapeutic doses of radiopharmaceutical to treat a disease.
- Advise pregnant staff and visitors to avoid prolonged patient contact for 24 to 48 hours after radioactive agent administration.

CLINICAL ALERT

- This test is contraindicated for those who are hemodynamically unstable. In these instances, angiography or surgery should be the procedure of choice.
- Recent blood transfusions may contraindicate this study.

GENETIC TESTING

Blood, Bone Marrow, Tissue, Skin, Placenta, Saliva

Genetics is concerned with the components and function of biologic inheritance. Genetic testing determines the presence, absence, or activity of genes in cells. With these tests, geneticists try to predict the course of a person's health state, especially if there is the possibility of deviation from normal, developmental problems and birth defects. Basic genetic technology counts chromosomes in a person's cells or measures the amount of specific gene-encoded proteins in the blood. Cellular DNA can be assayed with molecular probes to determine a specific genetic sequence among the billions of base pairs of genes that make up human DNA. Many disease states reflect hereditary components, even though general clinical studies usually focus on the specific disorder itself rather than on its genetic component. Chromosomal studies, linkage studies, and direct detection of abnormal genes (oncogenes or cancer) are common tests in this group. Molecular and biochemical tests are being done more and more often, primarily through detection of abnormal accumulation of proteins, abnormal cells, analytes, and other substances in body fluids and tissues.

Indications

- *Genetic counseling:* Done to address prognosis and diagnosis, as well as cause and recurrence risks in the context of the family and the individual.
- *Decisive diagnosis:* Differentiation and presymptomatic studies may be done to diagnose certain diseases related to chromosome or DNA studies in the unborn, newborn, children, or adults. Oncogene detection plays a part in the diagnosis of cancer.
- Newborn screening to detect preventable, common, or treatable disease.
- Investigation of fetal death, stillbirth, or miscarriage.
- Assignment of gender in the presence of ambiguous genitalia.

CLINICAL ALERT

- Many genetic diseases are far from rare.
- Tests are not performed purely for information's sake; instead, they should be ordered for conditions for which treatment is available. The best a predictive genetic test can offer is the degree of risk for acquiring the defect.
- All tests should be linked to genetic counseling so that patients understand the results and their implications.
- The patient should be able to use test results to make informed decisions about issues such as childbearing and medical treatment.
- Everyone is genetically defective to some degree. Most defects, however, do not impair a person's ability to function normally.
- Family history is a major tool in identifying genetic disorders and in recognizing and documenting dysmorphic features, growth problems, developmental delay, and adult mental retardation.

🖊 Chromosomal Analysis

Reference Values

Normal

- 46 chromosomes
- Women: 44 autosomes plus 2 X chromosomes; karyotype: 46,XX

• Men: 44 autosomes plus 1 X and 1 Y chromosome; karyotype; 46,XY

Clinical Implications

Many chromosomal abnormalities can be placed into one of two main classes.

ABNORMALITIES OF NUMBER

Example: Autosomes

    Trisomy 21 (Down's syndrome)
    Trisomy 18 (Edwards syndrome)
    Trisomy 13 (Patau syndrome)

Example: Sex Chromosomes

    Turner's syndrome (single X)
    Klinefelter's syndrome (XXY)
    XYY
    XXX

ABNORMALITIES OF STRUCTURE

Example: Deletions

Cystic fibrosis: F508 deletion

Example: Duplications

3q2 trisomy (Cornelia de Lange syndrome resemblance)

Translocations

Translocation of chromosomes 11 and 22: t(11;22)
Isochromosomes: A single chromosome with duplication of the long arm of the X chromosome; i(Xq) (ie, variant of Turner's syndrome)

Ring Chromosomes

Chromosome 13 with the ends of the long and short arms joined together, as in a ring: r(13)

Mosaicism

Two cell lines, one normal female and the other for Turner's syndrome: 46,X, 45,X

Indications

• Grow cells from fetal surface of placenta to determine cause of spontaneous abortion.
• Evaluate failure to thrive, mental retardation, recurrent miscarriages (especially with malformations), infertility, and delayed onset of puberty.

- Determine sex in the presence of ambiguous genitalia.
- Assess some forms of cancer and leukemias.

Procedure

Specimens for chromosome analyses are generally obtained as follows:

- Leukocytes from peripheral vascular blood samples are used most frequently because these are the most easily obtained cells. Laboratory preparation of the cells takes at least 3 days.
- Bone marrow analysis is often done to diagnose certain categories of leukemias. Bone marrow biopsies can sometimes be completed within 24 hours.
- Fibroblasts from skin or other surgical specimens can be grown and preserved in long-term culture mediums for future studies. Growth of a sufficient amount of the specimen for studies usually requires at least a week.
- Amniotic fluid obtained through amniocentesis requires at least a week to produce a sufficient amount of specimen for analysis.
- Chorionic villus sampling (CVS) can be done at earlier stages of pregnancy (about 9 weeks) than can amniocentesis. Some initial CVS studies can be done almost immediately after conception.
- The buccal smear for detecting sex chromosomes is taken from the inner cheek.

Nursing Interventions
▶ Pretest
- Some states require procurement of an informed, signed, and witnessed consent for genetic testing.
- Explain the purpose and procedure of genetic test, together with known risks.
- Provide information and referrals for appropriate genetic counseling, if necessary.

▶ Posttest
- If an amniotic fluid specimen is obtained for analysis, follow the precautions listed in the alphabetical listing.
- Provide timely information and compassionate support and guidance for parents, children, and significant others.

Special Chromosomal Studies

The fragile X syndrome is one of the most common genetic causes of mental retardation. An X-linked trait, it is most common in males.

Females may carry this gene without exhibiting any of its characteristics; however, they can also be as severely affected as males. In female carriers of this trait, the syndrome becomes harder to detect as the woman ages. Accurate detection of fragile X syndrome using molecular methods is available.

Rare conditions such as excess chromosome breakage (eg, Fanconi's anemia) or abnormal centromeres (eg, Roberts' syndrome) merit special analytic processes and procedures.

Direct Detection of Abnormal Genes by DNA Testing

In the past, abnormal genes were indirectly detected by the effects they produced. These effects typically presented themselves as biochemical or physical manifestations. Now it is possible to directly detect the specific sequence of DNA that causes an abnormality to occur.

Sometimes, detection of abnormal genes relies on the presence of what are called restriction sites. In this case, DNA can be "chopped" into pieces by the introduction of enzymes that attack specific sequences. Genetic maps of the genetic traits for a variety of structural and functional abnormalities can be obtained. Genes can contain several different DNA abnormalities.

Procedure
• Samples or specimens of body fluids or tissues are obtained.

Reference Values

Normal
• Normal genes in chromosomes 1 through 22, X, and Y.

Clinical Implications
• Genes related to abnormal structure and function have been located in each of chromosomes, and new ones are continually being discovered. The known numbers of gene defects related to structural and functional abnormalities for each chromosome are growing, and many others are under investigation. This has led to the improved diagnoses of several types of cancerous tumors (eg, hereditary colon cancer, nonpolypoid type, hereditary breast cancer [BRCA], leukemia, Philadelphia

chromosome, lymphomas, hereditary thyroid cancer, and retinoblastoma).
- Precise DNA tests can be performed for cystic fibrosis, sickle cell anemia, phenylketonuria, Duchenne-Becker muscular dystrophy, hemophilia, thalassemia, polycystic kidneys, alpha$_1$-antitrypsin deficiency, paternity testing, forensic testing, and identification of microbes in infectious diseases (ie, *Chlamydia*, cytomegalovirus, enterovirus, hepatitis B and C viruses, herpes simplex virus, HIV, Lyme disease bacteria *Borrelia burgdorferi*, and *Neisseria gonorrhoeae*).

Procedure
- Obtain venous blood samples from individuals to be studied.

Clinical Implications
- Ideally, related testing techniques (eg, nucleic acid–based detection tests, polymerase chain reaction [PCR]) can be used to detect certain gene disorders (eg, sickle cell anemia). These studies are more specific than linkage studies and may be performed on one individual, if appropriate.

GENITAL TRACT CULTURE AND VAGINAL SMEARS, VAGINAL TRACT AND KOH PREP, GRAM STAINS

Urethral and Vaginal Discharge

Genital tract cultures are obtained to isolate bacterial and viral organisms that may cause infection.

Indications
- Identify by culture microorganisms causing genital infections.
- Evaluate vaginal complaints to diagnose bacterial vaginalis.

Reference Values

Normal
- Growth of normal flora is detected; culture is negative for pathogenic *Neisseria* sp., *Chlamydia* sp., and viral organisms.

- Negative vaginal smears for trichomonal, candidal, and bacterial vaginalis.

Clinical Implications

- Possible pathogens include *Neisseria gonorrhoeae*, *Chlamydia trachomatis*, herpes simplex virus, *Haemophilus ducreyi*, *Trichomonas vaginalis* (a parasite), *Candida* sp., *Gardnerella vaginalis*, *Mycoplasma hominis*, and *Ureaplasma urealyticum*.

Procedure

- Culture specimens are usually collected on Dacron- or rayon-tipped swabs, which are then placed in a modified Stuart's transport medium for recovery of bacterial and yeast organisms. For recovery of *Chlamydia* sp. and herpes simplex virus, an additional swab should be placed in viral transport fluid. For recovery of *Mycoplasma* or *Ureaplasma*, an additional swab should be placed in *Mycoplasma* or *Ureaplasma* transport medium. Place the specimen in a biohazard bag.
- Other vaginal secretion specimens are obtained in the same manner as for culture. A wet prep of vaginal secretion is performed by adding a drop of saline to the vaginal smear, applying a coverslip, and examining the sample by light microscopy. The KOH prep is performed similarly, but a drop of 10% KOH is used instead of saline; the slide may be heated to allow direct visualization of fungus, hyphae, and spores.

Nursing Interventions
▶*Pretest*
- Assess the patient's knowledge about the test.
- Explain the purpose and specimen collection procedure.

▶*Intratest*
- Label specimens with the patient's name, date and time collected, and source of the specimen. Label the accompanying requisition form with the same information. Include the patient's symptoms, tests requested, and contact person or clinic for notification of positive results.

▶*Posttest*
- Promptly deliver specimens to the laboratory.
- Evaluate culture results and counsel the patient regarding the prevention of genital infections and possible treatment.

Gynecologic (GYN) Sonogram—Pelvic Ultrasound, Pelvic Uterine Mass Diagnosis, Intrauterine Device (IUD) Localization

Ultrasound Gynecologic and Bladder Imaging

This noninvasive study is used to visualize the soft tissue structures located in the pelvic cavity, including the urinary bladder, uterus, ovaries, and major pelvic blood vessels. The study examines the area from the umbilicus to the pubic bone in women.

Indications

• Determine the size and characteristics of a palpable pelvic mass and localize the position of an intrauterine contraceptive device.
• Evaluate postmenopausal bleeding.
• Rule out ectopic pregnancy.
• Monitor follicular development in women undergoing infertility treatment.
• Plan treatment and follow-up radiation therapy for gynecologic cancer.

Reference Values

Normal
• Normal pattern image and normal size of the urinary bladder, vagina, uterus, ovaries, and fallopian tubes.
• Normal Doppler flow pattern of major pelvic blood vessels.

Clinical Implications
Abnormal conditions include the following:

• Irregular shapes, enlargement (eg, swelling), change in thickness or thinness of walls
• Fibroids, bicornate uterus, ovarian cysts, metastatic ovarian tumors
• Distortion of the bladder (raises possibility of adjacent tumor)
• Mobility or immobility of pelvic mass

Interfering Factors
• Gas or barium in bowel overlying the pelvic contents obscures the image. Results may be compromised if the patient is obese or has a retroverted uterus.

• Success of transabdominal scans depends on the maintenance of a full bladder during the study.

Procedure
• The transabdominal approach requires a fully distended urinary bladder.
• A coupling gel is applied to area under study to promote transmission of sound. The active face of the transducer is placed in contact with the patient's skin and swept across the area being studied. The examination time is about 10 to 30 minutes.
• The transvaginal (endovaginal) approach does not require a full bladder.
• A small vaginal transducer, protected by a condom or sterile sheath, is lubricated and inserted into the vagina to a depth no greater than 8 cm. Some laboratories prefer that the patient insert the transducer herself. Scans are performed using slight rotational movements of the transducer handle. The examination time is about 10 to 30 minutes.

Nursing Interventions
▶ Pretest
• Explain the examination purpose and procedure. No radiation is used and the test generally is painless. Test preparation, in most cases, requires a full bladder, which generally requires 32 oz (930 mL) of water or clear fluid consumed 1 to 2 hours before the procedure. Instruct the patient not to void until the examination is completed. Discomfort associated with a very full bladder is expected.
• Under certain conditions, a transvaginal (endovaginal) approach is used, which does not require bladder filling. Determine whether the patient has a latex sensitivity and communicate such sensitivities to the examining laboratory.

CLINICAL ALERT

• For oral intake restrictions (NPO status) or in certain emergency situations, the patient may be catheterized to fill the bladder.
• The patient must agree to and sign a surgical consent form before any ultrasound-guided interventional technique, such as oocyte retrieval, is applied.

▶Intratest
- Encourage the patient if maintaining a distended bladder is difficult.

▶Posttest
- Remove or instruct the patient to remove any residual gel from her or his skin.
- Instruct the patient to empty the bladder frequently on completion of a full-bladder study.
- Evaluate outcomes and provide support and counseling as necessary.

HEART SONOGRAM (HEART ECHOGRAM, ECHOCARDIOGRAPHY, ECHOCARDIOGRAM, DOPPLER ECHOCARDIOGRAM)

Ultrasound Heart Imaging

This noninvasive examination of the heart visualizes cardiac structures and provides information about cardiac function.

Indications
- Monitor patients in congestive heart failure who rely on a left ventricular assist device (LVAD).
- Evaluate prosthetic and biologic valve dysfunction and disease; abnormalities of blood flow; and systemic and pulmonary artery hypertension.
- Evaluate myocardial disease.
- Monitor the cardiac patient over an extended period.

Reference Values

Normal
- Normal position, size, and movement of heart valves and chamber walls and normal velocity of blood flow as visualized in two-dimensional, M-mode, and color Doppler.

Clinical Implications
- Abnormal findings indicate valvular disease: stenosis, prolapse, dysfunction, function of prosthetic valves, pericardial effusion, tamponade, structural deformities (congenital and acquired), and aneurysms.

- Myocardial left ventricular dysfunction, hemodynamic disturbances, and cardiac lesions (eg, tumors, thrombi, and endocarditis).
- Congenital heart disease.

Interfering Factors

- Dysrhythmias and hyperinflation of the lungs with mechanical ventilation obscure visualization of cardiac anatomy.
- Marked obesity, chest trauma, and dressings may adversely affect examination outcomes.

Procedure

- The patient is positioned on an examining table in a slight side-lying position.
- An acoustic gel is applied to the skin over the chest and a transducer is moved over various regions of the chest and upper abdomen to obtain appropriate views of the heart.
- Leads may be applied for a simultaneous electrocardiogram.
- Examination time is 30 to 45 minutes.

Nursing Interventions

▶*Pretest*

- Explain the purpose, procedure, and benefits of the test.
- Assure the patient that although there is no pain involved, there may be some discomfort caused by lying quietly for a long period of time.
- Explain that the coupling gel is necessary to permit easier movement of the transducer and thus there may be a feeling of warmth or wetness.

▶*Posttest*

- Interpret test outcomes and counsel the patient appropriately about cardiac disorders and possible need for further testing or treatment (eg, medical, drugs, or surgical).

Helicobacter pylori (HPY) IgG Antibody (PY)

Blood, Breath, Stool

Traditionally, *H. pylori* has been detected by culturing gastric mucosal specimens obtained by endoscopy. These blood tests may be useful as a less-invasive screening test for *H. pylori* infection, with the breath test used to measure active infection. The *H. pylori* stool antigen (HpSa) test is used to monitor response during therapy and to test for cure after treatment.

Indications

- Screen for past or present *H. pylori* infection in persons with or without GI symptoms.
- Diagnose patients with peptic ulcer who are users of NSAIDs.
- Breath test detects gastric urease.

Reference Values

Normal

BLOOD AND STOOL

Negative: No detectable IgG antibody

BREATH

Negative for *H. pylori:* <50 disintegrations per minute (DPM)
  50–199 DPM is indeterminate
  >200 DPM is positive

Clinical Implications

- A positive result indicates the patient has antibodies to *H. pylori.* It does not necessarily indicate that existing symptoms are caused by *H. pylori* infection or colonization. It also does not differentiate between active and past infection.
- A negative result indicates that the patient does not have detectable levels of antibody to *H. pylori.* If a sample is taken too early in *H. pylori* colonization, IgG antibodies may not be present.

Procedure

- Serum (5 mL) in a red-top tube is obtained by venipuncture.
- This testing should be performed only on patients with gastrointestinal symptoms because of the large percentage of *H. pylori*–colonized individuals in the elderly population.
- A breath sample is obtained using a special kit. (See Chapter 2.)
- A random stool sample is obtained. (See Chapter 2.)

Nursing Interventions

▸*Pretest*

- Inform the patient about the test's usefulness as a noninvasive screening test for *H. pylori* infection.

▸*Posttest*

- Evaluate the results in light of the patient's history and other clinical and laboratory findings. Counsel the patient appropriately about treatment (antibodies and acid reducers) and other tests (eg, endoscopy).

HEPATITIS TESTS

Blood

Hepatitis A (HAV), Hepatitis B (HBV), Hepatitis C (HCV), Hepatitis D (HDV), Hepatitis E (HEV), and Hepatitis G (HGV)

These tests are performed to diagnose viral hepatitis. Viruses known to cause hepatitis are referred to by letters—A, B, C, D, E, and G. Abbreviations follow a similar pattern; for example, HAV stands for hepatitis A virus. New viruses, GBV-A, GBV-B, and GBV-C, may be causative agents in non-A through E hepatitis.

Indications

- Evaluate patients with jaundice and other symptoms of hepatitis.
- Aid in differentiation of various types of viral hepatitis, which is difficult because symptoms are similar.
- Evaluate blood products that have been donated for transfusion, as well as donated organs and patients who may have received contaminated blood.

Reference Values

Normal

- Negative (nonreactive) for hepatitis A (HAV), B (HBV), C (HCV), D (HDV), E (HEV), and G (HGV).
- Negative or undetected viral load (<0.01 pg/mL).

Clinical Implications

- Positive (reactive) for viral hepatitis markers.
- Positive for viral genome load (viral replication).

Interfering Factors
- Current methods of testing for hepatitis virus markers are not sensitive enough to detect all possible cases of hepatitis.

Procedure
- Serum (7 mL) is obtained by venipuncture by using a red-top tube or two lavender-top (EDTA) tubes.

Nursing Interventions
▶*Pretest*
- Assess the patient's social and clinical knowledge about the test and clinical symptoms and explain the blood test's purpose and procedure.
- Advise the patient that enteric, blood, and body fluid precautions will be followed until results of hepatitis testing are available.

▶*Posttest*
- Evaluate outcomes and counsel the patient appropriately about the presence of infection, recovery, and immunity. Provide information to the patient regarding precautions (body fluids and wastes) needed to avoid transmission of the virus to others.
- Continue precautions to avoid transmission of virus if test results are positive.
- Because acute hepatitis A is not followed by a chronic stage, no follow-up testing is required.
- Acute hepatitis B, C, and D infections may progress to chronic infections. This progression is suggested by persistent, elevated ALT levels and abnormal liver biopsy 6 months after the acute disease.

CLINICAL ALERT

- Most people are asymptomatic at the time of hepatitis diagnosis.
- Between 5% and 20% of hepatitis cases cannot be attributed to any known viruses. This entity, designated hepatitis X or non-A to E hepatitis, is not associated with toxic, metabolic, or genetic conditions.

TABLE 3.3 summarizes a differential diagnosis of viral hepatitis.

TABLE 3.3 INTERPRETATION OF HEPATITIS B SEROLOGY TESTS

HEPATITIS B SEROLOGY TESTS	TEST RESULTS	CLINICAL INTERPRETATION
HBsAg	Negative	Not infected with hepatitis B; susceptible
Anti-HBc	Negative	
Anti-HBs	Negative	
HBsAg	Negative	Immune due to natural infection
Anti-HBc	Positive	
Anti-HBs	Positive	
HBsAg	Negative	Immune due to hepatitis B vaccination
Anti-HBc	Negative	
Anti-HBs	Positive	
HBsAg	Positive	Acutely infected with hepatitis B
Anti-HBc	Positive	
Anti-HBc IgM	Positive	
Anti-HBs	Negative	
HBsAg	Positive	Chronically infected with hepatitis B
Anti-HBc	Positive	
Anti-HBc IgM	Negative	
Anti-HBs	Negative	
HBsAg	Negative	Interpretation unclear; four possibilities:
Anti-HBc	Positive	1. Resolved infection (most common)
Anti-HBs	Negative	2. False-positive anti-HBc; thus, susceptible
		3. "Low-level" chronic infection
		4. Resolving acute infection

HBsAg, hepatitis B surface antigen; Anti-HBc, total hepatitis B core antibody; Anti-HBc IgM, IgM antibody to hepatitis B core antigen; Anti-HBs, hepatitis B surface antibody.

HOLTER CONTINUOUS ELECTROCARDIOGRAPHIC (ECG) MONITORING

Special Study

For 24 to 48 hours or longer, Holter monitoring continuously records cardiac rhythms, unusual cardiac events, and patient activity.

Indications
- Document dysrhythmias.
- Evaluate chest pain or other symptoms such as syncope, palpitations, dyspnea, or lightheadedness.

- Evaluate cardiac status after acute MI, pacemaker function, and automatic, implantable, defibrillator function.
- Evaluate the effectiveness of drug therapy.

Reference Values

Normal
- Normal cardiac rhythms and heart rates.
- No hypoxic or ischemic ECG changes.

Clinical Implications
- Cardiac dysrhythmias such as premature ventricular contractions (PVCs), conduction defects, tachyarrhythmias, bradyarrhythmias, bradytachyrhythmia syndrome, and heart block.
- Hypoxic or ischemic changes.

Interfering Factors
- Smoking, eating, postural changes, and certain drugs.
- Incomplete diary or failure to "mark" symptoms.
- Interference with electrode placement and adhesion.
- Changes in normal daily routines or activities.

Procedure

- Apply electrodes and attach electrode wires to monitor and recorder pack. Make sure that everything is securely attached and that the recorder has fresh batteries before calibrating and turning it on.
- After the monitoring period is completed, the tape and diary are analyzed for patterns and variations in heart rhythm. The diary provides evidence of a possible correlation between symptoms and results.

Nursing Interventions

▶Pretest
- Explain the test purpose and procedure. Demonstrate how equipment may be attached to body and then removed after 24–48 hours.
- Encourage continuation of normal activities and emphasize diary entries related to activities and symptoms.
- Record time when the monitor is started.
- Do not get the recorder wet and avoid magnets and electric blankets.

▶Posttest
- Remove monitor and record time disconnected.
- Clean the electrode sites with mild soap and water and dry thoroughly.

• Evaluate outcomes and counsel the patient appropriately about further testing (eg, cardiac catheterization) and possible treatment (eg, medication).

CLINICAL ALERT

- The patient should avoid magnets, metal detectors, high-voltage environments, and electric blankets.
- "Itching" under electrodes is common. Do not readjust the placement sites.

HOMOCYSTEINE (THCY)

Fasting Blood, Urine

This test measures the blood plasma level of homocysteine and is used for biochemical analysis of inborn errors of methionine metabolism. Homocysteine probably plays a role in the development of vascular disease, and abnormal values are associated with risk of venous thrombosis and coronary artery disease.

Indications
- Evaluate the risk of premature atherosclerosis and thrombotic disorders associated with high homocysteine levels.
- Provide evidence of vitamin B_{12} and folate deficiency.
- Evaluate renal function in persons with homocystinuria.
- Evaluate risk for atherosclerotic vascular events in persons with end-stage renal disease if concentrations are lowered by hemodialysis.
- Detect cause of unexplained anemia, peripheral neuropathy, and myelopathy.
- Assess women who have recurrent spontaneous abortions or infertility.

Reference Values

Normal
- Plasma: 0.54–2.30 mg/L or 4.0–17.0 μmol/L
- Urine: 0–9 μmol/g or 0–1.0 μmol/mol of creatinine

Clinical Implications

- Increased levels occur in chronic renal failure, reduced renal function, inherited disorders of homocysteine metabolism, folate deficiency, and abnormal vitamin B_{12} metabolism and deficiency.
- Hyperhomocystinemia levels: mild, 2.3–4.0 mg/mL or 17–30 μmol/L; moderate, 4.2–13.5 mg/mL or 31–100 μmol/L; severe, >13.5 mg/mL or >100 μmol/L.

Interfering Factors

- Decreased levels occur after meals, delayed specimen processing, during storage, and in pregnancy (up to 50% decrease).
- Smoking, heavy coffee intake, hostility, and stress increase homocysteine levels.

Procedure

- Obtain a fasting venous blood sample by using a lavender-top (EDTA) tube.
- Place the specimen on ice immediately and transport to the lab in a biohazard bag.
- The choice of anticoagulant is important. Acidified sodium citrate (pH 4.3) stabilizes total homocysteine levels for up to 8 hours at room temperature.
- Obtain a random urine specimen after an overnight fast. Discard the first morning specimen, instruct patient to continue fasting, and collect the next random specimen (need 2 mL), or obtain 5 mL of a random specimen. Send it in a plastic tube on dry ice.

Nursing Interventions

▸Pretest

- Explain the homocysteine test purpose and blood-drawing procedure.
- Instruct the patient that fasting is required.

▸Posttest

- In collaboration with the physician, interpret test results and counsel the patient appropriately about possible relationship of homocysteine levels to coronary artery disease and end-stage renal disease.
- Evaluate other cardiovascular risk factors, compare test results, and monitor the patient appropriately for folic acid or vitamin B_{12} deficiency. Provide folic acid and vitamin B_{12} supplements as needed and promote lifestyle changes accordingly.

HUMAN LEUKOCYTE ANTIGEN (HLA) TYPING

Blood

The major histocompatibility antigens of humans that belong to the HLA system are present on all nucleated cells, but they can be detected most easily on lymphocytes. This test determines the type of leukocyte antigens present on human cell surfaces.

Indications
- Prevent transfusion reactions.
- Evaluate histocompatibility before organ transplantation to prevent transplant rejection.
- Determine parentage and identity.

Reference Values

Normal
- HLA requires clinical correlation with class I, class II, and class III gene regions.
- Match between transplant donor and recipient.

Clinical Implications
- Associations between particular HLAs and disease states include acute anterior ankylosing spondylitis (HLA-B27), multiple sclerosis (HLA-B27 + Dw2 + A3 + B18), myasthenia gravis (HLA-B8), psoriasis (HLA-A13 + B17), Reiter's syndrome (B27), juvenile insulin-dependent diabetes (Bw15 + B8), acute anterior uveitis (B27), Graves' disease (B27), juvenile rheumatoid arthritis (B27), celiac disease (B8), dermatitis herpetiformis (B*), and autoimmune chronic active hepatitis (B8).
- Four groups of cell surface antigens, HLA-A, HLA-B, HLA-C, and HLA-D, constitute the strongest barriers to tissue transplantation.
- In parentage determination, if a reputed father has a phenotype with no haplotype or antigen pair identical with one of the child's, he is excluded as the supposed father. If one of the reputed father's haplotypes is the same as one of the child's, he *may* be the father. The chances of his being accurately identified as the father increase in direct proportion to the rarity of the presenting haplotype in the general population.

Procedure

- A 10- to 24-mL heparinized (green-top tube) venous blood sample is obtained.
- The patient's HLA type is determined by testing the patient's lymphocytes against a panel of defined HLA antiserums directed against recognized HLAs. The HLAs are identified by letters and numbers. When viable human lymphocytes are incubated with a known HLA cytotoxic antibody, an antigen-antibody complex is formed on the cell surface. The addition of serum that contains complement kills the cells, which are then recognized as possessing a defined HLA.

Nursing Interventions

▶ Pretest

- Explain the test purpose and procedure.

▶ Posttest

- Interpret test outcomes and counsel the patient appropriately. HLA testing is best used as a diagnostic adjunct and should not be considered diagnostic in and of itself. Explain the need for possible further testing.

HUMAN T-CELL LYMPHOTROPHIC VIRUS TYPE 1 (HTLV-1) ANTIBODY

Blood

This test detects the presence of antibody to the human T-cell lymphocyte virus type 1 (HTLV-1), a retrovirus associated with adult T-cell leukemia and demyelinating neurologic disorders.

Indications

- Assess patients with clinical diagnosis of adult T-cell leukemia.
- Evaluate patients who have been exposed to the blood of HTLV-1–infected persons through transfusion or sharing of needles for drug use.
- Screen persons whose blood and plasma products are being donated for transfusion.

Reference Values

Normal
- Negative for antibody to HTLV-1.

Clinical Implications
- Positive results suggest HTLV-1 infection. HTLV-1 infection has been confirmed in persons with adult T-cell leukemia, intravenous drug users, and healthy persons.
- Positive results in an asymptomatic person exclude that person from donating blood; this finding does not mean that leukemia or a neurologic disorder will develop.

Procedure
- Serum (7 mL) is obtained by venipuncture using a red-top tube.

Nursing Interventions
▶*Pretest*
- Explain the purpose and procedure of the blood test.

▶*Posttest*
- If the test result is positive, advise the patient that HTLV-1 does not cause AIDS and that the finding of HTLV-1 antibody does not imply infection with HIV or a risk of developing AIDS.
- Provide counseling for the patient to minimize anxiety associated with positive test results.

5-Hydroxyindoleacetic Acid (5-HIAA), 5-Hydroxy-3-Serotonin

Timed Urine

This test is conducted to diagnose a functioning carcinoid tumor, which is indicated by a significant elevation of 5-HIAA, a major urinary metabolite of serotonin.

Indications
- Diagnose functioning carcinoid tumors, pancreatic or duodenal tumors, and biliary tumors.

Reference Values

Normal
- Quantitative: 2–7 mg/24 hours or 11–37 μmol/day

Clinical Implications
- *Levels higher than* 25 mg/24 hours or >130 μmol/day are indicative of carcinoid tumor, especially when metastatic.
- *Increased levels* are associated with celiac disease, Whipple's disease, cystic fibrosis, oat-cell cancer of bronchus, bronchial adenoma of the carcinoid type, chronic intestinal obstruction, sprue, and malabsorption.
- *Decreased levels* are associated with depressive illness, small intestine resection, mastocytosis, phenylketonuria (PKU), and Hartnup's disease.

Interfering Factors
- False-positive results can result if bananas, pineapples, plums, chocolate, walnuts, eggplant, tomatoes, and avocados are eaten within 48 hours of the test because they contain serotonin.
- False-positive results can result with drug use: phenacetin, salicylates, reserpine (Serpasil), and methamphetamine (Desoxyn).
- False-negative results can result with drug use: imipramine (Tofranil), methyldopa (Aldomet), MAO inhibitors, promethazine (Phenergan), phenothiazines, and naproxen (Anaprox).

Procedure
- Collect urine for 24 hours in a clean container; it may need an acid preservative (pH < 4.0). Refrigerate during collection.
- See the timed specimen collection guidelines in Chapter 2.

Nursing Interventions
▸ *Pretest*
- Assess the patient's compliance and knowledge base before explaining the test purpose and procedure. Note pertinent history of flushing, hepatomegaly, diarrhea, bronchospasm, and heart disorders.
- Ensure that the patient does not take drugs for 72 hours before the test, if possible, and does not eat foods listed previously for 48 hours before the test. Discontinue acetaminophen, naproxen, imipramine, and monoamine oxidase inhibitors for 48 hours.

▸ *Intratest*
- Accurate test results depend on proper collection, preservation, and labeling. Be sure to record the test start and completion times.

- Food and water are permitted, but ensure that foods high in serotonin content are not to be eaten during the test.

▸Posttest
- Evaluate the test outcome and provide counseling and support as appropriate about carcinoid tumors and depression.

25-Hydroxyvitamin D (25-OHD)

Blood

Vitamin D comes from two sources: produced in the skin upon exposure to sunlight and obtained from ingestion of food or oral supplements. This test measures the amount of vitamin D present to determine if there is vitamin D sufficiency.

Indications
- Assess for vitamin D deficiency or excess and monitor treatment.
- Assess for abnormal calcium, phosphorous, and/or parathyroid hormone levels.
- Assess for evidence of bone disease or bone weakness.
- Evaluate high-risk women (eg, elderly, malabsorption syndrome).

Reference Values

Normal
- 30–60 ng/mL or 75–150 nmol/L
- Optimal: 30 ng/mL or 75 nmol/L

Clinical Implications
- Decreased levels of 25-OHD may increase risk of some cancers, immune diseases, and cardiovascular disease.
- Increased levels of 25-OHD typically reflect excess intake and can potentially lead to kidney or blood vessel damage.

Interfering Factors
- Some drugs used to treat seizures (eg, Dilantin) can interfere with 25-OHD production.

Procedure
- Obtain serum (4.0 mL) by venipuncture using an SST or red-top tube.

- Place serum in a biohazard bag and transport to the clinical laboratory.

Nursing Interventions
▸*Pretest*
- Explain purpose and procedure of the test.

▸*Posttest*
- Evaluate outcomes and counsel patient for treatment, eg, vitamin D supplementation through dietary intake (cod liver oil, milk, fortified cereals, fruit juice) in deficient states. The current recommended dietary allowance (RDA) for adults is at least 2000 IU daily. Magnesium and calcium supplements may also be indicated in certain circumstances.

IgE Antibodies, Allergy Testing

Blood

A large number of substances have been found to have allergic potential. Measurements of IgE antibodies are useful to establish the presence of allergic diseases and to define the allergen specificity of immediate hypersensitivity reactions.

Indications
- Diagnose an allergy to a specific allergen (eg, mold, grasses, weeds, food, insects, animal dander, venoms, and dust mites).
- Identify specific allergens that cause asthma, hay fever, and atopic eczema.

Reference Values

Normal

Test results are reported as negative or positive by fluorescent enzyme immunoassay (FEIA), a laboratory method.

Negative: Class 0—rules out an allergy induced by a specific allergen
Positive: Class 1—equivocal
    Classes 2 to 3—positive
    Classes 4 to 6—strongly positive

Clinical Implications

- Detection of an allergen-specific IgE indicates immediate hypersensitivity to an allergen.
- A positive result is diagnostic of an allergy to a particular allergen or allergens, regardless of the total IgE level.

Procedure

- Serum (7 mL) is obtained by venipuncture in a red-top tube for each group of three panels.

Nursing Interventions

▶*Pretest*

- Assess the patient's history, hypersensitivity reactions, medication use, dietary history, environmental situations in relation to potential allergens, and history of localized itching (wheal and flare), ranging from anaphylactic shock to laryngeal edema to diarrhea.

▶*Posttest*

- Advise the patient that if the test is positive for a specific allergen, additional allergens may be tested from more than 100 categories.
- After the allergen is identified, instruct the patient what to avoid, such as specific medications, foods, animals, dust, and other allergens.
- If medication therapy is begun, instruct the patient regarding the therapy program.

IMMUNOGLOBULINS: IgG, IgA, AND IgM

Blood, Immune Disorders

Quantitative immunoglobulin measurements of IgG, IgA, and IgM can detect and monitor monoclonal gammopathies and immune deficiencies. This test is often ordered in conjunction with a serum protein electrophoresis (SPE). The gammaglobulin band as seen in conventional SPE consists of five immunoglobulins. In normal serum, approximately 80% (SI = 0.80) is IgG, 15% (SI = 0.15) is IgA, and 5% (SI = 0.05) belongs to the IgM class. There are only trace amounts of IgD and IgE.

Indications

- Investigate the suspicion of multiple myeloma and other myeloproliferative disorders.
- Assess the history of repeated infections, as may occur with congenital deficiencies.
- Monitor effectiveness of therapy through repeat testing.

Reference Values

Normal

Based on rate nephelometry, the normal immunoglobulin values for men and women 18 years or older are as follows:

IgG:	500–1500 mg/dL or 5.0–15.0 g/L
IgA:	100–490 mg/dL or 1.0–4.9 g/L
IgM:	50–300 mg/dL or 0.5–3.0 g/L
IgE:	<100 IU/mL or <100 kIU/L
IgD:	<3 U/mL or <3 kU/L

Total IgG (Males and Females)

0–4 months:	141–930 mg/dL or 1.4–9.3 g/L
5–8 months:	250–1190 mg/dL or 2.5–11.9 g/L
9–11 months:	320–1250 mg/dL or 3.2–12.5 g/L
1–3 years:	400–1250 mg/dL or 4.0–12.5 g/L
4–6 years:	560–1308 mg/dL or 5.6–13.0 g/L
7–9 years:	598–1379 mg/dL or 5.9–13.7 g/L
10–12 years:	638–1453 mg/dL or 6.3–14.5 g/L
13–15 years:	680–1531 mg/dL or 6.8–15.3 g/L
16–17 years:	724–1611 mg/dL or 7.2–16.1 g/L
>18 years:	700–1500 mg/dL or 7.0–15.0 g/L

IgA (Males and Females)

0–4 months:	5–64 mg/dL or 0.05–0.64 g/L
5–8 months:	10–87 mg/dL or 0.10–0.87 g/L
9–14 months:	17–94 mg/dL or 0.17–0.94 g/L
15–23 months:	22–178 mg/dL or 0.22–1.7 g/L
2–3 years:	24–192 mg/dL or 0.24–1.9 g/L
4–6 years:	26–232 mg/dL or 0.26–2.3 g/L
7–9 years:	33–258 mg/dL or 0.33–2.5 g/L
10–12 years:	45–285 mg/dL or 0.45–2.8 g/L
13–15 years:	47–317 mg/dL or 0.47–3.1 g/L
16–17 years:	55–377 mg/dL or 0.55–3.7 g/L
>18 years:	60–400 mg/dL or 0.60–4.0 g/L

IgM (Males and Females)

0–4 months:	14–142 mg/dL or 0.1–1.4 g/L
5–8 months:	24–167 mg/dL or 0.2–1.6 g/L
9–23 months:	35–242 mg/dL or 0.3–2.4 g/L
2–3 years:	41–242 mg/dL or 0.4–2.4 g/L
4–17 years:	56–242 mg/dL or 0.5–2.4 g/L
>18 years:	60–300 mg/dL or 0.6–3.0 g/L

IgE (Males and Females)

0–12 months:	<15 IU/mL or <15 kIU/L
1–5 years:	<60 IU/mL or <60 kIU/L
6–9 years:	<90 IU/mL or <90 kIU/L
10–16 years:	<200 IU/mL or <200 kIU/L
>16 years:	<100 IU/mL or <100 kIU/L

IgD (Males and Females)

All ages:	<3 U/mL or <3 kU/L

Clinical Implications: IgG

- *IgG levels increase* in infections of all types, hyperimmunization, liver disease, malnutrition (severe), dysproteinemia, disease associated with hypersensitivity granulomas, dermatologic disorders, IgG myeloma, and rheumatoid arthritis.
- *IgG levels decrease* in agammaglobulinemia, lymphoid aplasia, selective IgG or IgA deficiency, IgA myeloma, Bence Jones proteinuria, and chronic lymphoblastic leukemia.

Clinical Implications: IgA

- *IgA levels increase* in chronic, nonalcoholic liver diseases, primary biliary cirrhosis (PBC), obstructive jaundice, a wide range of conditions that affect mucosal surfaces, during exercise, with alcoholism, and in subacute and chronic infections.
- *IgA levels decrease* in ataxia-telangiectasia, chronic sinopulmonary disease, congenital defects, late pregnancy, prolonged exposure to benzene, immunosuppressive therapy, and protein-losing gastroenteropathies.

> **CLINICAL ALERT**
>
> - Persons with IgA deficiency are predisposed to autoimmune disorders and can develop antibody to IgA with possible anaphylaxis occurring if transfused with blood containing IgA.

Clinical Implications: IgM

- *IgM levels increase* in adults with Waldenström's macroglobuline-mia, trypanosomiasis, actinomycosis, Carrion's disease (ie, bartonellosis), malaria, infectious mononucleosis, SLE, rheuma-toid arthritis, and dysgammaglobulinemia (certain cases).
- *IgM levels decrease* in agammaglobulinemia, lymphoproliferative disorders (certain cases), lymphoid aplasia, IgG and IgA myeloma, dysgammaglobulinemia, and chronic lymphoblastic leukemia.

CLINICAL ALERT

- In the newborn, an IgM level higher than 20 mg/dL is an indication of in utero stimulation of the immune system by the rubella virus, and cytomegalovirus infection, syphilis, or toxoplasmosis.

Procedure

- Serum (5 mL) in the adult is obtained by venipuncture in a red-top tube.
- If a test is requested for a child, a 2- to 3-mL venous blood sample should prove sufficient to run the test by rate nephelometry.

Nursing Interventions

▶*Pretest*

- Explain that quantitative immunoglobulins are used for screening purposes to assess immune competence and provide base values.
- Explain that, depending on results, further confirmatory testing, such as SPE or immunofixation electrophoresis (IFE), may be needed.

▶*Posttest*

- Evaluate results and counsel the patient appropriately.

INFECTIOUS MONONUCLEOSIS (IM), RAPID SCREENING TEST (MONOSPOT) FOR HETEROPHILE ANTIBODY TITER, EPSTEIN-BARR (EB) ANTIBODIES TO VIRAL CAPSID NUCLEAR ANTIGENS (EBNA)

Blood

These tests measure heterophile antibodies and antibodies specific for Epstein-Barr virus (EBV).

Indications

- Evaluate patients with clinical symptoms (eg, fever, pharyngitis, and lymphadenopathy) of infectious mononucleosis and atypical lymphocytosis.
- Provide a differential diagnosis of chronic fatigue syndrome.
- Provide a differential diagnosis of acute lymphoblastic leukemia.

Reference Values

Normal

- Negative for infectious mononucleosis antibody titers, negative for infectious mononucleosis, and negative for EBV antibodies.

Clinical Implications

- Heterophile antibodies develop after the first week or two of illness in 90% of symptomatic young adults and remain elevated for 8 to 12 weeks after symptoms appear. If the heterophile test is negative for symptomatic individuals, tests for specific EBV antibodies are performed.
- The presence of heterophile antibodies (ie, Monospot), along with clinical signs and other positive blood work (eg, lymphocytes), is diagnostic for infectious mononucleosis.
- In chronic fatigue syndrome, EBV antibody levels stay elevated for the length of the disease.
- Ninety percent of adults are found to have antibodies to EBV.

Procedure

- Obtain a venous blood serum sample (7 mL) in a red-top tube.

Nursing Interventions

▶ *Pretest*

- Assess the patient's clinical history, symptoms, and knowledge about the test.
- Explain the purpose and procedure of the blood test. If preliminary tests are negative, follow-up tests may be necessary.

▶ *Posttest*

- Evaluate outcomes and monitor and counsel the patient appropriately.
- After primary exposure, a person is considered immune.

INTRAVENOUS PYELOGRAM (IVP)-EXCRETORY UROGRAPHY (EU); INTRAVENOUS UROGRAPHY (IVU); KIDNEY, URETER, AND BLADDER (KUB)-FLAT PLATE X-RAY

X-ray Abdomen (no contrast), Genitourinary (GU) System, and Renal Function with Contrast

These x-ray examinations are used to evaluate the anatomy of kidneys, ureters, and the bladder (KUB) by flat plate (without contrast) and indirectly demonstrate renal function following intravenous contrast agent injection.

Indications

- IVP—diagnose kidney and ureter disease and impaired renal function.
- KUB—rule out ascites, fluid collection, organ enlargement, rupture, calculi, masses, foreign bodies, and intestinal obstruction.
- Evaluate abdominal pain.
- Create preliminary film before contrast studies and surgery.

Reference Values

Normal
- Normal size, shape, and position of the KUB.
- Normal renal function.
- No residual urine on the postvoid film.

Clinical Implications
- Evidence of congenital deformities (eg, duplication of the pelvis or ureter, one kidney or more than two); renal or ureteral calculi, hydronephrosis, and masses (eg, cysts, tumors, hematomas, abscess); renal size deviations; disease of the urinary tract; and degree of renal injury from trauma, polycystic kidney disease, or obstruction.
- Kidney in the presence of failure (if a normal-size kidney, suggests acute rather than chronic disease process), irregular scarring of renal outlines in chronic pyelonephritis, and prostate enlargement (male).
- Delayed time of visualization of contrast media indicative of renal dysfunction. No contrast visualization may indicate very poor or no renal function.
- Evidence of ascites.

Interfering Factors

- Retained feces or intestinal gas can obscure visualization of the urinary tract.
- Retained barium can obscure optimal views of the kidneys. For this reason, barium tests should be scheduled after IVU and KUB x-rays should be scheduled before any barium tests.

Procedure

- For KUB alone, the patient lies on his or her back. Additional films may be taken with the patient standing or lying on his or her side.
- A preliminary abdominal x-ray film (KUB) is taken with the patient in a supine position to ensure that the bowel is empty and the kidney location can be visualized. A radiopaque iodine contrast agent is injected intravenously, usually into the antecubital vein. A series of three x-ray films is taken at predetermined intervals.
- After three films of the renal structures are taken, the patient is asked to void, to determine the ability of the bladder to empty, followed by a postvoid film.
- Total examination time is 45 to 60 minutes. Examination length may be increased if there is a physiologic delay that prevents rapid clearing of contrast by the kidneys.
- Computed tomography (CT) or plain tomography may be performed in conjunction with IVU to obtain better visualization of renal lesions. This increases the examination time. If a kidney CT scan or nephrotomograms are ordered separately, the procedure and preparation are the same as for IVU.

Nursing Interventions
▶*Pretest*

- Assess for test contraindications, including pregnancy, allergy or sensitivity to iodine contrast agents, severe renal or hepatic dysfunction, oliguria or anuria, multiple myeloma, advanced pulmonary tuberculosis, congestive heart failure, pheochromocytoma, and sickle cell anemia.
- Contraindications include medications received for chronic bronchitis, emphysema, or asthma; elevated BUN and creatinine levels; and food or beverage consumed 90 minutes before contrast administration.

CLINICAL ALERT

- If the patient has diabetes and takes oral drugs, special precautions may be necessary before and after the procedure.

- Observe iodine contrast test precautions. Assess for all allergies and determine any prior allergic reactions to contrast substances.
- Because a relative state of dehydration is necessary for contrast material to concentrate in the urinary tract, instruct the patient to abstain from all food, liquid, and medication for 12 hours before examination.

▶Intratest

- Encourage the patient to follow the breathing and positional instructions. Instruct the patient to breathe slowly and deeply during contrast administration. Have an emesis basin and tissue wipes available.
- Observe the patient closely for signs of allergic reaction (eg, hives, respiratory distress, palpitations, numbness, diaphoresis, changes in BP, convulsions). Be prepared with emergency drugs, equipment, and supplies.
- Assist the patient, if necessary, with voiding for the postvoid film.

▶Posttest

- Instruct the patient that he or she may resume the prescribed diet and activity after the test.
- Provide sufficient fluids to replace those lost during the pretest phase. Encourage rest as needed after the test.
- Observe the patient for evidence of mild reactions such as nausea, rashes, hives, and swelling of the parotid glands (iodonium). Oral antihistamines may relieve more severe symptoms. Document these reactions, and inform the physician.
- Evaluate outcomes and explain the need for further testing and possible treatment (eg, medication for tuberculosis, surgery for kidney masses).

IODINE-131 WHOLE-BODY (TOTAL-BODY) IMAGING; WHOLE-BODY IODINE IMAGING

Nuclear Medicine Scan, Endocrine Imaging

This study uses radioactive iodine to identify functioning thyroid tissue throughout the body and localize thyroid cancer.

Indications

- Localize metastatic thyroid cancer.
- Identify postthyroidectomy residual tissue.
- Monitor ^{131}I thyroid therapy for thyroid cancer.

Reference Values

Normal

- Normal whole-body ^{131}I image shows no evidence of abnormal radiopharmaceutical distribution.
- No functioning extrathyroidal tissue is found outside of the thyroid gland.

Clinical Implications

- Abnormal iodine uptake reveals areas of extrathyroidal tissue (ie, stroma ovarii, substernal thyroid, and sublingual thyroid).
- Metastatic thyroid cancer and residual tissue after thyroidectomy may be identified.

CLINICAL ALERT

- When possible, this test should be performed before any other nuclear medicine scans or radionuclide procedures and before administration of iodine contrast agents, surgical preparation, or other forms of iodine intake.
- The test is most effective when thyroid-stimulating hormone (TSH) levels are high to stimulate radionuclide uptake by metastatic neoplasms.

Procedure

- The radionuclide is administered orally in a capsule form.
- Imaging takes place 24 to 72 hours after administration and may take as long as 2 hours to complete.
- Sometimes, TSH is administered intravenously before the radionuclide is administered. This stimulates any residual thyroid tissue and enhances ^{131}I uptake.

Nursing Interventions

▸Pretest

- Explain the total-body imaging purpose, procedure, benefits, and risks.

- Advise the patient that the imaging process may take several hours. Assess for iodine allergies, document them, and treat the patient for possible reactions.

▶ *Posttest*

- Evaluate outcomes and counsel the patient appropriately regarding further tests, follow-up scans, and possible treatment.
- Monitor injection site for signs of infection or extravasation.

IRON TESTS

Blood, Fasting

Iron (Fe), Total Iron-Binding Capacity (TIBC), Transferrin Iron Saturation, Ferritin

These tests measure forms of iron storage in the body and are helpful in the differential diagnosis of anemia, in the assessment of iron deficiency anemia, and in the evaluation of thalassemia, hemochromatosis, and sideroblastic anemia.

Indications

- Evaluate iron absorption and ability of the body to deal with infection.
- Evaluate iron deficiency and blood loss.
- Aid in the diagnosis or differentiation of anemias.
- Evaluate iron poisoning and overload in renal dialysis patients.

Reference Values

Normal

Iron
    Men: 70–175 μg/dL or 12.5–31.3 μmol/L
    Women: 50–150 μg/dL or 8.9–26.8 μmol/L
    Newborns: 100–250 μg/dL or 17.9–44.8 μmol/L
    Children: 50–120 μg/dL or 8.9–21.5 μmol/L
Total iron-binding capacity (TIBC): 229–365 μg/dL or
    41.2–65.7 μmol/L
Transferrin: 215–375 mg/dL or 2.15–3.75 g/L
Transferrin iron saturation:
    Men: 10%–50%
    Women: 15%–50%

Ferritin
    Men: 18–270 ng/mL or μg/L
    Women: 18–160 ng/mL or μg/L
    Children: 7–140 ng/mL or μg/L
    Newborns: 25–200 ng/mL or μg/L

Critical Values

Iron
    Toxicity level: Children: 350–500 μg/dL or 63–90 μmol/L
    Severe poisoning: Children: 800–1000 μg/dL or 145–180 μmol/L
Ferritin
    <10 or >400 ng/mL or <10 or >400 μg/L

Clinical Implications: Transferrin

- *Transferrin levels increase* in iron deficiency anemia.
- *Transferrin levels decrease* in microcytic anemia of chronic disease, protein deficiency, liver and renal disease, genetic deficiency, and iron-overload states.

Interfering Factors: Transferrin

- Age (elevated in 2.5- to 10-year-olds), third-trimester pregnancy, some drugs (ie, chloramphenicol and fluorides), estrogen therapy, and contraceptives affect levels.

Clinical Implications: Iron

- Iron levels *increase* in hemolytic anemias, especially thalassemia, hepatitis, hemochromatosis, and lead poisoning.
- Iron levels *decrease* with iron deficiency anemia, chronic blood loss, insufficient dietary intake, inadequate absorption and impaired release of iron stores as in inflammation, infection, and chronic diseases and in the third trimester of pregnancy.

Interfering Factors: Iron

- Iron-chelating agents (eg, Desferal [deferoxamine]), antibiotics, aspirin, and testosterone decrease iron levels.
- Gross hemolysis of serum interferes with testing.
- Ethanol, estrogens, and oral contraceptives increase iron levels.
- Diurnal variation occurs, with high (normal) levels in the morning and low levels in the evening.

Clinical Implications: TIBC

- *TIBC decreases* in iron deficiency anemias, malignancies of the small intestines, anemia of infection and chronic disease, and iron neoplasms.

- *TIBC increases* in hemochromatosis, hemosiderosis, thalassemia, and iron overload.

Clinical Implications: Ferritin
- *Ferritin levels increase* with iron overload from hemochromatosis or hemosiderosis, acute or chronic liver disease, malignancies and chronic inflammatory diseases, acute myoplastic or lymphoblastic leukemia, hyperthyroidism, hemolytic anemia, megaloblastic anemia, and thalassemia.
- *Ferritin levels decrease* in iron deficiency anemia.

Interfering Factors: Ferritin
- Recently administered radiopharmaceuticals for nuclear scans cause spurious results.
- Oral contraceptives or hemolyzed blood interfere with testing.

Procedure
- A venous serum blood sample (10 mL) is obtained by using a red-top tube.
- Serum should be drawn from a patient fasting in the morning. Circadian rhythm affects the iron levels, which increase in the morning and decrease in the evening.

Nursing Interventions
▸Pretest
- Explain the purpose and procedure of the test.
- Draw fasting blood in the morning, when levels are higher.
- Draw samples before iron therapy or transfusion. The test must wait 4 days if a transfusion has been received.
- Note whether the patient is taking oral contraceptives or is on estrogen therapy or is pregnant.

▸Posttest
- Resume normal activities.
- Interpret test outcome and monitor appropriately. The combination of low serum iron, high TIBC, and high transferrin levels indicates iron deficiency. Diagnosis of iron deficiency may lead further to detection of adenocarcinoma of the gastrointestinal tract, a point that cannot be overemphasized. A significant minority of patients with megaloblastic anemias (20%–40%) have coexisting iron deficiency. Megaloblastic anemia can interfere with the interpretation of iron studies; repeat iron studies 1 to 3 months after folate or vitamin B_{12} replacement.

KIDNEY FUNCTION TESTS

Blood, Urine

Blood Urea Nitrogen (BUN), Uric Acid, Osmolality, Cystatin C

These tests are performed to measure kidney function, diagnose renal failure and kidney disease, and aid in kidney dialysis management.

Indications

- Measure BUN as an index of renal function, the production and excretion of urea, and creatinine level. BUN should be checked in patients who are confused, disoriented, or convulsing.
- Check uric acid levels to evaluate gout, renal failure, and the treatment of leukemia.
- Assess urine osmolality to evaluate its concentration, hydration, SIADH, and diabetes insipidus.
- Measure blood serum osmolality for toxic alcohol ingestion and to evaluate coma.
- Measure serum cystatin C (low-molecular-weight proteinase inhibitor) to assess glomerular filtration in the elderly.
- Note that creatinine clearance is usually performed with other tests of kidney function.

Reference Values

Normal

BUN

Adults: 7–18 mg/dL or 2.5–6.4 mmol/L
>60 years: 8–20 mg/dL or 2.9–7.5 mmol/L
Critical value for adults: BUN <2 mg/dL or >80 mg/dL (<0.71 or >28.6 mmol/L)
Children: 5–18 mg/dL or 1.8–6.4 mmol/L
BUN/Creatinine ratio: 10:1–20:1

BLOOD URIC ACID

Men: 3.4–7.0 mg/dL or 202–416 μmol/L
Women: 2.4–6.0 mg/dL or 143–357 μmol/L
Children: 2.0–5.5 mg/dL or 119–327 μmol/L

Urine

Normal diet: 250–750 mg/24 hours or 1.48–4.43 mmol/day
Purine-free diet: <400 mg/24 hours or <2.48 mmol/day
High-purine diet: <1000 mg/24 hours or <5.90 mmol/day

Osmolality, Serum

Adults: 275–295 mOsm/kg
Critical value for adults: <250 or >325 mOsm/kg
Newborns: As low as 266 mOsm/kg

Osmolality, Urine

Random: 50–1200 mOsm/kg of H_2O
24-hour specimen: 300–900 mOsm/kg of H_2O
After 12-hour fluid restriction: >850 mOsm/L
Ratio of serum/urine osmolality: 1:1–3:1
Ratio of serum/urine: >3:1 with overnight dehydration

Osmolality Gap

Serum: 5–10 mOsm/kg H_2O
Urine: 80–100 mOsm/kg H_2O

Cystatin C, Serum

Normal:
  Young adults: <0.70 mg/mL or <2.9 μmol/mL
  Elderly adults: <0.85 mg/mL or <3.5 μmol/mL

Clinical Implications: BUN

- *BUN increases* (ie, azotemia) in impaired renal function, acute renal disease, shock, dehydration, diabetes, ketoacidosis, acute MI, congestive heart failure, urinary tract obstruction, and excessive protein intake or protein catabolism, as occurs with burns or cancer.
- *BUN decreases* in liver failure and disease, malnutrition, acromegaly, anabolic steroid usage, celiac disease, and syndrome of inappropriate antidiuretic hormone (SIADH).

Interfering Factors: BUN

- *BUN decreases* with a low-protein and high-carbohydrate diet, in persons with smaller muscle mass, during early pregnancy, with many drugs, and with overhydration.
- *BUN increases* in late pregnancy, in older adults, and with many drugs.

Clinical Implications: Uric Acid

- *Uric acid levels are elevated* (ie, hyperuricemia) in renal failure, gout, leukemia, lymphoma, hemolytic anemia, severe eclampsia,

alcoholism, psoriasis, metabolic acidosis, lead poisoning, Down's syndrome, hypothyroidism, and hyperlipidemia.
- *Uric acid levels are decreased* (ie, hypouricemia) after treatment with uricosuric drugs (ie, allopurinol, probenecid, and sulfinpyrazone) and in Fanconi syndrome, Hodgkin's disease, some carcinomas, Wilson's disease, xanthinuria, and SIADH.

Interfering Factors: Uric Acid
- Stress, fasting, and strenuous exercise increase levels of uric acid.
- Many drugs (eg, long-term use of diuretics) and foods may affect levels.

Clinical Implications: Osmolality
- *Urine osmolality increases* (ie, hyperosmolality) are associated with dehydration, alcohol ingestion (eg, ethanol, methanol, and ethylene glycol), mannitol therapy, azotemia, inadequate water intake, chronic renal disease, amyloidosis, and Addison's disease.
- *Urine osmolality decreases* (ie, hypo-osmolality) are associated with loss of sodium with diuretics and a low-salt diet (ie, hyponatremia), hypokalemia, hypernatremia, SIADH (eg, trauma, lung cancer), excessive water replacement (eg, overhydration), panhypopituitarism, compulsive water drinking, diabetes insipidus, and hypercalcemia.

Clinical Implications: Osmolal Gap
- Abnormal values (>10 mOsm/kg) occur with methanol, ethanol, isopropyl alcohol, and mannitol and in severely ill patients, especially those in shock, with lactic acidosis, and with renal failure.
- Ethanol glycol, acetone, and paraldehyde have relatively small osmolal gaps, even at lethal levels.

Interfering Factors: Osmolality or Osmolal Gap
- *Decreases* are associated with altitude, diurnal variation with water retention at night, and some drugs.
- Some drugs increase values.
- Hypertriglyceridemia and hyperproteinemia elevate the osmolal gap value.

Clinical Implications: Cystatin C
- Cystatin C levels increase with impaired renal function.

Procedure
- A 24-hour specimen or random morning urine specimen is collected for osmolality after a high-protein diet for 3 days. Follow the guidelines in Chapter 2 for collection of blood and urine specimens.

- Serum (7 mL) is obtained by venipuncture by using a red-top tube.
- No fasting is required.

Nursing Interventions

▶ Pretest
- Explain the purpose and procedure of the test.
- The patient should avoid stress and strenuous exercise.

▶ Posttest
- Evaluate the outcome and monitor the patient appropriately.
- Make provision for further tests that may be needed to investigate impaired excretion of water, such as a water-loading antidiuretic hormone suppression test.

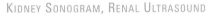

KIDNEY SONOGRAM, RENAL ULTRASOUND

Ultrasound Imaging, GU System

This noninvasive study is used to visualize the renal parenchyma, renal blood vessels, and associated structures. It is often performed after an intravenous pyelogram (IVP) to define and characterize mass lesions or the cause of a nonvisualized kidney.

Indications
- Characterize renal masses (ie, cystic or solid) and infectious processes, visualization of large calculi, and detection of ectopic or malformed kidneys.
- Provide guidance during biopsy, cyst aspiration, stent placement, and other invasive procedures.
- Monitor status of renal transplants and kidney development in children with congenital hydronephrosis.

Reference Values

Normal
- Normal pattern image indicating normal size and position of kidneys.
- Appropriate blood flow of renal vessels.

Clinical Implications
- Presence of space-occupying lesions, such as cysts, solid masses, hydronephrosis, or obstruction of ureters or calculi.

- Altered blood flow to or from the kidney.
- Size, site, and internal structure of nonfunctioning kidney.
- Spread of cancerous conditions from the kidney to the renal vein or inferior vena cava.

Interfering Factors

- Retained barium from prior radiographic studies may cause suboptimal results.
- Obesity adversely affects tissue visualization.

Procedure

- A coupling gel is applied to the exposed abdomen to promote transmission of sound.
- A handheld transducer is slowly moved across the skin during this imaging procedure. The patient is instructed to control the breathing pattern while imaging is performed. Both kidneys are routinely visualized.
- The examination time is 15–30 minutes.

Nursing Interventions

▶*Pretest*

- Explain the purpose and procedure of the examination.
- Limited preparation may be necessary. Some laboratories require patients to fast for 8 to 12 hours before the procedure.
- Explain that a coupling gel will be applied to skin. Although the couplant does not stain, advise the patient to avoid wearing nonwashable clothing.
- Doppler assessment of the renal blood vessels will yield a "swishing" sound that may be heard by the patient.

▶*Posttest*

- Evaluate the outcome and provide the patient with support and counseling about further testing (eg, CT scans, biopsies).

KLEIHAUER-BETKE TEST, FETAL HEMOGLOBIN STAIN

Blood at Time of Delivery of a Baby

The Kleihauer-Betke test is performed to determine the amount of fetomaternal hemorrhage in an Rh-D–negative mother and the amount of RhG (RhoGAM) necessary to prevent antibody production.

Indications
- Determine fetal-maternal hemorrhage in newborn.
- Diagnose certain types of anemia (HbF) in adults.
- Ascertain unexplained increased level of maternal alpha-fetoprotein (AFP).
- Diagnose intrauterine death.
- Find the cause of unexplained newborn anemia.
- Screen all Rh-negative women having a cesarean section (C-section) for fetal maternal hemorrhage and screen after amniocentesis and trauma.

Reference Values

Normal
- Negative: no fetal cells in the maternal circulation; no HbF in blood of adults.

Clinical Implications
- Abnormal results indicate moderate to great fetomaternal hemorrhage (50%–90% of fetal RBCs contain HbF).

Procedure
- A 7-mL maternal venous whole-blood sample (EDTA tube) is obtained during pregnancy, immediately after delivery, or after invasive procedures (amniocentesis), miscarriage, or trauma.
- The specimen should be examined immediately (<6 hours) or refrigerated.
- A cord blood specimen should also be obtained and tested for use as a positive control.

Nursing Interventions
▶*Pretest*
- Explain the test purpose and procedure to the mother or parents.

▶*Posttest*
- Interpret test outcomes and counsel parents appropriately regarding fetomaternal bleeding and RhIG to suppress the immunization of fetal red blood cells or whole-blood hemorrhage. (Overtreatment is better than undertreatment.)

LAPAROSCOPY (MEDICAL)—PELVISCOPY, PERITONEOSCOPY

Endoscopic Imaging, GYN Interventional Procedure

These minimally invasive procedures allow the intra-abdominal (greater curvature of the stomach or liver) and pelvic organs and cavities to be examined and tissue specimens to be obtained.

Indications

- Peritoneoscopy: Evaluate liver disease; obtain liver biopsy when liver is too small, when previous liver biopsy proves inadequate, and when liver cannot be properly palpated before a conventional liver biopsy (does away with the need to do *blind* liver biopsy); evaluate portal hypertension, unexplained ascites, ovarian carcinoma, for staging lymphomas or for evaluating other abdominal masses.
- Laparoscopy: Evaluate advanced chest, gastric, pancreatic, endometrial, or rectal tumors.
- Pelviscoscopy: Gynecologic laparoscopy: Diagnose cysts, adhesions, fibroids, malignancies, inflammatory process, and infections.
- Evaluate infertility.
- Perform tubal ligation and laser treatment of endometriosis.

Reference Values

Normal

Gynecologic: Uterus, ovaries, and fallopian tubes normal in size, shape, and appearance.

Intraabdominal: Liver, gallbladder, spleen, and greater curvature of stomach normal in size, shape, and appearance.

Clinical Implications

- Abnormal pelvic findings include evidence of endometriosis, ovarian cysts, pelvic inflammatory disease, carcinoma, metastatic sites, uterine fibroids, abscesses, hydrosalpinx (enlarged fallopian tubes), ectopic pregnancy, infection.
- Adhesions, ascites, cirrhosis, liver nodules (often a sign of cancer), engorged vasculature (portal hypertension).

Procedure

- Protocols for local, spinal, or general surgery are followed. Puncture sites are made near the umbilicus and in other areas so that the scope and other instruments may assess the operative site.

- Carbon dioxide or a nonconductive flushing solution (eg, glycerine) introduced into cavity causes organs and tissues to "push" out of the way so that better visualization and access are obtained.

- Access sites are closed with a few sutures or Steri-Strips and a small adhesive dressing is applied to the site.

Nursing Interventions

▶ Pretest

- Explain test purpose and procedure; assess patient's knowledge level.

> **⚠ CLINICAL ALERT**
>
> - Patient must be in a fasting state from midnight before unless otherwise ordered. Carry out bowel prep if ordered (enema and/or suppository).

▶ Intratest

- Position patient properly.
- Administer drugs and solutions as required.

▶ Posttest

- Recover patient according to protocols. Include frequent checks of vital signs and wounds.
- Administer pain medication as needed/ordered. Advise the patient that shoulder and abdominal discomfort may persist for a few days (because of residual CO_2 gas in abdominal cavity); semi-Fowler's position and mild oral analgesics may reduce discomfort.
- Observe for hemorrhage, bowel or bladder perforation, or infection.
- If urinary catheter has been removed, assess postoperative voiding within 8 hours.

> **⚠ CLINICAL ALERT**
>
> - These procedures may be contraindicated in persons with advanced abdominal carcinomas, severe respiratory or cardiac disease, intestinal obstruction, palpable abdominal mass, large hernia, tuberculosis, or a history of peritonitis.
> - Procedure may be interrupted in the event of massive bleeding or evidence of malignancy.
> - Be alert for postoperative signs of bladder or bowel perforation, hemorrhage, or infection.

LATEX ALLERGY TESTS (LATEX-SPECIFIC IgE)

Blood, Skin Tests

Testing for severe reactions to latex is performed more often because latex allergy has been more widely recognized and reports of ana-phylaxis due to latex-containing products are more widespread. This test measures IgE-mediated latex sensitivity.

Indications
- Evaluate high-risk groups for allergy to latex. Health care workers using latex gloves, patients with multiple surgeries, children with spina bifida or congenital abnormalities, respirating patients (ie, ventilators, tracheostomy, suctioning equipment), and workers with industrial latex exposure.
- Assess patients at risk for latex allergy, especially before medical procedures that would expose them to latex.

Reference Values

Normal

Negative: <0.35 IU/mL by enzyme immunoassay (EIA)

Clinical Implications
- Positive results are strongly associated with a latex allergy.
- In studies comparing latex-specific IgE results with clinical history, symptoms, and other confirmatory tests, the sensitivity has been >90% and the specificity >80%.

Procedure
- Obtain a 7-mL blood serum specimen in a red-top tube.

Nursing Interventions
▶*Pretest*
- Assess patient knowledge of test. Explain purpose and procedure.
- Obtain a specific patient history and document, including swelling or itching from latex exposure, hand eczema, previously unexplained anaphylaxis, oral itching from cross-reactive foods (eg, banana, kiwi, avocado, chestnuts), and multiple surgical procedures.

▶*Posttest*
- Evaluate test outcomes. Inform patient regarding meaning of positive test results and counsel appropriately. Teach patient what to avoid.

- If negative results are found by this test procedure, yet the patient is symptomatic, or if results are positive for this test, refer patient to an allergist.
- Review follow-up testing and treatment. In some instances of equivocal blood test results, a skin test is ordered.
- Treat all patients with positive latex history with latex-free procedures.
- Document *all* medical records for patients with positive results, including a clinical alert, ie, "flag chart" with "latex allergy."

LEAD (PB)

Blood and Urine

This test detects and measures the amount of lead as an indication of lead poisoning (plumbism).

Indications
- Detect lead poisoning in children. (See Display 3.6.)
- Screen for lead exposure or toxicity. In adults, the condition may be due to occupational hazard; in children, it may be due to eating old lead-containing paint chips.
- Monitor response to chelation therapy.

DISPLAY 3.6	**CDC Classification of Blood Lead Levels in Children**	
Class	*Blood Lead*	*Action*
I	<10 µg/dL (<0.48 µmol/L)	Not lead poisoned. In children, lead levels of >10 µg/dL is potentially dangerous
IIA	10–14 µg/dL (<0.48–0.68 µmol/L)	Rescreen frequently and consider prevention activities
IIB	15–19 µg/dL (<0.72–0.92 µmol/L)	Institute nutritional and educational interventions
III	20–44 µg/dL (<0.97–2.12 µmol/L)	Evaluate environment and consider chelation therapy
IV	45–69 µg/dL (<2.17–3.33 µmol/L)	Institute environmental interventions and chelation therapy
V	>69 µg/dL (>3.33 µmol/L)	A medical emergency

Reference Values

Normal

Blood: <10 μg/dL or <0.48 mmol/L
Urine: <50 μg/L or <241 nmol/L

Clinical Implications

- *Increased levels* occur with lead poisoning, industrial exposure, lead plumbing, leaded gasoline, fumes from heaters, lead-based paint, unglazed pottery, batteries, lead containers used for storage, contaminated cans, drinking water, hobbies such as stained-glass activities, lead dust that parents bring home on clothing to children.

Blood lead levels in adults:

- <10 μg/dL (<0.48 μmol/L) is normal without occupational exposure.
- <20 μg/dL (<0.97 μmol/L) is acceptable with occupational exposure.
- >25 μg/dL (>1.21 μmol/L): Report to State Occupational Agency.
- >60 μg/dL (>2.90 μmol/L): Remove from occupational exposure and begin chelation therapy.

Interfering Factors

- Failing to use lead-free blood collection tubes or lead-free urine collection bottles.

Procedure

- A fingerstick using lead-free heparinized capillary tubes or venous blood drawn in a 30-mL trace element–free tube (royal blue). Do not separate plasma from cells. Refrigerate.
- A random or 24-hour urine specimen may be requested for a quantitative test. Follow collection guidelines in Chapter 2 for handling instructions, using acid-washed lead-free plastic containers.

Nursing Interventions

▶*Pretest*

- Assess knowledge base and explain purpose and procedure for collection of specimen. Educate the patient regarding the importance of detecting high blood levels.

▶*Posttest*

- Evaluate patient outcomes and monitor and counsel appropriately.
- Monitor medical treatment of removing lead from body (chelation).

- Explain need for follow-up lead testing of blood, urine, hair, nails, or tissue biopsy.
- Counsel affected patient regarding the removal of lead source, which may be state mandated.

LEEP: LOOP ELECTROSURGICAL EXCISION PROCEDURE, CONE BIOPSY CERVICAL CONIZATION

Cervical Tissue GYN Biopsy

- These procedures are performed as a follow-up for an abnormal Pap smear and colposcopy findings and to enhance accuracy of colposcopy and to investigate squamous intraepithelial lesions (SIL).

Indications
- Exclude invasive cancer.
- Determine extent of noninvasive lesions.
- Treat (LEEP, cone biopsy) and remove abnormal cervical dysplasia, based on lesion size, distribution, and grade.
- Assess lack of correlation between Pap smear, previous biopsy, or colposcopy.

Reference Values

Normal
Findings reveal normal cervix cells, which flatten as they grow.

Clinical Implications
Abnormal findings include dysplasia and invasive cancer into deeper parts of the cervix.

Procedure
- The patient's feet are placed in stirrups and a speculum is inserted. A local anesthetic is applied to the cervix and a mild vinegar (acetic acid) or iodine may be applied, depending on the procedure type.
- LEEP procedure involves inserting a fine wire loop with a special high-frequency current to remove small piece of cervical tissue. A paste may be applied to the cervix to reduce bleeding. This causes a dark vaginal discharge.
- A laser or a cone biopsy may be one of the procedures.

> ## CLINICAL ALERT
>
> • Complications may include heavy bleeding, severe cramping, infection, and accidental cutting or burning of normal tissue.
> • Cervical stenosis may be an untoward effect of this procedure.

Nursing Interventions

♦ Pretest

• Explain purpose and procedure and equipment used for these procedures.
• Provide support and take measures to relieve fear and anxiety about possible diagnosis of cervical cancer.

♦ Posttest

• Instruct patient to call physician if heavy or bright-red bleeding or clots, fever, chills, aching, severe abdominal pain (not relieved by pain medication), foul-smelling discharge, or unusual swelling occurs.

LEUKOAGGLUTININ (TRANSFUSION REACTION) TEST

Blood, Transfusion

Leukoagglutinins are antibodies that react with *white blood cells* and sometimes cause *febrile, nonhemolytic transfusion reactions.* Patients who exhibit this type of transfusion reaction should receive leukocyte-poor blood for any subsequent transfusions.

Indications

• In patients with transfusion reactions.
• Before additional transfusions are administered.

Reference Values

Normal

• Negative for leukoagglutinins.

Clinical Implications

• Agglutinating antibodies may appear in the donor's plasma.
• When the agglutinating antibody appears in the recipient's plasma, febrile reactions are common; however, pulmonary manifestations do not occur.

• Febrile reactions are more common in pregnant women and those individuals with a history of multiple transfusions.

Procedure

• Obtain a 10-mL venous blood sample from the donor and the recipient. Observe standard and universal precautions.

CLINICAL ALERT

• Febrile reactions can be prevented by separating out white blood cells from the donor blood before transfusion. Patients whose blood contains leukoagglutinins should be instructed that they generally need to be transfused with leukocyte-reduced blood in order to minimize these reactions in the future.

Nursing Interventions

▶*Pretest*

• Assess patient's knowledge of test and symptoms and signs of transfusion reaction.
• Explain test purpose and procedure for transfusion reaction testing.

▶*Posttest*

• Interpret test outcome and counsel patient regarding future transfusion precautions.

LIVER FUNCTION TESTS

Blood and Timed Urine, Liver, Bone

Serum Glutamic-Oxaloacetic Transaminase (SGOT) or Aspartate Transaminase (AST), Serum Glutamic Pyruvic Transaminase (SGPT) or Alanine Amino Transferase (ALT), Gamma-Glutamyl Transferase (GGT), Ammonia, Bilirubin, Alkaline Phosphatase (ALP), Urobilinogen

These measurements are done primarily to evaluate liver function, assess bilirubin metabolism, and diagnose liver and bone diseases.

Indications

• Assess liver malfunction and detect alcohol-induced liver disease, hemolytic anemias, and hyperbilirubinemia in newborns.

- Evaluate progress of liver and pancreatic diseases and response to treatment.
- Measure GGT in differential diagnosis of liver disease in children and pregnant women and to detect alcohol-induced liver disease.
- Evaluate patients with jaundice.
- Monitor patients on hyperalimentation therapy using ammonia levels.
- Screen in geographic areas with a high prevalence of chronic viral hepatitis infection and those with chronic viral hepatitis (some homosexuals, intravenous drug abusers, and alcohol abusers).

Reference Values

Normal

There is a great deal of variation in reported values because of lab methods used.

ALT (SGPT)	AST (SGOT)	GGT
Adults: 10–60 U/L or 0.17–1.02 μkat/L	Adults: 8–20 U/L or 0.14–0.34 μkat/L	Women: 7–33 U/L or 0.12–0.55 μkat/L
Children: 5–30 U/L or 0.08–0.51 μkat/L	Children: 10–50 U/L or 0.17–0.85 μkat/L	Men: 11–51 U/L or 0.18–0.85 μkat/L
Newborns: 13–45 U/L or 0.22–0.76 μkat/L	Newborns: 25–75 U/L or 0.43–1.28 μkat/L	

BILIRUBIN	AMMONIA
Total: Adults: 0.2–1.3 mg/dL or 3.4–22.2 μmol/L	Adults: 15–56 μg/dL or 9–33 μmol/L
Conjugated direct: 0–0.2 mg/dL or 0–3.4 μmol/L	Children: 36–85 μg/dL or 21–50 μmol/L
Total: Newborns: 1.0–10.0 mg/dL or 17–170 μmol/L	Newborns: 109–182 μg/dL or 64–107 μmol/L
Conjugated direct: 0–0.8 mg/dL or 0–13.6 μmol/L	

ALKALINE PHOSPHATASE (ALP)

30–90 U/L or 0.50–1.50 μkat/L

UROBILINOGEN, URINE

2-hour specimen: 0.1–1.0 Ehrlich units/2 hours (SI units are the same); 24-hour specimen: 0.5–4.0 Ehrlich units/24 hours (SI units are the same)

Random: 0.1–1.0 Ehrlich unit (SI units are the same).

Clinical Implications: AST (SGOT)

- AST (SGOT) *increases* in hepatocellular disease, hepatitis, alcohol abuse, infectious mononucleosis and Reye's syndrome, and carcinoma.
- AST also *increases* in myocardial infarction, pancreatitis, dermatomycosis, polymyositis, recent brain trauma, crushing injuries, Duchenne's muscular dystrophy, pulmonary embolism, gangrene, malignant hypertension, hemolytic anemia, and congestive heart failure.
- AST levels are decreased in azotemia and chronic renal dysfunction.

Interfering Factors: AST

- Many drugs cause increased or decreased AST levels.
- Levels are falsely decreased in diabetic ketoacidosis, beriberi, severe liver disease, and uremia.
- AST decreases in pregnancy.

Clinical Implications: ALT

- *ALT (SGPT) increases* in hepatocellular disease and hepatitis, cirrhosis, metastatic liver tumor, obstructive jaundice and biliary obstruction, pancreatitis, myocardial infarction, infectious mononucleosis, burns, delirium tremens, and muscle trauma.
- *ALT decreases* in urinary tract infection and malnutrition.

Interfering Factors: ALT

- Many drugs falsely increase AST levels (salicylates high or low levels).

 CLINICAL ALERT

- Persons with elevated ALT levels should not donate blood because there is a correlation between elevated ALT and the abnormal antibodies to the hepatitis B core antigen.

Clinical Implications: GGT

- *GGT increases* in liver diseases, pancreatitis, pancreatic and liver cancers, cholestasis, and chronic use of alcohol and in hyperthyroidism, mononucleosis, and carcinoma of prostate, breast, and lung.
- *GGT decreases* in hypothyroidism.

Clinical Implications: Ammonia

- *Ammonia increases* in liver diseases, hepatic coma, transient elevated in newborns (may be fatal), GI hemorrhage, renal

disease, shock, certain inborn errors of metabolism, and Reye's syndrome.
- *Ammonia decreases* in hyperornithinemia.

Interfering Factors: Ammonia

- Levels vary with protein intake.
- Many drugs, exercise, or a tight fist or tight tourniquet can increase ammonia levels.

Clinical Implications: Adult Bilirubin

- *Bilirubin increases* accompanied by jaundice is due to hepatic, obstructive, or hemolytic causes such as viral hepatitis, cirrhosis and infectious mononucleosis, transfusion reactions, sickle cell anemia, and pernicious anemia.
- *Bilirubin indirect (nonconjugate) increases* in hemolytic anemias, large hematomas, hemorrhage, and pulmonary infarcts.
- *Bilirubin direct (conjugated) increases* in cancer of the head of the pancreas, choledocholithiasis, and Dubin-Johnson syndrome.
- *Bilirubin direct and indirect increase* (with direct more elevated) cholestasis secondary to drugs, cirrhosis, hepatitis and cancer of the head of the pancreas.

Clinical Implications: Neonatal Bilirubin

- *Elevated total bilirubin levels* (neonatal) occur in erythroblastosis fetalis; occur from blood incompatibility between the mother and the fetus; RH_0 (D) antibodies and other RH factors; ABO antibodies; other blood groups including KIDD, KELL, and DUFFY. Also, *increase* in galactosemia; sepsis; infectious diseases (eg, syphilis, toxoplasmosis, cytomegalovirus); and red cell enzyme abnormalities: G6PD, pyruvate kinase (PK) deficiency, spherocytosis, subdural hematoma, hemangiomas.
- *Elevated unconjugated* (indirect) neonatal bilirubin occurs in erythroblastosis fetalis, hypothyroidism, Crigler-Najjar syndrome, obstructive jaundice, and infants of diabetic mothers.
- *Elevated conjugated* (direct) occurs in biliary obstruction, neonatal hepatitis, and sepsis.

CLINICAL ALERT

- Adult critical value >12 mg/dL or >205 μmol/L; newborns critical value >15 mg/dL or >256 μmol/L; initiate exchange transfusion at once or mental retardation may result.

Interfering Factors: Bilirubin

* *Decreases* due to sunlight, contrast medium 24 hours before the test, high-fat meal, and drugs.
* *Increased* levels are seen during prolonged fasting.

Clinical Implications: ALP

* *Alkaline phosphatase (ALP) increases* in obstructive jaundice, cancer, abscesses of liver, and biliary and hepatocellular cirrhosis; moderate increases in hepatitis, infectious mononucleosis, cholestasis, diabetes mellitus, bone disease (increased calcium bone deposits); marked increases in Paget's disease and metastatic bone tumor; and moderate increases in osteomalacias, rickets, healing fractures, osteogenic sarcoma, hyperparathyroidism, pulmonary and myocardial infarction, Hodgkin's lymphoma, cancer of lung or pancreas, colitis, sarcoidosis, amyloidosis, and chronic renal failure.
* *ALP decreases* in malnutrition, scurvy, hypothyroidism, hypophosphatasia, magnesium deficiency, sprue, milk-alkali syndrome, and severe anemias.

Interfering Factors: ALP

* Increases in the presence of many drugs, age (young growing children, pregnant women, postmenopausal, older adults), and after IV albumin administration for several days.

Clinical Implications: Urobilinogen

* *Urinary urobilinogen increases* due to any condition that causes increase in production of bilirubin and due to any disease that prevents liver from normally removing reabsorbed urobilinogen from portal circulation whenever there is excessive destruction of red blood cells as in hemolytic anemias, pernicious anemia, malaria; also, in infectious and toxic hepatitis, pulmonary infarct, biliary disease, cholangitis, cirrhosis or viral and chemical exposures (chloroform, carbon tetrachloride), congestive heart failure.
* *Urinary urobilinogen decreases* or is absent when normal amounts of bilirubin are not excreted into the intestinal tract. This usually indicates partial or complete obstruction of bile ducts, as may occur in cholelithiasis, severe inflammatory disease, cancer of the head of the pancreas, during antibiotic therapy; suppression of normal gut flora may prevent breakdown of bilirubin to urobilinogen, leading to its absence in the urine.

Interfering Factors: Urobilinogen

* Peak excretion occurs from 12:00 PM to 4:00 PM. The amount of urobilinogen is subject to diurnal variation.

- Strong alkaline urine shows a higher value and strongly acidic urine shows a lower value. Intake of foods such as bananas may affect test outcome.
- False-negative results may be associated with high levels of nitrates in wine.
- Drugs that cause false-negative results include ascorbic acid, ammonium chloride, and antibiotics. Drugs that cause false-positive results include sodium bicarbonate, cascara, sulfonamides, phenothiazines, phenazopyridine (Pyridium), and methenamine mandelate (Mandelamine).

Procedure

- AST, alkaline phosphatase, ALT, and GGT procedure: Obtain serum (5 mL) by venipuncture in a red-top tube.
- Bilirubin procedure: Obtain fasting serum (5 mL) by venipuncture. Protect sample from sunlight. Allow no air bubbles or shaking of sample. Use red-top Vacutainer; store in a refrigerator or in darkness. In infants, blood can be collected from a heel puncture or cord blood.
- Ammonia procedure: A fasting plasma sample (3 mL) obtained by venipuncture in a green-top tube or heparinized syringe. Sample is placed in an iced container and examined within 20 minutes.
- Urobilinogen procedure: General instructions of a 24- or 2-hour specimen are followed depending on what has been ordered. See specimen collection guidelines in Chapter 2. The 2-hour timed collection is best done from 1:00 to 3 PM or 2:00 to 4 PM. Collect without preservatives. Record total amount of urine volume. Protect from light. Test immediately.

Nursing Interventions

▸Pretest
- Explain purpose and procedure of various liver function tests.

▸Intratest
- Accurate test results depend upon proper collection, preservation, and labeling. Be sure to include test start and completion times.

▸Posttest
- Evaluate outcomes, and monitor and counsel appropriately. Explain need for follow-up tests.
- Monitor neonatal bilirubin levels to determine indication for exchange transfusion.

LIVER/SPLEEN IMAGE

Nuclear Medicine Scan, GI Imaging

This nuclear test is used to assess the anatomy of the liver and spleen. Liver/spleen imaging is performed using SPECT, which gives three-dimensional images.

Indications
- Correlate with other imaging techniques.
- Evaluate functional liver and spleen diseases (cirrhosis and hepatitis).
- Localize site of metastatic disease.
- Provide a differential diagnosis for jaundice and identify hepatic or splenic lesions for biopsy.
- Evaluate ascites, fibrosis, infarction due to trauma, and effects from radiation therapy.
- Investigate unexplained upper right-quadrant pain.

Reference Values

Normal
Normal liver size, shape, and position within the abdomen.
Normal spleen size and blood flow.
Normally functioning liver and spleen reticuloendothelial system.

Clinical Implications
- Abnormal liver patterns occur in cirrhosis, hepatitis, hepatomas, sarcoidosis, metastasis, cysts, infarcts, perihepatic abscesses, hemangiomas, trauma, cancer, adenomas, ascites, unusual splenic size, infarction, ruptured spleen, accessory spleen, tumors, leukemia, Hodgkin's lymphoma.
- Spleens larger than 14 cm are considered enlarged; those less than 7 cm are considered small.
- About 30% of patients diagnosed with Hodgkin's lymphoma with splenic involvement will have a normal spleen scan.
- A cold spot in the liver may indicate a hepatic hemangioma.

Procedure
- Radiopharmaceutical (technetium-labeled sulfur colloid ^{99m}Tc) is injected intravenously.

- A SPECT study and planar images are acquired to give three-dimensional images of the radiopharmaceutical uptake.
- The study usually takes 60 minutes from injection to completion.

Nursing Interventions

♦ Pretest
- Explain purpose, procedure, benefits, and risks of liver/spleen imaging.

♦ Intratest
- Provide encouragement and support during the procedure.

♦ Posttest
- Evaluate patient outcomes. In collaboration with the physician, counsel about liver and spleen diseases and need for possible further tests and treatment. Monitor injection site. Observe for and treat (per order) mild reactions of skin, nausea, and vomiting.

LUNG IMAGING, V̇/Q̇ IMAGING, VENTILATION/PERFUSION IMAGING

Nuclear Medicine, Pulmonary Imaging

There are two phases of lung imaging: ventilation (V̇), to assess regional ventilation, and perfusion (Q̇), to assess pulmonary vascular supply.

Indications
- Rule out pulmonary emboli.
- Assess chest pain and respiratory distress.
- Pre- and postoperative evaluations of lung transplants. Pretest imaging is used to quantify lung function for transplant.
- Quantify lung function.
- Provide an estimate of regional pulmonary blood flow.
- Evaluate chronic obstructive pulmonary disease (COPD) and fibrosis.

Reference Values

Normal

Normal functioning lung: normal pulmonary ventilation and normal pulmonary perfusion.

Clinical Implications

- A study with normal ventilation and segmental perfusion defects indicates pulmonary embolism (PE). Other diseases may be detected: lung tumors and cancer, pneumonia, atelectasis, asthma, inflammatory fibrosis, and chronic obstructive pulmonary disease.

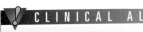

CLINICAL ALERT

- Pulmonary perfusion imaging is contraindicated in patients with primary pulmonary hypertension.

Interfering Factors

- False-positive results may occur in patients with vasculitis, thrombus, mitral stenosis, and pulmonary hypertension and when tumors obstruct a pulmonary artery with airway involvement, fatty tissues, and presence of parasites.
- False-negative results are associated with partially occluded vessels.

Procedure

- The patient is asked to inhale a radioactive gas (krypton, xenon, or aerosol technetium) through a mask or mouthpiece, using a commercial aerosol delivery system for approximately 1 to 4 minutes through a closed, nonpressurized ventilation system. During this time, a small amount of radioactive gas (^{99m}Tc DTPA or xenon^{133} gas with O_2) is administered into the system. The ventilation phase requires residual air in the lungs.
- Radioactive technetium macroaggregated albumin (MAA) particles are slowly injected intravenously while the patient is in a supine position. The perfusion scan visualizes blood supply to the lungs.
- The procedure lasts from 30 to 60 minutes.

CLINICAL ALERT

- During injection of MAA, care is taken that the patient's blood does not mix with the radiopharmaceutical in the syringe to prevent injecting coagulated clumps.

Nursing Interventions

▸*Pretest*

- Explain the purpose and procedure.
- Alleviate any fears the patient may have concerning the procedure.

▶*Intratest*
- Provide encouragement and support.
- Ensure that the patient is able to follow directions for breathing and holding his or her breath.

▶*Posttest*
- Evaluate procedure outcomes and counsel appropriately.

LYME DISEASE TEST

Blood, CSF, Infection

This test is used to diagnose Lyme disease (a multisystem disease) and measures antibodies caused by the spirochete *Borrelia burgdorferi* spread by tiny deer ticks that reside on deer and other wild animals.

Indications
- Evaluate infection with *B. burgdorferi* in patients lacking classic lesions of erythema chronicum migrans.
- Diagnose infection in patients outside an endemic area to identify antibodies to *B. burgdorferi*.

Reference Values

Normal
Indirect fluorescent antibody (IFA) titer <1:256; ELISA: Nonreactive to antibodies, negative for Lyme disease.

- Use Centers for Disease Control and Prevention (CDC) criteria for diagnosis: (a) isolation of *B. burgdorferi* from a clinical specimen, (b) IgM and IgG antibodies in blood or CSF, and (c) paired acute and convalescent blood samples showing significant response to *B. burgdorferi*.

Clinical Implications
- *Elevated levels* occur in 50% of patients with early Lyme disease and erythema chronicum migrans. Elevated levels do occur in most patients with later complications of carditis, neuritis, and arthritis. Elevated levels are seen in some patients in remission.

Interfering Factors
- False-positive results are seen in patients with antibodies to other spirochetes such as *Treponema pallidum*, the causative

agent of syphilis, and in persons with high levels of rheumatoid factor.

- Asymptomatic individuals in endemic areas may have already produced antibodies to *B. burgdorferi.*

Procedure
- Obtain serum (5 mL) by venipuncture in a red-top tube. Cerebrospinal fluid may be used.

Nursing Interventions
▶Pretest
- Assess patient's knowledge of test, clinical symptoms, exposure risk (highest transmission during spring, summer, and early fall; deer ticks reside on deer and other wild animals), and travel history to endemic areas.
- Explain the purpose and procedure of the blood test. No fasting is necessary.

▶Posttest
- Evaluate patient outcomes and counsel appropriately. Advise patient that if test results are not diagnostic, a repeat testing may be required.

MAGNETIC RESONANCE IMAGING (MRI, MR), FUNCTIONAL MRI (fMRI)

Special Imaging (Open and Closed) With IV/MR Contrast Agent

This diagnostic modality provides physiologic information and detailed anatomic views of tissues.

Indications
- To differentiate diseased tissue from healthy tissue and study blood flow.
- Evaluate multiple sclerosis, Alzheimer's disease, spine and cord abnormalities, neoplasms throughout the body, joint pathologies, cardiac function, and vascular pathologies.

Reference Values

Normal

- Normal soft tissue structures, brain, spinal cord, subarachnoid spaces (limbs, joints, fat, muscles, tendons, ligaments, nerves, blood vessels and marrow), heart, abdomen, and pelvis (particularly liver, pancreas, spleen, adrenals, kidneys, and reproductive organs).
- Blood vessels: normal size, anatomy, and hemodynamics.

Clinical Implications

- *MRI of brain* demonstrates white matter disease (multiple sclerosis, infections, AIDS), neoplasms, ischemia, cerebrovascular accident, aneurysms, hemorrhage; it is the test of choice to evaluate bone lesions and fractures.
- *MRI of spine* demonstrates disc herniation, degeneration, neoplasms (primary and metastatic), inflammatory disease, and congenital abnormalities. No spinal contrast is needed.
- *MRI of limbs and joints* demonstrates neoplasms, ligament or tendon damage, osteonecrosis, bone marrow disorders, and changes in blood flow.
- *MRI of heart* (cardiac MRI) demonstrates abnormal chamber size and myocardial thickness, valves and coronary vessels, tumors, congenital heart disorders, pericarditis, graft patency (cardiac), thrombic disorders, aortic dissection, and cardiac ischemias.
- *MRI of abdomen and pelvis* demonstrates neoplasms, especially useful in staging tumors, and tumor stage of abdominal organs, liver, pancreas, adrenals, spleen, kidneys, blood vessels, and abnormalities of renal transplants.
- *MRI angiography* (reference to noninvasive angiography) demonstrates aneurysms, stenosis, occlusions, graft patency, and vascular malformations.
- *Functional MRI* evaluates brain function while the patient is engaged in a task (eg, finger tapping) or auditory stimulus (eg, music) and may demonstrate abnormalities related to dementia, seizures, tumors, or strokes.

Procedure

- For closed-system imaging, the patient is positioned (supine) before the couch is moved into tunnel-shaped gantry. The patient is assured that there is sufficient air to breathe and that he or she will be monitored during entire procedure.
- Open MRI systems (less enclosed) may be used in some centers.

- In some instances, a noniodinated venous contrast is injected for better visualization of anatomy. The most commonly used contrast agents are gadolinium 50-DTPA, gadolinium manganese, or iron, which has very low toxicity and much fewer side effects than do iodine contrast agents. Gadolinium is generally used for examinations of the central nervous system (brain, vascular imaging, and spine).
- For abdominal or pelvic scans, glucagon may be administered to reduce bowel peristalsis.
- Exam time will vary between 60 and 90 minutes.

CLINICAL ALERT

- Safety concerns for patient and staff during MRI procedures are based on the interaction of strong magnetic fields with body tissues and metallic objects. These potential hazards are mainly due to *projectiles* (metallic objects can be displaced, giving rise to potentially dangerous projectiles); *torquing of metallic objects* (implanted surgical clips and other metallic structures can be torqued or twisted within the body when exposed to strong magnetic fields); *local heating* (exposure to radiofrequency (RF) pulses can cause heating of tissues or metallic objects within patient's body; for this reason, pregnant women are not routinely scanned since an increase in amniotic fluid/fetal temperature may be harmful); *interference with electromechanical implants* (electronic implants are at risk for damage from both magnetic fields and the radiofrequency (RF) pulses; consequently, those with cardiac pacemakers, implanted drug infusion pumps, cochlear implants, and similar devices should not be exposed to MRI procedures).

Nursing Interventions

▸*Pretest*
- Explain MRI purpose, procedure, benefits, and risks.
- Provide sedation if patient is claustrophobic or otherwise unable to lie still during procedure.
- Assure the patient that a two-way communication system between the patient and the operator will allow for continual monitoring and vocal feedback.
- Explain that fasting or drinking only clear liquids may be necessary for some MRI scans; also, no alcohol, nicotine, caffeine, or iron supplements may be taken before testing.

▸*Intratest*
- Provide reassurance during testing.

CLINICAL ALERT

- In the event of respiratory or cardiac arrest, the patient must be removed from the scanning room before resuscitation. Most general hospital equipment (eg, oxygen tanks, intravenous pumps, monitors) is not permitted in the MRI suite.

▶ *Posttest*
- Evaluate patient outcome and counsel appropriately.
- Monitor for sensitivity reactions and adverse reactions to contrast agent.
- Assess contrast injection site for signs of inflammation, bruising, irritation, or infection, as well as for extravasation of contrast agent.

MAMMOGRAPHY—BREAST X-RAY, SCREENING MAMMOGRAM, DIAGNOSTIC MAMMOGRAM

X-Ray Imaging and X-Ray–Guided Breast Biopsies

Mammography is an x-ray study of the soft tissues of the breasts that detects small abnormalities that could warn of cancer. The actual diagnosis of cancer is made by biopsy. Diagnosis by mammography is based on the x-ray appearance of gross anatomic structures.

Indications
- Evaluate known or suspected breast mass, skin (orange peel), skin retraction, nipple changes, nipple discharge, or breast pain.
- Screen for nonpalpable breast cancers in all women older than 35–40 years, younger women at high risk (family history), or those with history of breast cancer.
- Screen women of any age in whom genetic markers for breast cancer susceptibility (BRCA1 and/or BRCA2) are present.
- Guide for needle localization prior to biopsy.
- Survey "lumpy" breast, pendulous breast (difficult to examine), opposite breast after mastectomy.
- Perform as workup for adenocarcinoma of undetermined origin.
- Check for previous breast biopsies.

Reference Values

Normal

Essentially normal breast tissue. Calcification, if present, should be evenly distributed; normal ducts with gradual narrowing ductal system branches.

Clinical Implications

- Benign lesions push breast tissue aside as they spread, whereas malignant lesions may invade surrounding tissue.
- Abnormal findings may reveal abscesses, calcifications, cysts, tumors, or masses. A benign breast mass typically appears as a round, smooth mass with definite edges; if calcification present, they are usually coarse. A cancerous breast mass usually appears as an irregular shape with extension into adjacent tissue; increased numbers of blood vessels are present; and primary and secondary signs of breast cancer are apparent.
- Calcifications present in the malignant mass (duct carcinoma) or in adjacent tissue (lobular carcinoma) are described as innumerable punctate calcifications resembling fine grains of salt or rodlike calcifications that appear thin, branching, and curvilinear.
- The likelihood of malignancy increases with a greater number of calcifications in a cluster. However, a cluster with as few as three calcifications, particularly if they are irregular in shape or size, can occur in cancer.
- Typical parenchymal patterns are as follows: N_1, normal; P_1, mild duct prominence on less than one fourth of the breast; P_2, marked duct prominence; DY, dysplasia (some diagnosticians believe that the person who exhibits dysplasia is 22 times more likely to develop breast cancer than the person with normal results).
- Contrast mammography (ductogram, galactogram) is valuable for diagnosing intraductal papillomas. Mammary duct injection is used when cytologic examination of breast fluid or discharge is abnormal.

Procedure

- The breasts are exposed and positioned in a device used to compress the tissue. This brief, rigorous compression aids in visualization and also reduces the amount of radiation that needs to be applied to the breast. Generally, two images are obtained for each breast.
- Low-energy x-ray beams are used and applied to tightly restricted areas; consequently, significant radiation exposure to other body areas is not produced. The patient usually stands during the procedure.

- Tissue samples may be removed from the breast and radiographed using specialized mammographic techniques.
- Exam time is generally less than 30 minutes.

Procedure: Stereotactic X-Ray–Guided Core Biopsy

A sedative or local anesthetic is administered before the procedure. The patient is positioned on the abdomen with breasts protruding through an opening in a special table. Two stereo-view mammograms are then taken, allowing precise positioning of a needle into the breast tissue at specific locations. Multiple tissue samples are taken because tumors have both benign and malignant areas. A fine-needle aspiration biopsy (FNAB) uses a very thin needle to aspirate fluid and small amounts of tissue for cytologic evaluation.

A core needle biopsy (CNB) uses a larger, hollow core needle to extract cylindrical sample of tissue. After sampling, the breast is cleansed and sterile dressing is applied.

Procedure: Needle X-Ray Localization and Surgical Biopsy

This two-step process involves x-ray study and surgery after the patient has been administered a sedative and local anesthetic—in some instances, a general anesthetic may be used. With breast x-ray studies used as a guide, a needle that holds a fine wire is inserted. When the needle point is at the tip of the x-ray–defined abnormality, the guide wire is released. It stays there until the surgeon (guided by the wire) removes it along with the abnormal tissue. A small, plastic bandage–type dressing is applied after the procedure.

Nursing Interventions
▶Pretest
- Assess for test contraindications (ie, pregnancy).
- Explain exam purpose and procedure. Some discomfort is to be expected during breast compression.
- Make certain that jewelry and metallic objects are removed from the chest area.
- Advise patient to refrain from using underarm deodorants, powders, perfumes, or ointments before mammography because these agents may produce an image artifact.
- Instruct the patient to wash breasts before exam. Patients are most comfortable if they wear a two-piece outfit to the lab, which allows easy removal of upper-body clothing.
- Suggest that patients who have painful breasts refrain from coffee, tea, cola, and chocolate 5–7 days before the mammogram.

♦*Posttest*
- Evaluate patient outcome; provide support and counseling, especially important if findings of breast cancer appear.
- Anti-angiogenic drugs, e.g., vascular endothelial growth factor and epidermal growth factor receptor inhibitors, have recently been approved in the treatment of metastatic breast cancer.

CLINICAL ALERT

- Mammograms are compared with prior films to determine potential evolution of disease. It is important for the patient who changes imaging facilities to bring her old films to the new facility for comparison.
- All mammography facilities are required to send the patient results within 30 days of a normal mammogram or 5 days of an abnormal study.
- A mammogram detects abnormalities that could warn of cancer; the actual diagnosis of cancer is made by tissue biopsy (only one in five biopsies test positive for cancer).
- Several methods provide a breast tissue sample necessary for cancer diagnosis. Two of these are stereotactic core biopsy and surgical biopsy.

MECKEL'S DIVERTICULUM/MECKEL IMAGING

Nuclear Medicine, GI Imaging

This procedure is a very sensitive and specific test for identifying the congenital abnormality, Meckel's diverticulum. The diverticulum usually occurs in the ileum, about 2-ft proximal to the ileocecal valve.

Indications
- To detect a Meckel's diverticulum containing gastric mucosa in patients with recurrent lower abdominal pain.
- Performed often in young adults or pediatric patients who have suspected occult GI bleeding.
- To diagnose the congenital abnormality of the ileum, which sometimes continues to the umbilicus with ulcer formation and hemorrhage.

Reference Values

Normal

- Normal blood pool distribution; no increased biodistribution of the radiopharmaceutical agent in the right lower quadrant of the abdomen; and clearance of the radioactive tracer into the duodenum and jejunum.

Clinical Implications

- Abnormal radiopharmaceutical concentration and increased uptake in the right lower abdomen, in the ileum, and in the ectopic gastric mucosa of Meckel's diverticulum.
- No concentration of radionuclide in Meckel's diverticulum when no ectopic gastric mucosa is present; usually asymptomatic and test not helpful for diagnosing these situations.

Interfering Factors

- Inflammatory disease processes within the abdomen, such as appendicitis, Crohn's disease, or ectopic pregnancy, may simulate a Meckel's diverticulum on the image.
- This procedure is contraindicated if the patient has documented infection, is pregnant, or breast-feeding.
- Insufficient gastric mucosa within Meckel's diverticulum may produce negative results.
- A false-positive Meckel's image may occur when the source of gastrointestinal bleeding may be a carcinoid tumor.
- Other radionuclide procedures performed within the preceding 24 hours are a contraindication.
- Barium in the small or large intestines and prior proctoscopy may produce false-positive scan results.

Procedure

- The patient lies in a supine position and a nuclear gamma camera is placed over the abdomen.
- The radiopharmaceutical ^{99m}Tc pertechnetate is administered intravenously.
- During the imaging process, the patient may be asked to lie on the left side to minimize excretion of the radionuclide from the normal stomach and increase the concentration of the radioisotope in the intestine for visualizing Meckel's diverticulum.
- Glucagon may be given to decrease intestinal transit time and enhance identification.
- Gastrin may be given to increase the uptake of the radionuclide by the ectopic gastric mucosa.
- Total examining time is approximately 60 minutes.

Nursing Interventions

▸Pretest

- The patient should be instructed about Meckel's diverticulum imaging purpose and procedure. Prep requires an NPO status for at least 4 hours.
- Other diagnostic procedures of the gastrointestinal tract, as well as medications, should be avoided 2 to 3 days before the test. This is especially true of both lower and upper gastrointestinal x-ray procedures that often use barium.
- Cimetidine, a histamine H_2-receptor antagonist, may be administered 1 to 2 days before the test to inhibit acid secretion and allow for improved visualization of Meckel's diverticulum.

▸Intratest

- Reassure the patient that the test is proceeding normally.
- Instruct the patient that it is necessary to lie as still as possible during imaging.

▸Posttest

- Assess patient outcome and counsel appropriately.
- Observe for and treat (per orders) mild skin reactions, nausea, and vomiting.

MINERAL TESTING

Blood, Urine

Dietary minerals are inorganic elements that are essential for life. Unlike vitamins, the source for minerals comes from nonliving, naturally occurring elements, such as mineral salts in the soil or water. Minerals become a part of the chemical constituents of food via their extraction from the soil by plants and subsequent ingestion by animals, or they are dissolved in ocean water and ingested by fish and then enter the human food chain. Mineral concentrations in blood, urine, and certain body tissues can be measured and reflect the nutritional status of the patient. Minerals can be classified as macronutrients (major or essential) or micronutrients (trace, ultratrace, or nonessential). Measurements of minerals are used to assess occupational exposure and toxicity, monitor effectiveness of treatment, and evaluate mineral status along with other laboratory levels to verify deficiencies or excesses.

(text continues on page 414)

Reference Values

SUBSTANCE TESTED (SPECIMEN NEEDED), REFERENCE RANGE (RR), CRITICAL TOXIC RANGE (CR), AND DIETARY REFERENCE INTAKES (DRIs) IF AVAILABLE	SUBSTANCE FUNCTION AND INDICATIONS FOR TEST	CLINICAL IMPLICATIONS	
		INCREASED	DECREASED
Aluminum (Al)	No metabolic role.	Aluminum absorption with	
(serum)	Metal used in other forms	citrate-containing drugs	
RR: 20–550 µg/L	as an astringent (Burrow's	(effervescent or analgesics).	
(0.74–20.4 µmol/L)	solution) and as an antacid.	Use of aluminum-containing	
dialysis patients.	Assess for occupational	astringents hydroxide gels,	
(urine)	exposure and toxicity from	aluminum-containing	
RR: 5–30 µg/L	antacids; monitor chronic	phosphate binders.	
(0.19–1.11 µmol/L).	renal failure and dialysis	Excessive occupational	
Collect urine in acid-washed polypropylene container.	patients who readily accumulate aluminum from medications and dialysate.	exposure. *Toxicity:* Aluminosis (lung disease) Aluminum-induced encephalopathy.	

Hypophosphatemia.
Dialysis dementia.
Iron-resistant microcytic anemia.
Aluminum-related osteomalacia.

Note: Aluminum is a neurotoxin. The primary symptom is motor dysfunction leading to dysarthria, myoclonus, or epilepsy. Aluminum toxicity is not related to Alzheimer's disease. Aluminum can be found in laboratory solutions used with tissue samples and in laboratory dust. New testing methods are being adopted to rule out contamination.

(continued)

Substance Tested (Specimen Needed), Reference Range (RR), Critical Toxic Range (CR), and Dietary Reference Intakes (DRIs) if Available	Substance Function and Indications for Test	Clinical Implications	
		Increased	Decreased
Antimony (Sb) (24-hour urine) RR: <10 μg/L (<82 nmol/L) CR: >1 mg/L (plasma) RR: 0.03–0.07 μg/dL (2.5–5.7 nmol/L)	No metabolic role. Compounds are used in alloys, medicines, poisons. Assess for occupational exposure and toxicity.	Excessive occupational exposure (ore from mining, bronze ceramics). Ingested compounds (drugs used in parasitic infections). *Toxicity:* Acrid metallic taste, gastrointestinal pain (as in arsenic poisoning), throat constriction, dysphagia, pulmonary edema, liver and renal failure. *Lethal dose:* 5–50 mg/kg body weight (>1 mg/L)	

Arsenic (As)
(hair or nails)
<1.0 µg/g of hair or nails
Acute poisoning (serum)
≥5 µg/mL (≥0.07 µmol/L)
(2-hour urine)
Normal concentration, <100 µg per specimen
Toxic concentration, ≥5000 µg per specimen
(24-hour urine)
5–50 µg/day (0.07–0.67 µmol/L)

Ultratrace mineral; no function.
Found in pesticides, paints, weed killer.
Used as a homicidal poison.
High selectivity.
Assess for occupational exposure, exposure from pesticides and herbicides, and intentional poisoning.

Dermatoses (hyperpigmentation, hyperkeratosis, desquamation, and hair loss); hematopoietic for hair and nails.
Depression.
Liver damage characterized by jaundice.
Peripheral neuropathy.
Accidental or intentional poisoning.
Excessive occupational exposure (ceramics, agriculture).
Toxicity: Metallic taste, burning pain in gastrointestinal tract, bloody diarrhea, pulmonary edema, and liver failure.

(continued)

Substance Tested (Specimen Needed), Reference Range (RR), Critical Toxic Range (CR), and Dietary Reference Intakes (DRIs) if Available	Substance Function and Indications for Test	Clinical Implications	
		Increased	Decreased
		Lethal dose: 5–50 mg/kg body weight Arsenic trioxide (As/kg body weight): 0.35–0.91 µmol or 10.2–26 nmol	
Beryllium (Be) (24-hour urine) RR: <1.0 µg/day CR: >20 µg/L (>2.22 µmol/L)	No metabolic role. Assess for occupational exposure and toxicity.	Acute beryllium disease (a chemical pneumonitis). Excessive occupational exposure (metal extraction, refinery, rocket base, nuclear plant, extensive coal burning); secondary polycythemia.	

Bismuth (Bi)
(24-hour urine)
Collect urine in a metal-free acid-washed polypropylene container.
RR: 0.3–4.6 µg/L (1.40–22.0 nmol/L)
(plasma)
RR: 0.1–3.5 µg/L (0.5–16.7 nmol/L)

No metabolic role. Workers exposed in cosmetics, disinfectants, pigments, and solder industries.
Used in some drugs; poisoning as a consequence of therapy for syphilis.
Assess for occupational exposure, toxicity, and medication levels.

Used as treatment of syphilis in a growing child when mother has been treated during pregnancy
Treatment of peptic ulcer with bismuth-containing drug.
Bismuth subcarbonate, subgallate, and subnitrate compounds.
Toxicity: Ulcerative stomatitis, anorexia, headache, rash, renal tubular damage, resembles lead poisoning without the blood changes and paralysis, rheumatic-like pain.

(continued)

SUBSTANCE TESTED (SPECIMEN NEEDED), REFERENCE RANGE (RR), CRITICAL TOXIC RANGE (CR), AND DIETARY REFERENCE INTAKES (DRIs) IF AVAILABLE	SUBSTANCE FUNCTION AND INDICATIONS FOR TEST	CLINICAL IMPLICATIONS	
		INCREASED	DECREASED
Boron (B) (blood, 4-mL serum) RR (total): 1 mg/dL CR: 10–20 mg/dL (plasma) RR: 200 ng/mL (24-hour urine, 5-mL aliquot) RR: 0.3 µg/dL UL (tolerable upper intake level): Adults: 20 mg/day	Ultratrace mineral; a nonmetallic element, found as a compound such as boric acid or borax. Assess for exposure and toxicity, ingestion of boric acid, and unexpected absorption of boric acid from diapers or infant pacifier dipped in borax preparation and honey.	Increase in total plasma calcium concentrations and urinary excretions of calcium and magnesium. *Toxicity:* Lethargy; gastrointestinal symptoms; bright-red rash; shock. *Infants:* reports of scanty hair; patchy, dry erythema; anemia; seizure disorders. *Lethal dose* (adults): boric acid or borate salts, 50–500 mg/kg body weight.	Decreased serum concentrations of 17-beta-estradiol, testosterone, and iodized calcium. Depressed mental alertness.

Bromine (Br), Bromide
(serum)
RR: 20–120 mg/dL
(2.5–15.0 mmol/L)
(plasma)
RR: 1000–2000 mg/L
(12.5–25.0 mmol/L)

Ultratrace mineral; acts as a central nervous system depressant.
Bromine: liquid, nonmetallic element obtained from natural brines from wells and seawater. Compounds used in medicine and photography.
Assess for occupational exposure to bromide in medicine or photography.

Bromide acne.
Neurologic disturbances.
Increased spinal fluid.
Toxicity: Bromism or brominism.

Lethal dose: 500–5000 mg/kg body weight.

Cadmium (Cd)
(blood)
Use metal-free tubes.
RR: 0.3–1.2 µg/L
(2.7–10.7 nmol/L)
urine preferred (100 mL)
0–5.0 µg/24 hours
(0–44 nmol/day)

Ultratrace mineral; a metallic element in zinc ores.

Used in electroplating and in atomic reactors. Its salts are poisonous.

In tissue, in prostatic and renal cancer.

In urine, in hypertension, industrial exposure (electroplating, atomic

(continued)

Substance Tested (Specimen Needed), Reference Range (RR), Critical Toxic Range (CR), and Dietary Reference Intakes (DRIs) if Available	Substance Function and Indications for Test	Clinical Implications	
		Increased	Decreased
Refrigerate or ice.	Assess for occupational exposure, environmental poisoning. Check hair for evidence of chronic poisoning (nape and neck). Place in envelope or plastic petri dish.	reactors, zinc ores, cadmium solder), inhalation of cadmium dust and fumes, goods grown in soil heavily fertilized with superphosphate. *Toxicity:* Severe gastroenteritis, mild liver damage, acute renal failure; pulmonary edema; cough; duck-like gait; brown urine. *Lethal dose:* Several hundred mg/kg body weight.	

Chromium (Cr) (plasma)

RR: 0.3 µg/L (0.5 ng/mL)

Men
Aged 14–50: 35 µg/day
Aged ≥ 51: 30 µg/day
Women
Aged 14–50: 25 µg/day
Aged >51: 20 µg/day

Required for normal glucose metabolism; affects cholesterol synthesis.

Serum Cr levels are highest in the morning and fall after each meal.

Cr deficiency may be a factor in the development of diabetes in iron-overloaded persons with hemochromatosis.

Assess for occupational exposure, poor diet, long-term unsupplemented total parenteral nutrition (TPN), the elderly at risk. Severe trauma and stress increase need.

Evaluate toxic Cr exposure. Monitor patients on TPN receiving Cr therapy.

Excessive industrial exposure (carcinogenic).
Renal damage.

Insulin resistance (hyperinsulinemia).
Impaired glucose.
Increased risk for congestive heart disease.
Hypercholesterolemia.
Decreased fertility.

(continued)

SUBSTANCE TESTED (SPECIMEN NEEDED), REFERENCE RANGE (RR), CRITICAL TOXIC RANGE (CR), AND DIETARY REFERENCE INTAKES (DRIs) IF AVAILABLE	SUBSTANCE FUNCTION AND INDICATIONS FOR TEST	CLINICAL IMPLICATIONS	
		INCREASED	DECREASED
Cobalt (Co) (serum) 0.11–0.45 µg/L (1.9–7.6 nmol/L) (part of the vitamin B_{12} molecule) (plasma) RR: 0.007–6 µg/dL (0.1–0.4 ng/mL) (urine) RR: 1–2 µg/L (17–34 nmol/L)	Essential element in vitamin B_{12}—stimulates production of red blood cells. Assess for occupational exposure and monitor dialysis.	Cardiomyopathy after industrial exposure, during maintenance dialysis, and after drinking beer contaminated with cobalt during processing.	Cobalamin (vitamin B_{12}) deficiency.
Copper (Cu) (serum, 3 mL) RR (total): 85–150 µg/dL (0.7–1.5 µg/mL;	Required for hemoglobin synthesis; essential component of several	T-cell proliferation. Hepatic glutathione.	Rheumatoid arthritis. Menkes' steely hair disease:

Reference Range / Requirement	Clinical Significance	Associated Conditions	Effects
11–24 μmol/L (24-hour urine)	enzyme systems; present in the liver and excreted by the kidneys and in bile.	Wilson's disease (hepatolenticular degeneration).	Lack of pigmentation of skin and hair.
RR: 3–35 μg/24 hours (0.047–0.55 μmol/day)		Ingestion of solutions of copper salts.	Collagen abnormalities, osteoporosis.
Use acid-washed plastic container. (plasma/500 RBCs)	Assess for excessive antacid intake, nephrotic malabsorptive disorder, hemodialysis, and consumption of water high in copper content by infants.	Contaminated water or dialysis fluids.	Ataxia
RR: 0.47–0.0067 mg/g		Indian childhood cirrhosis.	Hypochromic anemia unresponsive to iron therapy.
Ceruloplasmin is an indirect test for copper:	Screen for Wilson's disease.	Female rheumatoid arthritis.	Hypercholesterolemia.
RR: 21–53 mg/dL (210–530 mg/L) (neonates: 5–18 mg/dL; 50–180 mg/L)	Diagnose copper deficiency and acute copper toxicity.	Oral contraceptive use.	Impaired cardiovascular system.
		Inflammatory conditions.	Oversupplementation of zinc.
		Cancer at injection sites or muscles.	Altered interleukin-2 production.
EAR (estimated average requirement) Adults: 900 μg/day		*Toxicity:* Hepatic or renal failure.	Neutropenia; leukopenia.
		Lethal dose: 50–500 mg/kg body weight	Liver disease; kidney disease.
			Lack of pigmentation of skin and hair.

(continued)

Substance Tested (Specimen Needed), Reference Range (RR), Critical Toxic Range (CR), and Dietary Reference Intakes (DRIs) if Available	Substance Function and Indications for Test	Clinical Implications	
		Increased	Decreased
Cyanide (Cn Radical) (blood, 5 mL) RR: <0.2 µg/mL (0.004 mg/L or 0.15 µmol/L)	No metabolic role. The most common and most deadly poison—stops cellular respiration by inhibiting the actions of cytochrome oxidase, carbonic anhydrase, and other enzyme systems.	Industrial exposure (pesticides, metallurgy). Inhalation of hydrocyanic acid and fumes from burning nitrogen-containing products.	
Nonsmokers: Toxic: ≥0.1 mg/L (>3.8 µmol/L)	Toxicity comes from inhalation or ingestion, a hazard to firefighters. Assess for industrial exposure, inhalation, or accidental poisoning from ingestion.	*Toxicity:* Lethal dose is <5 mg/kg body weight (small child); fatal dose = 5–25 seeds. Death within 5 minutes of ingestion/inhalation. Side effects are	

Fluorine (F)			
Fluorine (F) (plasma) RR: 0.01–0.2 µg/mL (0.5–10.5 µmol/L) (urine) RR: 0.2–3.2 µg/mL (10.5–168 µmol/L) DRI flouride: Men: 4 mg/day Women: 3 mg/day	Gaseous chemical found in combination with calcium. Used as a compound (fluoride) in toothpaste and dental products. Assess for excess ingestion; evaluate dental caries or mottling.	dizziness, weakness, mental and motor impairment, and sudden death. Fluorosis (excess fluorine use: >4 ppm in water; treatment of osteoporosis, multiple myeloma, or Paget's disease). Osteosclerosis. Exostoses of spine and genuvalgum. Excess ingestion from swallowing fluoridated toothpaste. *Toxicity:* Hemorrhagic gastroenteritis; hypoglycemia; central nervous system depression; renal failure.	Marginal to deficient dietary intake from deficiencies in geochemical environments. Dental caries. Skeletal changes, especially in long bones.

(continued)

Substance Tested (Specimen Needed), Reference Range (RR), Critical Toxic Range (CR), and Dietary Reference Intakes (DRIs) if Available	Substance Function and Indications for Test	Clinical Implications	
		Increased	Decreased
Gold (Au) (colloidal gold in fluid) RR: minute amount (serum) RR: 0–0.1 mg/L Therapeutic range: 1.0–2.0 mg/L Collect in a metal-free container.	No metabolic role; a metallic element. Salts used in early rheumatoid arthritis and in nondisseminated lupus erythematosus. Detectable in serum 10 months after the cessation of treatment. Assess for toxicity in the treatment of rheumatoid arthritis.	*Lethal dose:* 50–500 mg/kg body weight; 5–10 g sodium fluoride. Rheumatoid arthritis if gold sodium thiomalate or gold thioglucose (aurothioglucose) is given parenterally; oral gold compound. *Toxicity:* At least 35% of patients undergoing chrysotherapy develop some degree of toxicity. Pruritus, dermatitis, stomatitis, albuminuria	

with or without nephrotic syndrome, agranulocytosis, thrombocytopenic purpura, and aplastic anemia.

Adverse reactions:
Enterocolitis, intrahepatic cholestasis, peripheral neuropathy, and pulmonary infiltrates.

Prolonged excessive intake of iodine leading to iodide goiter and myxedema (common with pre-existing Hashimoto's thyroiditis).

Hypothyroidism in autoimmune thyroid diseases.

Toxicity: Mucous membranes stained brown; burning pain in mouth and esophagus; laryngeal

Simple, endemic, colloid, or euthyroid goiter.

Endemic cretinism (neurologic and/or myxedematous).

Children/teenager: impaired mental function, retarded physical development.

(continued)

Iodine (I)
(plasma)

RR: 2–4 μg/dL (157–315 nmol/L)

Deficiency: iodine deficiency disorders (IDDs)
(daily urine)

Mild IDD RR: 50–100 μg/day (median urine, 3.5 μg/dL)

Nonmetallic element belonging to the halogen group.

Aids in the development and function of the thyroid gland, formation of thyroxine, and prevention of goiter.

Assess for goiter.

Substance Tested (Specimen Needed), Reference Range (RR), Critical Toxic Range (CR), and Dietary Reference Intakes (DRIs) if Available	Substance Function and Indications for Test	Clinical Implications	
		Increased	Decreased
Moderate IDD RR: 25–49 μg/day (median urine, 2–3.4 μg/dL) Severe IDD RR: <25 μg/day (median urine, 0–1.9 μg/dL) DRI: Adults: 150 μg/day		edema; shock; nephritis; circulatory collapse. Lethal dose: 5–50 mg/kg body weight.	Adults: Hypothyroidism or hyperthyroidism; impaired mental function.
Iron (Fe) (serum, 5 mL, diurnal; morning specimen shows higher values) RR: 35–140 μg/day Toxic: >300 μg/dL Iron RR values: Males: 60–175 μg/dL	Essential for hemoglobin formation, transportation of oxygen, and cellular respiration. Plays a role in the nutrition of epithelial tissues.	Diets high in heme iron. Excessive iron absorption: hereditary hemochromatosis; prolonged therapeutic administration of iron to subjects not iron deficient; chronic alcoholism or	Iron-deficiency anemia; inadequate diet (grossly iron deficient). Koilonychia (spoon-shaped nails).

(11.6–31.3 µmol/L) Females: 50–170 µg/dL (9.0–30.4 µmol/L) Newborns: 100–250 µg/dL (17.9–44.8 µmol/L) Children: 50–120 µg/dL (9.0–21.5 µmol/L) *Total iron-binding capacity* *(TIBC) RR values:* 250–400 µg/dL *Transferrin RR values:* Adults: 250–380 µg/dL (45–68 µmol/L) Newborns: 130–275 µg/dL (23–49 µmol/L) Children: 203–360 µg/dL (36–64 µmol/L) DRI: Men: 8 mg/day Women: Aged 19–50: 18 mg/day	Assess for ingestion of iron pills or vitamin and mineral pills (toxicity). Populations at risk for deficiency are infants and children 0.5–4.0 years, early adolescents, and women who are pregnant.	liver disease; pancreatic insufficiency potential; severe anemia with ineffective erythropoiesis and increased hemolysis; diabetes in 80% of patients. Transfusional hemosiderosis. *Other:* Cancers (primary hepatic carcinoma, acute leukemia, early breast cancer); demyelinating disease; Alzheimer's disease.	Excessive menstrual loss. Pregnancy, lactation. Recent blood donors. Malabsorption syndromes, chronic diarrhea, gastrectomy. Turner's syndrome. Angiodysplasia. Ménière's disease. Zollinger-Ellison syndrome, pseudo–Zollinger-Ellison syndrome (hypersecretion of gastric HCl). Drugs (aspirin and ethanol), adreno-corticosteroids

(continued)

Substance Tested (Specimen Needed), Reference Range (RR), Critical Toxic Range (CR), and Dietary Reference Intakes (DRIs) if Available	Substance Function and Indications for Test	Clinical Implications	
		Increased	Decreased
Aged ≥51: 8 mg/day			or nonsteroidal anti-inflammatory agents. Sports anemia. Patterson-Kelly (Plummer-Vinson) syndrome. Factitia iron-deficiency anemia (Lasthenie de Ferjol syndrome—self-induced bloodletting). Transferrin: Severe protein-energy malnutrition

Iron sequestration—
chronic disease
with inability to
metabolize iron from
reticuloendothelial
cell deposits.

Lead (Pb)

(blood, preferred 2 mL,
collect with oxalate-
fluoride mixture)

RR: 0–9 µg/dL (0–0.43
µmol/L) in children
and in most adults
without occupational
exposure

CR: >30 µg/dL
(>1.45 µmol/L)
in adults

If blood levels are
>60 µg/dL (>2.9
µmol/L), the patient
should be admitted to a
hospital for treatment.

Ultratrace mineral; a
metallic element—its
compounds are poisonous,
and any level of lead in
blood is abnormal.

Lead oxides are used in
paint pigment; lead
additives in gasoline are
air pollutants.

Earthenware made of clay
rich in lead salts; lead
in some insecticides.

Assess for environmental
or occupational
contaminants and toxic
exposure.

Children: Irreversible
cognitive deficits; acute
encephalopathy.

Adults: Progressive,
irreversible renal disease;
toxic psychosis from
inhalation of tetraethyl or
tetramethyl lead.

Children and adults:
Hypochromic microcytic
anemia.

Lead sources: Ingested or
inhaled leaded paint
(renovation dust);
contaminated soil;
contaminated water

(continued)

Substance Tested (Specimen Needed), Reference Range (RR), Critical Toxic Range (CR), and Dietary Reference Intakes (DRIs) if Available	Substance Function and Indications for Test	Clinical Implications	
		Increased	Decreased
(24-hour urine) RR: up to 500 µg/24 hours (2413 nmol/day) CR: >400 µg/L (>1.93 µmol/L) (hair) RR: <5 µg/g (<24 nmol/g) CR: >2 µg/g (>9.6 nmol/g) Collect specimen in a lead-free container and avoid airborne contaminants. Use specifically monitored tubes for blood lead collection.		(lead pipes, lead solder on copper pipes, softened water); retention of a lead object in the stomach or joint, contaminated acidic foods and beverages (storage in lead-glazed ceramics, leaded crystal, or galvanized pots); inhalation of leaded gas fumes; occupational exposure.	

Lithium (Li) (serum) Use lavender-topped EDTA tube; do not refrigerate. RR: 0.0055 µg/mL (plasma) RR: 11 ng/mL (1.0–1.5 mEq/L or mmol/L) Therapeutic range: Serum: 0.6–1.5 mEq/L or mmol/L Serum CR: >1.5 mEq/L or >1.5 mmol/L Lethal: >2.0 mEq/L or mmol/L	Ultratrace mineral; a metallic element used as a drug to treat manic phase of manic-depressive illness. Assess psychotherapeutic drug levels.	Therapy for bipolar disorder. Diabetes insipidus. Renal failure; weight gain.	High dietary caffeine and/or sodium intake.
Manganese (Mn) (serum) RR: 0.40–0.85 ng/mL (7.2–15.5 nmol/L)	Essential for lipid and carbohydrate metabolism, bone and tissue formation, and reproductive processes.	Chronic inhalation of airborne manganese. "Manganic madness," permanent, crippling	Certain types of epilepsy, impaired bone metabolism, weak bone in

(continued)

Substance Tested (Specimen Needed), Reference Range (RR), Critical Toxic Range (CR), and Dietary Reference Intakes (DRIs) if Available	Substance Function and Indications for Test	Clinical Implications	
		Increased	Decreased
CR: >100 ng/mL (>1820 nmol/L) (24-hour urine) RR: <0.3 μg per specimen (urine) CR: >10 μg per specimen ESAI (estimated safe and adequate intake): 2–5 mg/day DRI: Men: 2.3 mg/day Women: 1.8 mg/day	Assess for occupational exposure and evaluate certain diseases.	neurologic disorder of the extrapyramidal system (similar to lesions in Parkinson's disease). Increased urine levels in acute hepatitis, myocardial infarction, and rheumatoid arthritis.	association with low concentrations of copper and zinc; possible result of alcohol abuse.

Mercury (Hg)
(24-hour urine)

RR: 0–50 µg/24 hours (<99.8 nmol/L/day)

Whole blood—dark-blue–top container; refrigerate.

RR: 0–5 µg/dL (3.0–294.4 nmol/L)

CR: >150 µg/L (>48.5 nmol/L)

Use acid-washed, leakproof container; keep specimen on ice. Blood is recommended specimen for organic mercury measurement, and urine is recommended specimen for inorganic mercury measurement.

No metabolic role. Mercury is the only metal that is liquid at ordinary temperatures. Primarily absorbed by inhalation but can also be absorbed through the skin and gastrointestinal tract. It is then distributed to the central nervous system and kidneys and excreted in the urine.

Evaluate for mercury toxicity, neurologic findings related to inorganic or organic mercurials, inhalation of mercury vapors.

Assess for occupational exposure, toxicity, and poisoning from contaminated fish.

Mercury poisoning: occupational activities (smelters, miners, gilders, hatters, and factory workers); hobbies (painting, ceramics, target shooting); home renovation; auto repair.

Most common nonindustrial mercury poisoning is the consumption of methylmercury-contaminated fish.

Iodine-containing drugs may cause false low levels.

Organic mercury poisoning is more serious because it develops quickly.

Inhalation of mercury vapors may lead to pneumonitis, cough, fever, and other pulmonary symptoms.

(continued)

Substance Tested (Specimen Needed), Reference Range (RR), Critical Toxic Range (CR), and Dietary Reference Intakes (DRIs) if Available	Substance Function and Indications for Test	Clinical Implications	
		Increased	Decreased
	Clinical Alert: A gum-chewing habit will release mercury from dental fillings.	Acute and chronic mercury poisoning affects kidneys, central nervous system, and gastrointestinal tract.	
Molybdenum (Mo) (plasma) RR: 1.3 µg/dL (0.1–3.0 µg/L or 1.0–31.3 mmol/L) (blood, mainly within red blood cells) RR: 2–6 ng/mL DRI: Adults: 45 µg/day	A trace element, associated with the inborn error of molybdenum metabolism. Assess for genetic molybdenum deficiency and parenteral nutrition deficiency.	Massive ingestion of tungsten (W). Occupational and high dietary intake (elevated uric acid blood concentration, gout). Sulfur amino acid toxicity. Growth depression and anemia similar to copper deficiency.	Sulfite oxidase deficiency (lethal inborn error of metabolism deranges cysteine metabolism). Prolonged total parenteral nutrition ("acquired molybdenum deficiency"). Interference with copper metabolism.

Nickel (Ni)	Ultratrace mineral; metallic	Consistent in alcoholic	Lack in diet, depressed
(serum or plasma)	element.	liver disease.	iron absorption.
RR: 1–2 ng/mL	Nickel carbonyl is an	Nickel dermatitis.	
(0.14–1.0 µg/L or	industrial chemical	Inhalation of nickel	
2.4–17 nmol/L)	used in plating metals.	carbonyl (predisposes	
UL:	It is toxic when inhaled,	to lung cancer).	
Adults: 1 mg/day	causes pulmonary edema,		
(urine)	results in lesions in liver,		
RR: 0.1–10 µg/dL	kidney, adrenal glands,		
(2–170 nmol/day)	and spleen.		
	Assess for occupational		
	exposure.		
Selenium (Se)	A chemical element	Endemic selenosis.	Keshan disease,
(component of the	resembling sulfur,	Nail and hair loss.	osteoarthritis
enzyme glutathione	found in soil.	Increased dietary intake	endemic.
peroxidase, isolated	Has a role in the metab-	owing to high-soil	Decreased dietary
from human red	olism of enzymes.	concentrations.	intake owing
blood cells)			

(continued)

405

Substance Tested (Specimen Needed), Reference Range (RR), Critical Toxic Range (CR), and Dietary Reference Intakes (DRIs) if Available	Substance Function and Indications for Test	Clinical Implications	
		Increased	Decreased
(plasma) RR: 100–300 ng/mL (1.27–3.81 μmol/L) DRI: Adults: 55 μg/day	Determine the cause for loss of pigmentation of hair and skin. Toxic >400 ng/mL (>5.08 μmol/L). Monitor selenium nutritional status, toxic exposure, acute toxicity, long-term parenteral nutrition.	Changes in nail beds.	to low-soil concentrations, aspermatogenesis. Long-term total parenteral nutrition (cardiomyopathy). Duchenne's muscular dystrophy, cataracts, tumor development. Whitening of nail beds, loss of pigmentation of hair and skin, muscle pain and weakness.

Silicon (Si)—silicic acid (H₂SiO₃)

(plasma)
RR: 500 μg/dL
(serum or plasma)
RR: 0.4–10.0 μg/mL
(0.13–0.15 mg/L
or 4.6–5.3 μmol/L)

Ultratrace mineral; nonmetallic element in soil.

Occurs in traces in skeletal structures (bones and teeth).

Necessary for the formation of collagen, bones, and connective tissue; healthy nails, skin, and hair; and calcium absorption in early stages of bone formation.

Needed to maintain flexible arteries and major role in cardiovascular disease.

Important in the prevention of Alzheimer's disease and osteoporosis; inhibits aging process in tissues.

Long-term antacid therapy (magnesium trisilicate).

Siliceous renal calculi.

Blood or tissue increased levels correlate with the presence of breast implants but not with symptoms of joint disease.

(continued)

Substance Tested (Specimen Needed), Reference Range (RR), Critical Toxic Range (CR), and Dietary Reference Intakes (DRIs) if Available	Substance Function and Indications for Test	Clinical Implications	
		Increased	Decreased
	Assess for toxicity, which may be related to asbestos-contaminated dust. Evaluate renal stone etiology.		
Silver (Ag) (serum) RR: 0.21 ± 0.15 mg/dL (19.47 ± 13.90 nmol/L) (urine): Negative	No metabolic role. Salts used as antiseptic and bacteriostatic agents. In normal individuals, silver slowly accumulates in body tissue with age but causes no apparent harm.	Chemical conjunctivitis from silver nitrate. Gastroenteritis. Argyria (bluish-gray skin) associated with growth retardation and blood, heart, liver, and kidney diseases.	

	Assess for occupational exposure or toxicity from medicinal uses of silver.	Silvadene applied topically for burns. Silver nitrates (as antiseptic). *Lethal dose:* 3.5–35.0 g total dose.
Thallium (Tl) (serum) <0.5 µg/dL (<24.5 nmol/L) (blood) RR: 0–2.0 µg/dL CR: 10–800 µg/dL (0.5–39.1 µmol/L) (urine) RR: 0–2.0 µg/L/ 24 hours CR: 1.0–20.0 mg/L (4.9–97.8 µmol/L) Collect urine in metal-free container. Red-top metal-free tube.	No metabolic role. Used in medications, cosmetics, and pesticides. Poisoning occurs from ingestion or from absorption through intact skin and mucous membranes; accumulates in liver, kidneys, bone, and muscle tissue. Assess for toxicity from either accidental ingestion or exposure to insecticides or rat poison.	Formerly used in ant, rat, and roach poisons. *Toxicity:* Thallitoxicosis or thallotoxicosis (ingestion of pesticides) causes vomiting, hair loss, delirium, coma, ataxia, pulmonary edema, paralysis, death. Poisoning results in blindness, facial paralysis, paresthesias, peripheral neuropathy, and liver and renal damage. *Lethal dose:* 1 g

(continued)

Substance Tested (Specimen Needed), Reference Range (RR), Critical Toxic Range (CR), and Dietary Reference Intakes (DRIs) if Available	Substance Function and Indications for Test	Clinical Implications	
		Increased	Decreased
Tin (Sn) (plasma) RR: 23 ng/mL (serum) RR: 24–50 μg/L (202–421 nmol/L) Collect in a metal-free container.	Ultratrace mineral. Used in the manufacturing of alloys, plating, food containers. Assess for industrial exposure.	Diet high in canned fruits/juices. Zinc balance negatively affected at 50-mg intakes; industrial exposure to organic tin compounds and dust. Tin salts used in calico printing. Organic compounds found in polyvinyl plastics, chlorinated rubber paints, fungicides, insecticides, and anthelmintics.	

Vanadium (V)
(plasma or serum)
RR: 0.02–10 ng/mL
(2–24 µg/L)
(hair)
RR: 0.01–2.2 µg/g
(0.2–10 mg/mL)
(urine)
RR: 0–10 µg/day
Collect in a metal-free container.

Ultratrace mineral (found in all tissues).
Used in the steel industry and to a lesser degree in photography and in the manufacturing of insecticides, dyes, inks, paints, and varnish.
Assess for occupational exposure.
Determine acute overdose, toxicity, and need for decontamination and enhanced elimination.

Occupational inhalation, hemorrhagic endotheliotoxic with leukocytotactic and hematotoxic components.
Toxicity: Industrial processes (sore eyes and bronchi), dermatitis, gastrointestinal distress, cardiac palpitation, kidney damage, central nervous system disturbances, green tongue.

Zinc (Zn)
(plasma)
RR: 78–136 µg/dL
(12–21 µmol/L)
Fasting morning specimen

Plays a role in protein synthesis: Critical for growth and sexual maturation.
Important in wound healing and sensory perception (particularly taste and smell).

Zinc therapy for Wilson's disease.
Long-term ingestion of excessive zinc supplements

Decreased intake (chronic): Diarrhea.
Decreased circulatory and splenic T lymphocytes.

(continued)

411

Substance Tested (Specimen Needed), Reference Range (RR), Critical Toxic Range (CR), and Dietary Reference Intakes (DRIs) if Available	Substance Function and Indications for Test	Clinical Implications	
		Increased	Decreased
(serum) RR: 55–150 µg/dL (decreases with aging) (8–23 µmol/L) (24-hour urine) RR: 300–600 µg/24 hours (4.6–9.2 µmol/day) (serum or plasma) RR: <70 µg/dL (<11 µmol/L) (deficiency)	Important in activating certain serum enzymes and in insulin and porphyrin metabolism. Assess population that may have increased needs for zinc intake. Monitor zinc therapy. Evaluate zinc toxicity and poisoning. Monitor for inadequate nutritional status during enteral and parenteral	>150 mg/day(secondary copper deficiency). Low-serum, high-density lipoprotein. Gastric erosion. Depressed immune system. Lethargy in dialysis patients. Hyperzincuria increasing with the severity of diabetes. Inhalation of zinc oxide fumes causes neurologic	Decrease in absorption of tetracyclines. Rheumatic diseases. Infection. Growth retardation (dwarfism). Male hypogonadism and hypospermism. Nyctalopia (night blindness). Hypogeusia (blunting of sense of taste). Impaired wound healing, long-term total

DRI:
Men: 11 mg/day
Women: 8 mg/day

nutrition in critical illness, in the treatment of burn patients, and in the treatment of persons with diabetes or cirrhosis.

damage (metal fume fever, brass founders' ague, zinc shakes), metallic taste, bloody diarrhea.

parenteral nutrition without zinc supplement.
Chronic liver disease.
Acrodermatitis enteropathica.
Parasitism (Egypt).
Compromised immune function.
Low facteur thymique serique (FTS).
Impaired embryogenesis.
Behavioral disturbances (impaired hedonic tone).
Skeletal abnormalities, defective collagen synthesis, alopecia, impaired protein synthesis.
Some cancers.

MONKEYPOX VIRUS

Blood, Lesion, Oropharyngeal

Individuals exposed to exotic pets (eg, prairie dog and Gambian giant rat) and have complained about a rash and fever should be tested for the monkeypox virus (Orthopoxvirus). The primary route of transmission is via close contact or a bite from an infected animal.

Indications
- Assess for virus following bite from an infected animal.
- Evaluate for close contact with an infected individual.

Reference Values

Normal
- Negative for Orthopoxvirus.

Clinical Implications
- Detection of the virus after the onset of symptoms is evidence of the disease.

Procedure
- An oropharyngeal, scab lesion, or blood specimen can be used.
- An oropharyngeal specimen can be obtained by swabbing or brushing the posterior tonsillar tissue. The swab should then be placed into a 2.0-mL screw-capped tube.
- For a scab lesion, cleanse the site with an alcohol wipe. Using either a scalpel or sterile 26-gauge needle, remove the top of the vesicle or pustule. Place the specimen in a 2.0-mL sterile screw-capped plastic tube. Also, the base of the vesicle or pustule should be scraped with a swab or the wooden end of an applicator stick and smeared onto a glass microscope slide. *Note:* The microscope slide can be applied directly to the vesicular fluid for "touch prep."
- For a serum sample, obtain 7.0–10.0 mL of venous blood in a marble-topped or yellow-topped serum separator tube, centrifuge the sample, and collect the serum.
- For a whole-blood sample, obtain 3.0–5.0 mL of venous blood in a purple-topped tube and mix it with an anticoagulant.
- Place specimens in a biohazard bag.

Nursing Interventions

▶ Pretest
- Explain the necessity, purpose, and procedure of testing.
- Keep in mind that questions regarding contact with wild or exotic mammalian pets or with suspected human cases are important.

▶ Intratest
- Follow standard precautions, considering the monkeypox virus can be spread by direct contact with body fluids or contaminated items (eg, clothing, bedding) of an infected person.

▶ Posttest
- Counsel, monitor, and treat the patient appropriately.
- Report cases of human monkeypox virus to local, state, and federal health departments.

MULTIGATED ACQUISITION (MUGA) IMAGING: REST AND STRESS EJECTION FRACTION/GATED EQUILIBRIUM IMAGING

Nuclear Medicine, Cardiac Imaging

The primary purpose of this test is to evaluate ventricular function at either rest or stress. The term "gated" refers to the synchronizing of the imaging equipment and computer with the patient's own ECG to assess left ventricular function. Wall motion of the ventricles can be shown in a cinematic mode to visualize contraction and relaxation of the heart.

Indications
- Obtain information about cardiac output, end-systolic volume, end-diastolic volume, ejection fraction, ejection velocity, and regional wall motion of the ventricles.
- Diagnose coronary artery disease.
- Evaluate pre- and post–heart transplant.
- Evaluate effects of cardiotoxic chemotherapy.

Reference Values

Normal

Normal myocardial wall motion, ejection fractions, cardiac output, and filling volumes.

Clinical Implications

Abnormal MUGA results are associated with abnormal quantitative data, for example, cardiac output and ejection fraction, congestive heart failure, change in ventricular function due to infarction, persistent arrhythmias from poor ventricular function, regurgitation due to valvular disease, ventricular aneurysm formation, and regional wall motion abnormalities.

Interfering Factors

• Arrhythmias may inhibit the ability to capture the appropriate EKG.

Procedure

• Electrodes are placed on the patient's chest.
• This procedure may be performed during stress or at rest.
• A blood sample of the patient's own red blood cells is labeled with ^{99m}Tc technetium stannous pyrophosphate. The ^{99m}Tc-labeled red blood cells are reinjected through an intravenous line.
• An ECG captures the patient's R-wave and signals the computer and the camera to acquire several image frames for each cardiac cycle.
• The procedure takes about 90 minutes.

Nursing Interventions

▶Pretest

• Instruct patient about MUGA study, purpose, procedure, benefits, and risks.
• Instruct the patient to fast for 4 hours prior to the procedure. There are no medication restrictions.

▶Intratest

• Provide encouragement and support during procedure.
• Monitor children for effects of sedation and analgesia.

▶Posttest

• Interpret MUGA outcomes (in collaboration with the physician) and monitor appropriately for cardiac disease.
• Resume medications as ordered.

MYOCARDIAL INFARCTION IMAGING

Nuclear Medicine, Cardiac Imaging

This test is used to demonstrate general location, size, and extent of myocardial infarction (MI) 24–96 hours after suspected myocardial infarction.

Indications
- Differentiate between old and new areas of infarct (12 hours to 7 days after its occurrence).
- Detect full-thickness (Q-wave) infarction.

Reference Values

Normal
- Normal distribution of radiopharmaceutical in sternum, ribs, and other bone structures. No myocardial uptake.

Clinical Implications
- Normal imaging indicates that the myocardium is viable.
- Myocardial uptake of the pyrophosphate (PYP) is compared with the ribs (2+) and sternum (4+). Higher uptake levels (4+) reflect greater myocardial damage.
- Larger defects have a poorer prognosis than do small defects.
- Acute infarction is associated with an area of increased radioactivity and "hot spot" on the myocardial image.

Interfering Factors
- False-positive PYP infarct scans in the presence of chest wall trauma, recent cardioversion, and unstable angina.
- Some drugs that may interfere with results include aminophylline, theophylline, caffeine, and pentoxifylline.

Procedure
- The patient is injected with the radioactive imaging agent ^{99m}Tc pyrophosphate (PYP).
- There is a 4- to 6-hour delay after the injection of the radionuclide before imaging can begin.
- The imaging procedure takes 15 to 30 minutes, during which time the patient must lie still on a scanning table.

Nursing Interventions
▶Pretest
- Assess for infarct signs and symptoms.
- Explain nuclear scan purpose, procedure, benefits, and risks.
- Imaging must occur within a 12-hour to 7-day period following the onset of infarct symptoms; otherwise, false-negative results may be reported.

▶Intratest
- The patient may resume pretest activity level after the injection and during the waiting period for the imaging procedure.

▶ Posttest

- Interpret test outcome and monitor appropriately. If surgery is needed, counsel about follow-up testing after surgery.
- Monitor injection site for extravasation or infiltration of radiopharmaceutical agent.
- Observe and treat mild reactions: pruritus, rashes, and flushing 2–24 hours after injection; sometimes nausea and vomiting may occur.

MYOCARDIAL PERFUSION

Nuclear Medicine, Cardiac Imaging

This test is used to diagnose ischemic heart disease, allow differentiation of ischemia and infarction, and quantitate the degree and location of ischemia. The procedure involves two phases—rest and stress—and reveals myocardial wall defects and heart pump performance during increased oxygen demands.

Indications

- Identify coronary artery disease and estimate the progress of disease.
- Assess for coronary artery thrombosis.
- Evaluate patency of coronary artery bypass graft and angioplasty.
- Monitor effectiveness of treatment.

Indications for Drug-Induced Stress

- Predict cardiovascular death, reinfarction, and risk of postoperative ischemic event.
- Re-evaluate unstable angina.
- Candidates are those with lung disease, peripheral vascular disease with claudication, amputation, spinal cord injury, multiple sclerosis, and morbid obesity.
- Ensure quantitative evaluation of the degree and location of ischemia.
- Evaluate patient with potential false-positive stress electrocardiogram (EKG).

Pediatric Indications

- Evaluate for ventricular septal defects and congenital heart disease.
- Assess postsurgical evaluation of congenital heart disease.

Reference Values

Normal
- Normal test: Electrocardiogram and blood pressure are normal.
- Normal uptake; myocardial perfusion and blood flow under both rest and stress conditions; no ischemic areas.

Interfering Factors
- Inadequate cardiac stress.
- Caffeine intake.
- Certain medications may contraindicate the study.

Procedure

- The patient is monitored by a cardiologist and either an RN, electrophysiologist, nuclear medicine technologist, or EKG technician during the cardiac stress test.
- For the rest scan, the patient is injected with the radiopharmaceutical, and 30–60 minutes later, single photon emission computed tomography (SPECT) imaging is performed.
- For the stress scan, the patient begins walking on the treadmill. When the patient has reached 85%–95% of the maximum heart rate, the radiopharmaceutical is injected and the exercise is terminated. A SPECT imaging is performed 30 minutes later.
- Radiopharmaceutical agents used include ^{99m}Tc sestamibi (Cardiolite), thallium-201 (^{201}Tl), and ^{99m}Tc tetrofosmin (Myoview).
- Dipyridamole (DPY or Persantine) or adenosine may be administered to adults or children who are unable to exercise to the desired levels.
- There are many protocols for myocardial perfusion imaging.

Nursing Interventions

▸*Pretest*
- Explain myocardial perfusion scan purpose and procedure.
- Caffeine- and theophylline-containing medications and beta-blockers should be withheld, if possible, for 2 days. Nitrates, eg, Viagra should be discontinued for 48 hours in case nitroglycerin is needed (which, if given to patients on Viagra, can cause fatal hypotension).
- Patients should be fasting for at least 6 hours before the stress test and are advised to avoid tobacco and chocolate products for at least 24 hours before the test. Check with physician about discontinuing prescribed medication 12–24 hours before the test.
- Blood pressure, heart rate, and ECGs are monitored for any changes during dipyridamole infusion. Aminophylline may be given to reverse the effects of the dipyridamole if there is a rapid change in vital signs.

> ## CLINICAL ALERT
>
> - The stress study is contraindicated on patients who
>   - have a combination of right and left bundle branch block.
>   - have left ventricular hypertrophy.
>   - are using digitalis and quinidine.
>   - are hypokalemic (because the results are difficult to evaluate).
> - Adverse short-term effects of dipyridamole (DPY) may include nausea, headache, dizziness, facial flush, angina, ST-segment depression, ventricular arrhythmia, or pain. Aminophylline may be given to reverse or alleviate these symptoms.

♦ Intratest

- Reassure the patient that the test is proceeding normally.

♦ Posttest

- Monitor injection site for extravasation or infiltration of radiopharmaceutical agent.
- Observe and treat mild reactions (per orders): pruritus, rashes, and flushing 2–24 hours after injection; sometimes nausea and vomiting may occur.
- Interpret test outcomes and counsel appropriately about further tests and possible treatments.

NEONATAL THYROXINE (T4)

Blood, Thyroid

This test measures thyroxine (T_4) activity in the newborn.

Indications

Screen for hypothyroidism after 24 hours of life, preferably within first week.

Reference Values

Normal

1–5 days: 12–22 μg/dL or 152–292 nmol/L
1–2 weeks: 10–17 μg/dL or 126–214 nmol/L
1–4 months: 7–14 μg/dL or 93–186 nmol/L

Reference range for newborn screening are laboratory dependent.

Clinical Implications
- *Decreased T_4 values occur in hypothyroidism.*
- *Alert limits:*
  1–5 days: ≤4.9 μg/dL (≤63 nmol/L)
  6–8 days: ≤4 μg/dL (≤52 nmol/L)
  9–11 days: ≤3.5 μg/dL (≤45 nmol/L)
  12–120 days: ≤3 μg/dL (≤39 nmol/L)
- 6%–12% of infants with hypothyroidism have normal screening results.

Procedure
- Obtain blood sample by skin puncture, following specimen collection guidelines in Chapter 2. The circles of the filter paper must be completely filled. This is best done by placing one side of the filter paper against infant's heel and waiting for blood to appear on front side of paper and completely fill the circle.
- Air dry for 1 hour; fill in all requested information and send to laboratory immediately. Protect from heat and light.

Nursing Interventions
▶ *Pretest*
- Assess parent knowledge base before explaining the purpose of the test and procedure.

▶ *Posttest*
- Evaluate patient outcome. Notify physician and parents of positive results within 24 hours.
- Advise regarding need for follow-up neonatal thyrotropin-releasing hormone (TRH) test and possible treatment.

Newborn Screening Panel

Dried Blood on Filter Paper

All North American states and provinces, and most industrialized countries of the world, require screening of newborns to detect congenital and metabolic disorders within the first week of life (eg, before discharge from hospital or maternity home or after a home birth). See Display 3.7. Providing follow-up on all abnormal results is the responsibility of state health departments. Some state health departments also provide the required types of dietary treatments, genetic counseling, and long-term care.

(text continues on page 426)

DISPLAY 3.7 **Newborn Screening Blood Disorders**

Biotinidase

Substance measured	Biotinidase enzyme activity
Abnormal	No enzyme activity
Interfering factors	Transfusions may cause a false-negative result
Treatment	Biotin—daily supplements
Clinical symptoms (not treated):	Seizures, dermatitis, hair loss

Congenital Adrenal Hyperplasia (CAH)

Substance measured	17-Hydroxyprogesterone (17-OHP)
Abnormal (cutoff)	Elevated 17-OHP; cutoffs will vary on the basis of birth weights and/or specimen collection age
Interfering factors	False-positive results can be expected in low-birth-weight babies and early sample collections ($<$24 hours). False-negative results in mothers on glucocorticoid replacement
Treatment	Glucocorticoid replacement, 9-alpha-fluorohydrocortisone
Clinical symptoms (not treated)	Salt-losing crisis in males that often results in death. Virilization (ambiguous genitalia) in females

Congenital Hypothyroidism

Substance measured	Thyroid-stimulating hormone (TSH) and/or thyroxine (T_4)
Abnormal (cutoff)	Elevated TSH: typical cutoff range: 20–50 μI/mL (258–645 nmol/L) (program dependent)
	Decreased T_4: typical cutoff range: 6–8 μg/dL (77–103 nmol/L) (program dependent)
Interfering factors	False positives can be expected in early ($<$24 hours) discharges. False negatives can occur in very low-birth-weight babies
Treatment	Synthroid—daily supplements
Clinical symptoms (not treated):	Mental retardation, cretinism, liver failure

Cystic Fibrosis (CF)

Substance measured	Immunoreactive trypsinogen (IRT)
	Mutant alleles

Interfering factors	False-negative results can occur because some CF genotypes may not cause an IRT elevation
Abnormal (cutoff)	Elevated IRT: typical cutoff range: 140–180 ng/mL (program dependent)
	Mutation analysis: detection of one or two mutant alleles
Treatment	Care at a CF foundation–approved center
Clinical symptoms (not treated):	Persistent diarrhea, malnutrition, chronic cough, respiratory diseases (infections)

Hemoglobinopathies (Sickle Cell Disease)

Substance measured	Hemoglobin fractions (eg, fetal, sickle, adult, hemoglobin C)
Abnormal	Detection of hemoglobin(s) other than fetal and adult
Interfering factors	Transfusions will invalidate testing for up to 60 days
Treatment	Penicillin—daily supplements
Clinical symptoms (not treated)	Sepsis, pain crisis, death (25% of babies)

Fatty Acid Oxidation (FAO) Disorders

Substance measured	Acylcarnitines
Abnormal	Each FAO disorder has a distinctive acylcarnitine profile
	The exact profile is program dependent
Interfering factors	False-negative results may occur if specimen collection is delayed (>14 days)
Treatment	Diet restrictions that are disorder dependent
Clinical symptoms (not treated)	Vomiting, lethargy, hypoglycemia, hypotonia; sudden death or permanent neurologic damage can occur

Galactosemia

Substance measured	Total metabolites (galactose and galactose-1-phosphate) and/or galactose-1-phosphate uridyl transferase (GALT)
Abnormal (cutoff)	Elevated metabolites
	Typical cutoff range: 10–15 mg/dL or 555–832 μmol/L (program dependent)
	No GALT activity

(display continues on page 424)

DISPLAY 3.7 (continued)

Interfering factors	False-negative results may occur if there has not been a lactose load before specimen collection. Transfusions may also cause false-negative results
Treatment	Lactose restriction diet
Clinical symptoms (not treated)	Sepsis, milk intolerance; mental retardation, sudden death can occur

Organic Acidemias (OA) disorders

Substance measured	Acylcarnitines
Determined by	Tandem mass spectrometry
Abnormal	Each OA disorder has a distinctive acylcarnitine profile
	The exact profile is program dependent
Interfering factors	False-negative results may occur if specimen collection is delayed (>14 days)
Diagnostic testing	Consult with a certified biochemical geneticist. Urine organic acids; mutation analysis
Treatment	Diet restrictions that are disorder dependent
Clinical symptoms (not treated)	Vomiting, lethargy, hypoglycemia, hypotonia, sudden death, or permanent neurologic damage can occur

Phenylketonuria (PKU)

Substance measured	Phenylalanine
Abnormal (cutoff)	Elevated phenylalanine: typical cutoff range: 2.0–4.0 mg/dL or 121.1–242.2 µmol/L (program dependent)
Interfering factors	False-negative results may occur because of lack of protein
Treatment	Dietary restriction of phenylalanine
Clinical symptoms (not treated)	Mental retardation

Maple Syrup Urine Disease (MSUD)

Substance measured	Leucine, isoleucine, valine
Abnormal (cutoff)	Elevated leucine/isoleucine/valine. Typical cutoff range: 4.0–6.0 mg/dL or 304.9–457.4 µmol/L (program dependent)
	Elevated valine: Typical cutoff: 2.0 mg/dL (250 µmol/L)
Interfering factors	False-negative results may occur because of lack of protein

Treatment	Dietary restrictions of branched-chain amino acids
Clinical symptoms (not treated)	Lethargy, vomiting, coma, mental retardation

Homocystinuria

Substance measured	Methionine
Abnormal (cutoff)	Elevated methionine. Typical cutoff range: 1.0–2.0 mg/dL or 67–134 μmol/L (program dependent)
Interfering factors	False-negative results may occur because of lack of protein
Treatment	Dietary restrictions of methionine. Cystine supplementation, folic acid, betaine
Clinical symptoms (not treated)	Dislocated lenses, cataracts, muscle weakness, arterial and venous thrombosis, developmental delay

Tyrosinemia

Substance measured	Tyrosine
Abnormal (cutoff)	Elevated tyrosine: typical cutoff range: 4.0–6.0 mg/dL or 220.8–331.0 μmol/L (program dependent)
Interfering factors	False-negative results may occur because of lack of protein
Treatment	Dietary restrictions of phenylalanine and tyrosine
	Liver transplantation
Clinical symptoms (not treated)	Vomiting, diarrhea, renal dysfunction, chronic liver disease, speech delays

Citrullinemia/Argininosuccinic Acidemia

Substance measured	Citrulline
Abnormal (cutoff)	Elevated citrulline: typical cutoff range: 1.0–2.0 mg/dL or 57.1–114.2 μmol/L (program dependent)
Interfering factors	False-negative results may occur because of lack of protein
Treatment	Dietary protein restriction of arginine
Clinical symptoms (not treated)	Vomiting, lethargy, coma, seizures, anorexia, death, ataxia, progressive neurologic deterioration

Adapted from Watson, M. S., Lloyd-Puryear, M. A., Mann, M. Y., Rinaldo P., & Howell R. R. (2006). Newborn screening: Toward a uniform screening panel and system *Genetics in medicine* 8(5) 1S–252S.

◢ Blood Collection Procedure

- Sample newborn blood by a heelstick procedure. A special filter paper blood collection card obtained from the screening laboratory is used.
- Complete all data fields on the form attached to the blood collection card.
- Select puncture site and cleanse with 70% isopropanol.
- Use a sterile, disposable lancet with a 2.0-mm or less point to perform a swift, clean puncture.
- Keep heel in a horizontal position (heel down) at or below heart level.
- Wipe away first blood drop.
- Allow a second *large* blood drop to form and apply to the surface of one filter paper circles. Use subsequent blood drops to fill the additional circles on the filter paper.

Note: Heparin capillaries can be used to apply blood to the filter paper. Apply blood immediately upon filling the capillary and do *not* touch the filter paper surface with the capillary. *Do not* use blood collection devices that contain EDTA.

- *Fill* all required circles. Fill from only one side of the filter paper. Circles must be completely filled when observed from both sides of the filter paper.
- Dry specimen at room temperature for 3–4 hours in a *horizontal* position. Do not allow the blood-soaked portion of the collection card to come in contact with another surface (eg, desktop, absorbent paper).

Note: Be sure the attached cover slip (if present) does not come in contact with the blood until completely dry.

- *Improperly* collected specimens will be rejected and a redraw will be requested.
- Send specimens (courier or United States Postal Service [USPS]) to the state laboratory as soon after drying as possible.

◢ Blood Collection Guidelines

- If initial specimen was collected before 24 hours of age, obtain repeat specimen in about 14 days as recommended by the American Academy of Pediatrics.
- For home or out-of-hospital births, specimens are collected before 24 and 48 hours of life.
- For premature or sick infants, specimens are collected at the time of admission to the neonatal intensive care unit (NICU) if possible.

Some state screening programs have repeat testing guidelines while the baby is in the NICU. In the absence of retesting guidelines, a repeat blood specimen should be collected at discharge.

- Initial specimen should be collected before transfusion, if possible. If collected before transfusion and less than 24 hours of age, repeat testing at 30 and 60 days of life. If initial specimen was collected posttransfusion, testing should be done at 6, 30, and 60 days of life. Always list date of most recent transfusion on the data collection form of the blood collection card.

Newborn Hearing Screening

Most hospitals have implemented (voluntary or by state mandate) hearing screening before discharge from the hospital. Generally, one of two techniques is used to determine the risk of hearing loss in babies.

- The first technique is called otoacoustic emissions (OAEs). The process consists of placing an earphone in the inner ear canal and measuring the response to certain clicks or tones.
- The second technique is called auditory brainstem response (ABR). In addition to an earphone placed in the inner ear, electrodes are placed on the infant's head, neck, and shoulder to record neural activity.
- Abnormal test results are recorded as *refer* or *pass* for each ear. Those babies with *refer* results are retested, and if a potential hearing loss is still suspected, then consultation with an audiologist is recommended.
- Newborn hearing results are forwarded to the state's Early Hearing Detection and Intervention (EDHI) program for appropriate tracking and follow-up.

Nursing Interventions
▶*Pretest*
- Explain importance and timing of newborn screening to the parents.
- Inform parents of their option(s) to refuse the newborn screening testing.
- Complete the data form on the blood collection card. Be sure the name on the blood collection card matches the baby whose blood is being drawn.
- Prepare the baby for the hearing testing.
- Collect the newborn screening specimen before hospital discharge.

- Be familiar with local newborn screening program guidelines for initial and repeat testing.
- Record the date the specimen was sent to the screening laboratory.

▸*Posttest*

- Record the receipt and review of the report from the screening laboratory. If no report has been received within 10 days of the specimen being sent, contact the newborn screening laboratory.
- For those test results that require further testing, contact the baby's health care provider to make necessary arrangements.
- Make sure that the newborn screening test results are entered into the baby's medical record.
- Forward the hearing test results to the state EDHI program.

CLINICAL ALERT

- If there is a family history of one of the disorders screened for, notify the newborn screening laboratory so that a specialist can be alerted.
- The most frequent reason for a retest is that the first specimen was not collected properly (inadequate amount of blood, improper use of a capillary, etc.).
- Be sure the baby undergoes the newborn screen before hospital discharge or by the seventh day of life for extended hospital stays.
- Ensure a positive correlation between the name written on the blood collection card and the name of the baby whose blood is being drawn.
- Ensure there is a newborn screen test report in the medical record.
- Check newborn screening results on babies readmitted to hospital with severe jaundice, anemia, failure to thrive, seizures, etc.

OBSTETRIC SONOGRAM—OB ULTRASOUND, FETAL AGE DETERMINATION, FETAL ECHOCARDIOGRAPHY

Ultrasound Pregnancy and Fetal Imaging

These noninvasive ultrasound procedures of the obstetric patient are used to visualize and document fetal, placental, and maternal structures and to estimate fetal age and weight; confirm multiple pregnancy; locate placenta; and identify postmature pregnancy (increased amniotic fluid and degree of placental calcification). Ultrasonography has become the method of choice for evaluating the fetus and placenta, eliminating the need for the potentially injurious radiographic studies that were used previously.

Indications

- Confirm presence and position of intrauterine gestation and rule out ectopic pregnancy; clarify size or date discrepancy (large or small for dates) and rule out suspected fetal pathology; and assess maternal pathologies (fibroids, cysts).
- Guide for amniocentesis, chorionic villi sampling, and invasive procedures.

Reference Values

Normal

Normal fetal, maternal, and placental anatomy; fetal viability; and adequate amniotic fluid volumes.

Clinical Implications

- During the *first trimester*, the following information can be obtained:
  - Number, size, and location of gestational sacs
  - Presence or absence of fetal cardiac activity and body movement
  - Presence or absence of uterine abnormalities (eg, bicornuate uterus, fibroids) or ovarian masses (eg, ovarian cyst, ectopic pregnancy)
  - Pregnancy dating (eg, biparietal diameter, crown-rump length)
  - Presence and location of an intrauterine device
- During the *second* and *third trimesters*, ultrasound can be performed to obtain the following information:
  - Fetal viability, number, position, gestational age, growth pattern, and structural abnormalities
  - Amniotic fluid volume
  - Placental location, maturity, and abnormalities
  - Uterine fibroids and anomalies
  - Adnexal masses
- Early diagnosis of fetal structural abnormalities makes the following choices possible:
  - Intrauterine surgery or other prenatal therapy, if possible.
  - Preparation of the family for care of a child with a disorder or planning of other options.
- *Fetal viability:* Fetal heart activity can be demonstrated as early as 5 weeks of gestation in most cases. This information is helpful in establishing dates and in the management of vaginal bleeding. Molar pregnancies and incomplete, complete, and missed abortions can be differentiated.

- *Gestational age:* Indications for gestational age evaluation include uncertain dates for the last menstrual period, recent discontinuation of oral hormonal suppression of ovulation, bleeding episode during the first trimester, amenorrhea of at least 3 months' duration, uterine size that does not agree with dates, previous cesarean birth, and other high-risk conditions.

- *Fetal growth:* The conditions that serve as indicators for ultrasound assessment of fetal growth include poor maternal weight gain or pattern of weight gain, previous intrauterine growth retardation (IUGR), chronic infection, ingestion of drugs such as anticonvulsants, "street drugs," or heroin, maternal diabetes, pregnancy-induced or other hypertension, multiple pregnancy, and other medical or surgical complications.

- *Fetal anatomy:* Depending on the gestational age, the following structures may be identified: intracranial anatomy, neck, spine, heart, stomach, small bowel, liver, kidneys, bladder, and extremities. Structural defects may be identified before delivery. The following are examples of structural defects that may be diagnosed by ultrasound: Hydrocephaly, anencephaly, and myelomeningocele are often associated with polyhydramnios. Potter's syndrome (renal agenesis) is associated with oligohydramnios. These can be diagnosed before 20 weeks of gestation, as can skeletal defects (dwarfism, achondroplasia, osteogenesis imperfecta) and diaphragmatic hernias. Other structural anomalies that can be diagnosed by ultrasound are pleural effusion (after 20 weeks), intestinal atresias or obstructions (early pregnancy to second trimester), hydronephrosis, and bladder outlet obstruction (second trimester to term with fetal surgery available). Two-dimensional studies of the heart, together with echocardiography, allow diagnosis of congenital cardiac lesions and prenatal treatment of cardiac arrhythmias.

- *Detection of fetal death:* Inability to visualize the fetal heart beating and separation or overlap of bones in the fetal head are signs of death. With real-time scanning, the absence of cardiac motion for 3 minutes is diagnostic of fetal demise.

- *Placental position and function:* The site of implantation (eg, anterior, posterior, fundal, in lower segment) can be described, as can the location of the placenta on the other side of midline. The pattern of uterine and placental growth and the fullness of the bladder influence the apparent location of the placenta. For example, when ultrasound scanning is performed in the second trimester, the placenta seems to be overlying the os in 15%–20% of all pregnancies. At term, however, the evidence of placenta previa is only 0.5%. Therefore, the diagnosis of placenta previa can seldom be confirmed until the third trimester. Abruptio placentae (premature separation of placenta) can also be identified.

- *Fetal well-being:* The following physiologic measurements can be accomplished with ultrasound: heart rate and regularity, fetal breathing movements, urine production (after serial measurements of bladder volume), fetal limb and head movements, and analysis of vascular wave forms from fetal circulation. Fetal breathing movements decrease with maternal smoking and alcohol use and increase with hyperglycemia. Fetal limb and head movements serve as an index of neurologic development. Identification of amniotic fluid pockets is also used to evaluate fetal status. A pocket of amniotic fluid measuring at least 1 cm is associated with normal fetal status. The presence of one pocket measuring <1 cm or the absence of a pocket is abnormal; it is associated with increased risk of perinatal death.

- *Assessment of multiple pregnancies:* Two or more gestational sacs, each containing an embryo, may be seen after 6 weeks. Routine ultrasound cannot totally be relied on to exclude the possibility of triplets or quadruplets, instead of only twins.

- If the fetal position and amniotic fluid volumes are favorable, fetal sex can be determined by visualization of the genitalia. It must be cautioned, however, that sex determination is not the purpose of obstetric sonography.

- Abnormalities detected during fetal echocardiography include cardiac arrhythmias, cardiac tumors, septal defects (including tetralogy of Fallot), hypoplastic heart syndrome, valvular abnormalities (including Ebstein's anomaly), and vessel abnormalities (eg, coarctation of the aorta, transposition and truncus arteriosus).

Interfering Factors

- Gas overlying pelvic structures in early first trimester may compromise ultrasound study. Obesity adversely affects ultrasonic visualization of tissues. Posterior placentas may be obscured by overlying fetal anatomy.

Procedure
Obstetric Sonogram

- The patient lies supine with abdomen exposed during the procedure. First- and second-trimester scans generally require patient to have a full bladder when scanning transabdominally. Scans performed to evaluate placental location also require a full bladder in most cases. Scans of first-trimester pregnancy may be performed with a transvaginal approach. In this procedure, a slim, lubricated transducer is inserted directly into woman's vaginal vault.

- A coupling medium, generally gel, is applied to exposed abdomen or pelvis in order to promote transmission of sound. A handheld transducer is slowly moved across the skin during this imaging procedure.
- Exam time is about 30–60 minutes.
- A full bladder may not be needed or desired for patients in the late stages of pregnancy or active labor. However, if a full bladder is required and the woman has not been instructed to report with a full bladder, at least another hour of waiting time may be needed before the examination can begin.
- A transvaginal (endovaginal) scan does not require the patient to have a full bladder.
- Endovaginal studies typically involve the use of a latex condom to sheath the transducer before it is inserted into the vaginal vault.
- Fetal age determinations are most accurate during the crown-rump stage in the first trimester. The next most accurate time for age estimation is during the second trimester. Sonographic dating during the third trimester has a large margin of error (up to ±3 weeks).

Fetal Echocardiography

- The fetal echocardiogram is performed in the same manner as a routine obstetric scan and requires similar patient preparation—unless, combined with an obstetric sonogram, the fetal echocardiogram does not require the mother to have a full bladder.
- The pregnant woman lies on her back with the abdomen exposed. Couplant is applied to the skin and a transducer is moved across the abdomen.

Nursing Interventions
▶*Pretest*

- Explain exam purpose and procedure; no radiation is employed, and test is painless. Emphasize test preparation. In most cases, a full-bladder study is performed that will require the patient to consume approximately 32 oz (950 mL) of clear fluid (preferably water) 1–2 hours before the procedure. The patient is instructed not to void until examination is completed. Discomfort associated with a very full bladder is to be expected.
- Explain that a liberal coating of coupling agent must be applied to the skin so that there is no air between the skin and the transducer and to allow for easy movement of the transducer over the skin. A sensation of warmth or wetness may be felt. Although the acoustic couplant does not stain, advise the patient not to wear nonwashable clothing for the examination.

▶*Intratest*
• Because maintenance of a distended bladder may be quite difficult, offer encouragement to the patient. If supine hypotension syndrome is experienced, instruct the patient to turn on her right side and breathe slowly and deeply.

▶*Posttest*
• Remove or instruct the patient to remove any residual gel from the skin. Instruct the patient to empty bladder frequently on completion of full-bladder study.
• Evaluate patient outcome; provide support and counseling as required.

ORTHOPEDIC X-RAY: BONES, JOINTS, AND SUPPORTING STRUCTURES

X-Ray Imaging—Bones and Joints

Diagnostic x-ray studies can be performed on a certain bone or bony part such as the extremities (eg, hand, wrist, shoulder, foot, knee, hip), group of bones (eg, thorax, ribs, sternum, clavicle, spine), the head and skull, and all of the joints.

Indications
• Rule out fracture (trauma).
• Detect masses, foreign bodies, arthritis, or other bone or joint pathologies (eg, tumors).

Reference Values

Normal
Normal osseous (bone) and normal soft tissue structures.

Clinical Implications
• Traumatic changes (fractures, dislocations), degenerative changes (arthritis, gout, osteoporosis, aseptic necrosis), bone tumors (benign, malignant, metastatic), osteomyelitis, abscess infarcts, and osteochondrosis (eg, Osgood-Schlatter disease, Legg-Calve-Perthes disease).
• Abnormal soft tissues, such as swelling or calcification.

Interfering Factors
• Jewelry, metallic objects, buttons, and other foreign bodies that may overlie the area to be studied interfere with visualization

of the bony part. Radiographic examination of the lower abdomen and pelvic region may be obscured owing to retained barium.

Procedure

• Patient may be instructed to sit, lie on the exam table, or stand, depending on the body part being examined. Some manipulation of body part will occur to provide a minimum of two radiographic views. On occasion, restraints or other stabilizing hardware must be removed, requiring nursing assistance.

Nursing Interventions

▶*Pretest*
• Explain exam purpose and procedure.
• Assess for test contraindication: pregnancy. If the procedure is medically necessary for a pregnant woman, the application of lead shielding can minimize radiation exposure to the fetus.

▶*Intratest*
• Encourage patient to follow positional instructions.

▶*Posttest*
• Evaluate patient outcomes; provide support and counseling about bone and joint pathologies and fractures. Instruct regarding need for future x-rays to monitor response to treatment.

CLINICAL ALERT

• Although orthopedic x-ray study can readily be used to diagnose bony disease, general radiography is inadequate to assess the condition of cartilage, tendons, or ligaments.
• Portable x-ray machines can be taken to the nursing unit if the patient cannot be transported to radiology.

OSTEOCALCIN (BONE G1A PROTEIN)

Blood

This test is used to screen for osteoporosis in postmenopausal women.

Indications
* Assess risk for fractures.
* Monitor treatment of osteoporosis.

Reference Values

Normal
Osteocalcin: 8.1 ± 4.6 μg/L or 1.4 ± 0.8 nmol/L
Carboxylated osteocalcin: 9.9 ± 0.5 μg/L or 1.7 ± 0.1 nmol/L
Undercarboxylated osteocalcin: 3.7 ± 1.0 μg/L or 0.6 ± 0.2 nmol/L

Normal Using Radioimmunoassay (RIA)
Adult male: 3.0–13.0 ng/mL or 3.0–13.0 μg/L
Premenopausal female: 0.4–8.2 ng/mL or 0.4–8.2 μg/L
Postmenopausal female: 1.5–11.0 ng/mL or 1.5–11.0 μg/L

Clinical Implications
* *Increased levels* indicate increased bone formation in persons with hyperparathyroidism, fractures, and acromegaly.
* *Decreased levels* are associated with hypoparathyroidism, deficiency of growth hormone, and medications (eg, glucocorticoids, bisphosphonates, and calcitonin).

Interfering Factors
* Increased during bed rest and no increase in bone formation.
* Increased with impaired renal function and no increase in bone formation.

Procedure
* A venous blood sample of serum is collected on ice, separated within 1 hour, and immediately frozen. (Avoid a freeze-thaw cycle.)

Nursing Interventions
▶Pretest
* Explain the purpose and the procedure of the test.
* Record the patient's age and menopausal state.
* Obtain a pertinent family and personal history of osteoporotic fractures, falls, etc.

▶Posttest
* Interpret test outcomes and counsel the patient regarding further tests.

PANCREATIC FUNCTION TESTS

Blood and Urine Enzymes, Pancreas, Salivary Glands

These tests are ordered to detect inflammation of the pancreas or salivary glands and to recognize recurrent attacks of acute pancreatitis in persons who exhibit severe abdominal pain.

Indications
- Assess pancreatic and salivary gland function and malfunction.
- Differentiate acute pancreatitis from peptic ulcer and other disorders in which amylase is increased.
- Monitor treatment of pancreatitis.
- Provide workup of abdominal pain, nausea, and vomiting.

Reference Values

Normal

AMYLASE

Adults: 25–130 U/L or 0.42–2.17 μkat/L (blood); elderly: 21–160 U/L or 0.35–2.67 μkat/L; newborns: 6–65 U/L or 0.10–1.08 μkat/L

AMYLASE RANDOM URINE

Check with laboratory; values depend upon the method used.

AMYLASE 2-HOUR URINE

Adults: 2–34 U/hour or 16–284 nkat/hour

AMYLASE/CREATININE CLEARANCE SERUM

Adults: 1%–4% or 0.01–0.04 (ratio of urine and serum amylase/creatinine)

AMYLASE 24-HOUR URINE

24–408 U/24 hours or 400–6800 nkat/day

LIPASE

10–140 U/L or 0.17–2.33 μkat/L; elderly: 18–180 U/L or 0.30–3.00 μkat/L
Critical value: lipase >600 U/L or >10.0 μkat/L

Clinical Implications: Amylase/Creatinine Ratio

- *Urine amylase increases* in acute pancreatitis, parotitis, peritonitis, biliary tract disease, intestinal obstruction, and renal insufficiency.

- *Amylase/creatinine clearance increases* in pancreatitis, diabetic ketoacidosis, burns, and renal insufficiency.
- *Amylase/creatinine ratio decreases* (<1%) in macroamylasemia (a relatively benign condition).
- *Blood amylase increases* in acute pancreatitis and other pancreatic disorders, cholecystitis, perforated peptic ulcer, cerebral trauma, salivary gland disease (parotitis), ruptured tubal pregnancy, ruptured aortic aneurysm, alcohol poisoning, and macroamylasia.
- *Blood amylase decreases* in marked destruction of pancreas (pancreatectomy), severe liver disease, traumas of pregnancy, and advanced cystic fibrosis.
- *Lipase increases* in pancreatitis, pancreatic duct and high intestinal obstructions, pancreatic cancer, acute cholecystitis, peritonitis, and organ transplant complications.
- Lipase elevation occurs 24–36 hours after the onset of illness and persists for approximately 14 days. Lipase may still be elevated when amylase is back to normal.
- Lipase is usually normal with increased amylase in peptic ulcer, mumps, inflammatory bowel disease, and intestinal obstructions and macroamylasemia.

Interfering Factors: Amylase
- Anticoagulated blood gives lower results.
- Lipemic serum interferes with test.
- Increased levels are found in alcoholism, pregnancy, and diabetic ketoacidosis.
- Many drugs, including morphine, interfere with test results.
- Newborns have little or no amylase. By the end of their first year, amylase rises to adult levels.

Procedure
- A venous blood sample (5.0 mL) using a red-top tube may be collected at the same time a random urine specimen is obtained.
- A random, 2-hour or 24-hour timed urine specimen is ordered. A 2-hour specimen is usually collected. Collect urine in a clean container; keep refrigerated. See specimen collection guidelines in Chapter 2.

Nursing Interventions
▸Pretest
- Assess patient compliance and patient knowledge base before explaining test purpose and procedure.

♦Intratest

- Encourage fluids during test if fluids are not restricted for other medical reasons.
- Accurate test results depend on proper collection, preservation, and labeling. Be sure to include start and completion times of the test.

♦Posttest

- Evaluate patient outcomes. Provide counseling and support as appropriate.

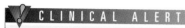

> ## CLINICAL ALERT
>
> - A 2-hour amylase excretion in the urine is a more sensitive test than either the serum amylase or lipase test. In patients with acute pancreatitis, the urine often shows a prolonged elevation of amylase compared with the short-lived peak in the blood.

PAPANICOLAOU (PAP) SMEAR, MATURATION INDEX, CELL (CYTOLOGIC) STUDY OF FEMALE GENITAL TRACT, VULVA, VAGINA, AND CERVIX

Special Genital Cell Study

This test examines cells from the vagina, cervix, endocervix, and posterior fornix; it is used for early detection of cervical cancer, for the diagnosis of precancers and cancerous conditions of female genital tract, and for the diagnosis of inflammatory disease.

Indications

- Screen for early detection of cervical cancer and human papillomavirus (HPV).
- Assess hormone cytology (especially in relation to ovarian function) and inflammatory and infectious diseases.
- Screen all women with Pap smears diagnostic of atypical squamous cells of undetermined significance (ASCUS) for HPV.

Reference Values

Normal
No abnormal or atypical cells.
No inflammation, no infection, no partially obscuring blood.

Major cell types within normal limits.
Negative for intraepithelial cell abnormality of malignancy.
Negative for HPV.

Clinical Implications

- Abnormal Pap cytologic responses include atypical squamous cells of undetermined significance (ASCUS) and can be classified as protective, destructive, reparative (regenerative), or neoplastic. (See DISPLAY 3.8.)
- Inflammatory reactions and microbes (*Trichomonas vaginalis* and *Monilia*, *Coccobacillus*, *Candida*, and *Actinomyces* species, cells indicative of herpes simplex virus [HSV]) can be identified to help in the diagnosis of vaginal diseases and for the evidence of *Chlamydia trachomatis* and *Neisseria gonorrhoeae.*
- Reactive cells associated with inflammation, typical surgical repair, radiation, intrauterine contraception devices (IUDs), posthysterectomy glandular cells, atrophy, and endometrial cells in women 40 years or older.
- Positive DNA test for HPV.
- Precancerous and cancerous lesions of the cervix can be identified.

Interfering Factors

- Medications (tetracycline, digitalis), use of lubricating vaginal jelly, recent douching, infection, and heavy menstrual flow and blood affect outcomes.

Procedure

- Ask the patient to remove clothing from the waist down.
- Place the patient in a lithotomy position on an examining table.
- Gently insert an appropriately sized bivalve speculum, lubricated and warmed only with water, into the vagina to expose the cervix.
- Observe standard precautions (see the Appendix).
- If a conventional Pap smear, as opposed to liquid base, is being taken, scrape the posterior fornix and the external os of the cervix with a wooden spatula, a cytobrush, or a cytobroom. Smear material obtained on glass slides and place immediately in 95% alcohol or spray fixative before air drying occurs.
- If a ThinPrep Pap smear is being taken, use a broomlike collection device. Insert the central bristles of the broom into the endocervical canal deep enough to allow the short bristles to contact the ectocervix fully. Push gently and rotate the broom in a clockwise direction five times. Rinse the broom with a PreservCyt solution vial by pushing the broom into the bottom of the vial 10 times, forcing the bristles apart. As a final step, swirl the broom vigorously

Display 3.8 Bethesda System—2001

Specimen type: Indicate conventional [Pap] versus liquid versus other
Specimen Adequacy
- Satisfactory for evaluation (describe presence or absence of endocervical/transformation zone component and any other quality indicators)
- Unsatisfactory for evaluation (specify reason):
  - Specimen rejected but processed (specify reason)
  - Specimen processed and examined but unsatisfactory for the evaluation of epithelial abnormality because of (specify reason)

General Categorization
- Negative for intraepithelial lesion or malignancy
- Epithelial cell abnormality (followed by interpretation)
- Other: see interpretation/result

Interpretation/Result
Negative for intraepithelial lesion or malignancy
Organisms:
- *Trichomonas vaginalis*
- Fungal organisms morphologically consistent with *Candida* species
- Shift in flora suggestive of bacterial vaginosis (coccobacillus)
- Bacteria morphologically consistent with *Actinomyces* species
- Cellular changes consistent with herpes simplex virus

Other nonneoplastic findings:
- Reactive changes associated with inflammation (includes repair), radiation, IUD, atrophy, glandular cells status after hysterectomy, or endometrial cells (in women >40 years of age)

Epithelial Cell Abnormalities Squamous Cell Type
Squamous cells:
- ASCUS, cannot exclude high-grade squamous intraepithelial lesion (HSIL) (ASC-H)
- LSIL encompassing human papillomavirus (HPV), mild dysplasia, cervical intraepithelial neoplasm (CIN) grade 1 (low-grade precursor)
- HSIL encompassing moderate, severe, CIS/CIN 2 and CIN 3 (grades 2 and 3 are high-grade precursors)
- Squamous cell carcinoma

Glandular Cell Lesions
- Atypical
  - Endocervical cells (NOS or specify in comments)
  - Endometrial cells (NOS or specify in comments)

(display continues on page 441)

DISPLAY 3.8 (continued)

- ○ Glandular cells (NOS or specify in comments)
- ○ Endocervical cells, favor neoplastic
- ○ Glandular cells, favor neoplastic
- Endocervical adenocarcinoma in situ
- Adenocarcinoma
  - ○ Endocervical
  - ○ Endometrial
  - ○ Extrauterine
  - ○ NOS (not otherwise specified)

to release material. Discard the collection device. Tighten the cap on the solution container so that the torque line on the cap passes the torque line on the vial.

- Label the specimen properly with the patient's name and identifying number (if appropriate) and the area from which the specimen was obtained and send it to the laboratory with a properly completed information sheet, including date of collection, patient's date of birth, date of last menstrual period, and pertinent clinical history.
- Examination takes about 5 minutes.

FURTHER TESTING AND MANAGEMENT AFTER ABNORMAL RESULTS OF PAP TESTING

ADOLESCENTS—LSIL	ASCUS	HSIL
Repeat cytology at 12 months—if positive, proceed to colposcopy, and if negative, repeat cytology at 1 year.	Repeat cytology at 6 and 12 months—if both negative, continue with routine screening, and if positive, proceed to colposcopy.	Colposcopy with endocervical assessment.
If repeat cytology is positive, proceed to colposcopy, and if negative, continue with routine screening.	Colposcopy preferred in women with no lesions and if either the 6- or 12-month cytology is positive.	If no CIN, review cytology, colposcopy, and histology (an amended report may be necessary), or perform colposcopy and cytology at 6 and 12 months, or perform an excisional procedure.

If colposcopic exam is negative for CIN, perform cytology at 6 and 12 months or HPV DNA testing at 12 months. (If results of these follow-up procedures are negative, to proceed routine screening, and if positive, repeat colposcopy.)

If colposocopic exam is positive for CIN, manage per ASCCP guidelines.

Manage and treat per ASCCP guidelines.

HPV DNA testing preferred if liquid-based cytology is available—if positive, manage same as in women with LSIL, and if negative, repeat cytology at 12 months.

Manage and treat per ASCCP guidelines.

If colposcopy and cytology are negative at 6 and 12 months, continue with routine screening. If positive at either 6 or 12 months, perform biopsy.

Manage and treat per ASCCP guidelines.

LSIL, low-grade squamous intraepithelial lesions; ASCUS, atypical squamous cells of undetermined significance; HSIL, high-grade squamous intraepithelial lesions; CIN, cervical intraepithelial neoplasm; ASCCP, American Society for Colposcopy and Cervical Pathology. (Adapted from 2006 Consensus Guidelines for the Management of Women with Abnormal Cervical Cancer Screening Tests. (2007). *American Journal of Obstetrics & Gynecology, 197*(4):346–355.)

Nursing Interventions
▶ *Pretest*
- Explain the purpose and procedure of Pap test. Obtain a pertinent history. No douching, vaginal suppositories for 2–3 days before test. Empty bladder and rectum before exam.

▶ *Intratest*
- Help the patient to relax, protect modesty, and provide support.
- Consider all specimens infected until fixed with a germicidal preservative.

▶ *Posttest*
- Evaluate patient outcomes and counsel appropriately regarding repeat testing and need for follow-up biopsies and possible colposcopy.

PARATHYROID HORMONE ASSAY

Blood Hormone, Fasting

This test measures the parathyroid hormone in the blood—a major factor in calcium metabolism—and is used to detect primary and secondary diseases of the parathyroid glands.

Indications
- Diagnose hyperparathyroid and hypoparathyroid diseases.
- Distinguish nonparathyroid from parathyroid causes of hypercalcemia, as renal failure or vitamin D deficiency, compensatory responses to hypercalcemia in metastatic bone tumors.

Reference Values

Normal

Varies greatly with method used—necessary to check with the laboratory regarding test results.

Parathyroid hormone (PTH): Intact: 10–65 pg/mL or 10–65 ng/L

Calcium: 8.5–10.9 mg/dL or 2.12–2.72 mmol/L

Clinical Implications
- PTH should always be interpreted along with total calcium.
- *Increased parathyroid hormone values:* Primary hyperparathyroidism, secondary hyperparathyroidism (chronic renal failure), pseudohyperparathyroidism (slight increase). Intact PTH is often within the reference range in mild primary hyperparathyroidism but is inappropriately elevated for the total calcium concentration.
- *Decreased parathyroid hormone values:* Nonparathyroid hypercalcemia (eg, hypercalcemia of malignancy), primary hypoparathyroidism, secondary hypoparathyroidism (surgical), magnesium deficiency and DiGeorge's syndrome, and hyperthyroidism.

Interfering Factors
- Recent injection of radiopharmaceuticals.
- Elevated blood lipids and hemolysis interfere with testing methods.
- Milk-alkali syndrome may falsely lower levels.
- Vitamin D deficiency increases PTH levels.

- Increases after meals and in obesity.
- Decreases occur with exercise, high-protein diet, and ethanol.

Procedure
- Ensure a 10-hour fasting test—NPO after midnight except water.
- Obtain morning specimen—diurnal rhythm affects PTH levels (check with laboratory if the patient normally works night shift).
- Obtain 10 mL of venous blood in a red-top tube. Chill on ice immediately.
- Obtain serum calcium–level determination at the same time, if ordered. The serum PTH and serum calcium levels are important for meaningful clinical interpretation.

Nursing Interventions
▶ *Pretest*
- Explain purpose and blood test procedure, including fasting for test.
- Assess patient regarding sleep and work patterns, because the test outcome is related to diurnal rhythm; highest at 4:00 PM, lowest at 8:00 AM.

▶ *Posttest*
- Advise patient if results are abnormal and that repeat testing may be necessary.
- In collaboration with the physician, compare parathyroid hormone during test outcome with those of serum calcium levels to aid differential diagnosis.

PARATHYROID IMAGING

Nuclear Medicine, Endocrine Imaging

This test is used to evaluate patients with hyperparathyroidism, elevated calcium and inappropriately high parathyroid hormone levels to demonstrate the location of parathyroid adenomas before surgery.

Indications
- Differentiate between intrinsic and extrinsic parathyroid adenomas.

- Localize parathyroid adenomas in patients with primary hyperthyroidism.
- In children, verify the presence of the parathyroid gland after thyroidectomy.

Reference Values

Normal
- No areas of increased perfusion or uptake in the parathyroid and thyroid glands.

Clinical Implications
- Abnormal concentrations reveal intrinsic and extrinsic parathyroid adenomas. Benign parathyroid disease *cannot* be differentiated from malignant parathyroid disease; computer subtraction of one image from another results in visualization of adenoma.

Procedure
- Administer radiolabeled iodine (^{123}I) intravenously. The neck is imaged about 4 hours later.
- Position the patient with the neck hyperextended and head secured on the head rest.
- Inject ^{99m}Tc sestamibi without moving the patient, and after 10 minutes, acquire additional images.
- Inform the patient that the imaging may take 1 hour.

Nursing Interventions
▶ Pretest
- Explain parathyroid imaging purpose and procedure.
- Note that recent ingestion of iodine in food, thyroid medication, and recent tests with iodine could affect the study.

▶ Intratest
- Provide support and encouragement during the procedure.
- Instruct the patient to remain absolutely still during the procedure.

▶ Posttest
- Evaluate patient outcome and counsel appropriately about scan outcomes.
- Monitor injection site for extravasation or infiltration of radiopharmaceutical agent.
- Observe and treat mild reactions (per orders): pruritus, rashes, and flushing 2–24 hours after injection; sometimes nausea and vomiting may occur.

PAROTID (SALIVARY) GLAND IMAGING

Nuclear Medicine, GI Imaging

This test is performed to evaluate swelling masses in the parotid region and to determine size, location, and function of salivary glands.

Indications

- Detect blocked ducts of the parotid and submaxillary glands.
- Assess tumors of parotid or salivary glands.
- Diagnose Sjögren's syndrome in patients with rheumatoid arthritis.
- Evaluate xerostomia (dryness of mouth) associated with thyroiditis and collagen vascular diseases.

Reference Values

Normal

Normal size, shape, and position of glands and lack of evidence of tumor-type activity or blockage of ducts.

Clinical Implications

- "Hot nodule" (increased uptake of radionuclide) within normal tissue is associated with inflammation, as in Warthin's tumor, oncocytoma, and mucoepidermoid tumor.
- "Cold nodule" (decreased uptake of radionuclide) within normal tissue is associated with benign tumors, abscesses, or cysts, indicated by smooth shape–defined outlines, and, in adenocarcinomas, indicated by ragged, irregular outlines.
- Diffuse *decreased* activity occurs in obstructions, Sjögren's syndrome, and chronic sialadenitis.
- Diffuse *increased* activity as in acute parietis.

Procedure

- The radiopharmaceutical ^{99m}Tc pertechnetate is injected intravenously and imaging begins immediately. The patient is examined in a seated position and imaging takes place every few seconds for 2–3 minutes. There are three imaging phases: (a) blood flow; (b) uptake or trapping; and (c) secretions.
- If a secreting function test is being performed to detect salivary duct blockage, three-fourths of the way through the test, the patient is asked to suck on a lemon slice. If the salivary duct is normal, this

causes the gland to empty. This phase is *not* performed in studies for tumor detection.
- Total test time is 45–60 minutes.

Nursing Interventions
▶*Pretest*
- Explain parotid scan purpose, benefits, risks, and procedure. No discomfort or pain is involved.

▶*Intratest*
- Provide encouragement and support during the procedure.

▶*Posttest*
- Evaluate patient outcomes and counsel appropriately about inflammation, obstruction, abscesses, or cysts. Monitor IV site for signs of extravasation, infiltration, or infection.
- Advise pregnant staff and visitors to avoid prolonged contact for 24–48 hours after radioactive administration.
- Observe and treat mild reactions such as pruritus, rashes, and flushing for 2–24 hours after injection; sometimes nausea and vomiting may occur.

PHENYLKETONURIA (PKU)

Blood and Urine

Routine blood and urine tests are performed on newborns to detect PKU, a genetic disease characterized by a lack of enzyme that converts phenylalanine to tyrosine, which can lead to mental retardation and brain damage if left untreated.

Indications
- Screening neonatal period to detect genetic hepatic enzyme deficiency. May be state mandated.

Reference Values

Normal
- Blood phenylalanine: <2 mg/dL or <121.0 μmol/L (2–5 days after birth)
- Urine: Negative dipstick; no observed color change
  Note: Cord blood cannot be used.

Clinical Implications

- PKU is increased in sepsis, severe burns, and transient tyrosinemia of the newborn.

Interfering Factors

- Premature infants, infants weighing less than 11 kg (5 lb), may have elevated phenylalanine and tyrosine levels without having the genetic disease.
- Large amounts of ketones in the urine produce an atypical color reaction.
- Antibiotics interfere with the assay and the results cannot be interpreted.

Procedure

Collecting Blood Sample

- After skin is cleansed with an antiseptic, infant's heel is punctured with a sterile disposable lancet. If bleeding is slow, it is helpful to hold baby so that blood flows with the help of gravity. Circles on filter paper must be filled completely. This can best be done by placing one side of the filter paper against infant's heel and watching for blood to appear on front side of the paper and completely fill circle. Do not expose filter paper to extreme heat or light.
- Refer to guidelines for specimen collection in Chapter 2.

Collecting Urine Samples

- The reagent strip is either dipped into a fresh sample of urine or pressed against a wet diaper. Follow the manufacturer's directions exactly. Refer to guidelines for specimen collection in Chapter 2.

Nursing Interventions

♦Pretest

- Assess parent knowledge base before explaining test purpose and procedure.

♦Intratest

- Accurate test results depend on proper collection, following manufacturer's directions, and labeling.

♦Posttest

- Evaluate patient outcome. Provide genetic counseling and support to parent as appropriate.

CLINICAL ALERT

- PKU studies should be done on all infants weighing 5 lb or more.
- The blood test must be performed at least 3 days after birth or after the child has had a chance to ingest protein (milk) for a period of 24–48 hours. Urine testing is done at the 4- or 6-week checkup if a blood sample was not obtained.

PLATELET ANTIBODY DETECTION TESTS (PLAI) (ALTP) (PAIgG)

Blood, Platelet Disorders

This test is performed to detect platelet antibodies.

Indications

- Diagnose posttransfusion purpura, alloimmune neonatal thrombocytopenic purpura, idiopathic thrombocytopenia purpura, paroxysmal hemoglobinuria, and drug-induced immunologic thrombocytopenia.
- Diagnose neonatal thrombocytopenia purpura.
- Evaluate drug-induced immunologic thrombocytopenia.
- Assess posttransfusion purpura.

Reference Values

Normal
- Platelet-associated IgG (PLAI): Negative platelet hyperlysibility: Negative.
- Antiplatelet-antibody (ALTP): Negative drug-dependent platelet antibodies: Negative.
- Platelet-bound IgG (PAIgG): Negative.

Clinical Implications
- Presence of antibodies to platelet antigens: There are two types: Autoantibodies develop in response to one's own platelets, as in idiopathic thrombocytopenic purpura, and alloantibodies, following exposure to foreign platelets posttransfusion.
- Antiplatelet antibody, usually having anti-PLAI specificity, occurs in posttransfusion purpura.

- A persistent or rising antibody titer during pregnancy is associated with neonatal thrombocytopenia.
- PLAI incompatibility between the mother and the fetus appears to account for more than 60% of alloimmune neonatal thrombocytopenic purpura. A finding of a PLAI-negative mother and a PLAI-positive father provides presumptive diagnostic evidence.
- Platelet-associated IgG antibody is present in 95% of idiopathic (autoimmune) thrombocytopenic purpura (both acute and chronic) cases. Patients responding to steroid therapy or undergoing spontaneous remission show increased circulatory times that correlate with decreased PAIgG levels.
- The platelet hyperlysibility assay measures the sensitivity of platelets to lysis. This test is positive in and specific for paroxysmal hemoglobinuria.
- In drug-induced immunologic thrombocytopenia, antibodies that react only in the presence of the inciting drug can be detected. Quinidine, quinine, chlordiazepoxide, sulfa drugs, and diphenylhydantoin most commonly cause this type of thrombocytopenia. Gold-dependent antibodies and heparin-dependent platelet IgG antibodies can be detected by direct assay. (Approximately 1% of persons receiving gold therapy develop thrombocytopenia as a side effect.) Thrombocytopenia is also a well-known side effect of heparin.

Interfering Factors

- Alloantibodies formed in response to previous blood transfusions during pregnancies may produce positive reactions. Such antibodies are usually specific for human leukocyte antigens (HLAs) found in platelets and other cells. Whenever possible, obtain samples for platelet antibody testing before transfusion is performed.

Procedure

- A 10- to 30-mL venous blood sample is required; these procedures are not well standardized. Required tubes depend upon the method used.
- Blood specimen requirements: 30 mL of venous blood when platelet count is 50,000 to 100,000/mm^3 or (50–100) $\times$ 10^9/L; 20 mL of venous blood when platelet count is 100,000 to 150,000/mm^3 or (100–150) $\times$ 10^9/L; 10 mL of venous blood when platelet count is >150,000/mm^3 or >150 $\times$ 10^9/L.

Nursing Interventions

♦ *Pretest*

• Explain test purpose and procedure. The large amount of blood required for platelet isolation may make the test impractical in children or anemic adults.

♦ *Posttest*

• Interpret test outcomes, counsel, and monitor appropriately for bleeding tendencies. Assess for prescribed medications as cause of purpura.

PORPHYRINS, PORPHOBILINOGENS (PBG), AND DELTA-AMINOLEVULINIC ACID (ALA)

Random and Timed Urine

This test measures cyclic compounds formed from delta-aminolevulinic acid (ALA), which are important for the formation of hemoglobin and other hemoproteins that function as carriers of oxygen in the blood and tissues.

Indications

• Diagnose acute intermittent porphyria (AIP).
• Assess porphyria in persons with unexplained neurologic manifestations, unexplained abdominal pain, cutaneous blisters, photosensitivity, and relevant family history.
• Evaluate lead poisoning and pellagra.
• Investigate both dark and red urine in newborns.

Reference Values

Normal

Porphobilinogen (urine): <3.4 mg/24 hours or <15 µmol/day; random: <2.0 mg/L or <8.8 mmol/L

	µG/24 HOURS	SI UNITS (NMOL/DAY)
MALE		
Uroporphyrin	8–44	9.6–53
Coproporphyrin	10–109	15–166
Heptacarboxyporphyrin	0–12	0–15
Pentacarboxyporphyrin	0–4	0–6
Hexacarboxyporphyrin	0–5	0–7
Total porphyrins	8–149	9.6–179

	µG/24 HOURS	SI UNITS (NMOL/DAY)
FEMALE		
Uroporphyrin	4–22	4.8–26
Coproporphyrin	3–56	4.6–85
Heptacarboxyporphyrin	0–9	0–11
Pentacarboxyporphyrin	0–3	0–4
Hexacarboxyporphyrin	0–5	0–7
Total porphyrins	3–78	3.6–94

Delta-aminolevulinic acid (Δ-ALA): 0–7.5 mg/24 hours (57.2 µmol/day); random: <4.5 mg/L or <34 µmol/L

Clinical Implications

* *Increased porphobilinogen* in porphyria; during crisis in acute inter-mittent porphyria, variegate porphyria, and hereditary coproporphyria.
* *Increased porphyrins* (fractionated) in acute intermittent porphyria, congenital erythropoietic porphyria, hereditary coproporphyria, var-iegate porphyria, and chemical porphyria; caused by heavy metal poisoning, carbon tetrachloride and lead poisoning; other conditions with increased porphyria: viral hepatitis, cirrhosis, and the newborn of a mother with porphyria.
* Porphobilinogen (PBG) is not increased in lead poisoning. PPG is the hallmark of an acute attack of porphyria found in a random urine test; 24-hour test is used for confirmation.
* *Increased delta-aminolevulinic acid (Δ-ALA)* in acute intermittent porphyria, acute variegate porphyria, hereditary coproporphyria, lead poisoning (remains elevated months after treatment), and dia-betic acidosis.
* *Decreased Δ-ALA* is seen in alcoholic liver disease.

Interfering Factors

* Oral contraceptives and diazepam can cause acute porphyria attacks in susceptible patients.
* Alcohol must be avoided during the test.
* Certain drugs interfere with the test, especially phenothiazines, procaine sulfamethoxazole, and the tetracyclines.

Procedure

* Collect urine in a clean, dark container; refrigeration is usually required. The specimen is kept protected from exposure to light and must be covered. See specimen collection and handling guide-lines in Chapter 2. Check with your lab.
* Five grams of sodium bicarbonate is usually added to the container before collection.

- For random urine tests, 2:00–4:00 PM is the best time because more porphyrins are excreted at this time.

Nursing Interventions

▶ *Pretest*

- Assess patient compliance.
- Assess patient knowledge base before explaining test purpose and procedure.
- If possible, discontinue all drugs for 2–4 weeks before the test so that results are accurate.

> ### CLINICAL ALERT
>
> - This test should not be ordered for patients receiving Donnatal (belladonna/phenobarbital) or other barbiturate preparations. If intermittent porphyrin is suspected, the patient should take these medications according to prescribed protocols because these drugs may provoke an attack of porphyria. If signs and symptoms occur, notify the physician and record them.

▶ *Intratest*

- Food and fluids are permitted; alcohol and excessive fluid intake during collection should be avoided.
- Accurate test results depend on proper collection, preservation, and labeling. Be sure to include test start and completion times.
- Observe and record color of urine. If porphyrins are present, urine may have a grossly recognizable amber red or burgundy color. It may vary from pale pink to almost black. Some patients excrete urine of normal color that turns dark after standing in the light.

▶ *Posttest*

- The patient may resume normal activities and preparations.
- Interpret test outcomes and counsel appropriately.

POSITRON EMISSION TOMOGRAPHY (PET)

Nuclear Medicine, PET Imaging

Positron emission tomography (PET) is the combined use of IV-administered, positron-emitting isotopes (carbon[11], nitrogen[13], oxygen[15], and fluorine[18]) and emission-computed axial tomography to image physiologic tissue function: perfusion, metabolism, and neuron activity. Unlike MRI and CT imaging, PET provides physiologic, anatomic, and biochemical data.

Indications

- Assess blood flow and tissue metabolism.
- Evaluate epilepsy, dementia, stroke, schizophrenia, and brain tumors.
- Determine cardiac tissue viability, myocardial perfusion, and coronary artery disease.
- Detect and stage early tumors; distinguish between recurrent tumor, active tumor, and necrotic masses in soft tissue; monitor therapy.
- Differentiate Alzheimer's disease from Huntington's disease and Parkinson's disease.

Reference Values

Normal

- Normal patterns of tissue metabolism and body metabolism based on oxygen, glucose, fatty acid utilization, and protein synthesis.
- Normal blood flow and tissue perfusion.

Clinical Implications

- In *epilepsy*, focal areas with increased metabolism have been visualized during actual stage of epilepsy with decreased oxygen use and blood flow during interictal stage.
- In *stroke*, an extremely complex pathophysiologic picture is revealed: anaerobic glycolysis, depressed oxygen use, and decreased blood flow.
- In *dementia*, decreased glucose consumption (hypometabolic activity) is revealed by PET imaging.
- In *schizophrenia*, some studies using labeled glucose indicate reduced metabolic activity in the frontal region.
- In *brain tumors*, data have been collected concerning oxygen use and blood-flow relationships for these tumors.
- With *coronary artery disease*, areas of decreased blood flow or perfusion, or both, occur and indicate myocardial tissue that is no longer viable; transient ischemia (using both stress and rest imaging) can be determined.
- In cases of suspected tumor recurrence after therapy, PET differentiates any new growth from necrotic tissue. (Abnormal glucose metabolism determines tumor growth.) Tumor grading can be assessed by the rate of increases in glucose metabolism.

Procedure

- Specific procedures vary depending on the imaging equipment and physician preference. The most commonly used positron-emitting radiopharmaceutical is F-18 fluorodeoxyglucose (FDG) or fluorine[18].
- The patient is positioned on the table and a background transmission imaging is obtained.
- The radioactive drug is administered intravenously. The patient must wait 30–45 minutes, usually on the table, and then the area of interest is imaged.
- Total procedure time can be 1–2 hours.

Nursing Interventions

◆ *Pretest*

- *For neurology (brain PET image):* Advise patient that lying as still as possible during imaging is necessary. However, the patient is not allowed to fall asleep or count to pass the time.
- Use measures, such as progressive relaxation and breathing techniques, to reduce anxiety and help patient manage stress.
- *For cardiology:* An intravenous line is established. Smoking and certain medications may be restricted before imaging. Consult with the referring physician or the nuclear imaging department.
- *For colon cancer or kidney procedures:* A urinary catheter may be inserted.

◆ *Intratest*

- Blood pressure is often monitored. Sometimes, fasting blood glucose samples are obtained. If blood glucose levels are too high, insulin may be ordered and administered. Insulin suppresses glucose tissue uptake. Insulin also suppresses FDG tissue uptake, which affects the quality of the resulting scan.
- For neurology, it is important to maintain a quiet environment.
- For cardiology, it may be necessary to place ECG leads on patient.

◆ *Posttest*

- Evaluate image outcomes, and in collaboration with physician, counsel appropriately.

PREALBUMIN (TRANSTHYRETIN)

Blood, Proteins

Prealbumin (PAB) testing offers the specificity and precision to detect daily changes in patient's protein status caused by nutritional support or metabolic derangements. It is the best index of total parenteral nutrition because of its short half-life (1–2 days).

Indications

- Assess nutritional status; monitor response to nutritional support of acutely ill patient and patients at risk for protein calorie malnutrition (PCM).
- Monitor low-birth-weight neonates and those with certain congenital abnormalities.
- Screen hospital admissions and presurgical, trauma, septic, and GI patients.

Reference Values

Normal

- Adult normal range is 10–40 mg/dL or 100–400 mg/L by rate nephelometry.

Note: Levels are *decreased* in pregnancy, after age 60 (approximately up to 20%), and in premenopausal women.

Clinical Implications

- Prealbumin value of 0–5 mg/dL or 0–50 mg/L indicates severe protein depletion; 5–10 mg/dL or 50–100 mg/L, moderate protein depletion; and 10–15 mg/dL or 100–150 mg/L, mild protein depletion.
- Decreased levels occur in malnutrition, acute inflammatory processes, and hepatic disease and nephrotic syndrome.

Interfering Factors

- Many drugs affect results. *Increases* occur with androgens and oral contraceptives. *Decreases* occur with amiodarone and estrogens.

Procedure

- Serum (5 mL) is obtained by venipuncture in a red-top tube. A fasting sample is recommended. Place specimen in a biohazard bag.
- If test is requested on a child, a venous blood sample of 2–3 mL should prove sufficient to run the test by rate nephelometry.

Nursing Interventions

▶ Pretest

- Explain prealbumin's usefulness as a screening tool to determine nutritional status.

▶*Posttest*
- Evaluate patient results and counsel appropriately about nutritional status.
- Prepare patient for possibility of repeat testing to monitor response to nutritional support.

PREGNANCY TESTS—HUMAN CHORIONIC GONADOTROPIN BETA-SUBUNIT (BETA-HCG)

Blood and Urine

All pregnancy tests are designed to detect the presence of human chorionic gonadotropin (hCG). The quantitative beta-subunit of hCG is the most sensitive and specific test for early pregnancy, gestational age, ectopic pregnancy, or threatened abortion; it is also used in the management of testicular tumors.

Indications
- Confirm pregnancy and estimate gestational age through serial measurements.
- Detect trophoblastic and testicular tumors in men.
- Evaluate ectopic pregnancy and miscarriage.
- Monitor treatment of chorioendocarcinoma.

Reference Values

Normal

BLOOD AND URINE (QUALITATIVE)

Nonpregnant women and men: Negative
Commercial, over-the-counter pregnancy kits are available. Usually test can be performed 5–7 days after missed menstrual period.

SERUM (QUANTITATIVE)

Nonpregnant women and men: <5 mIU/mL or <5 IU/L
Pregnant women: 1–12 weeks: 50–220,000 mIU/mL or 50–220,000 IU/L

Clinical Implications
- *Increased or positive urine* levels usually indicate pregnancy but are also present in choriocarcinoma, hydatidiform mole, testicular

tumors, chorioepithelioma, chorioadenoma destruens, some ectopic pregnancies, multiple gestations, and some neoplasms of lung, stomach, colon, and liver.

- *Decreased or negative urine* levels indicate fetal death or an incomplete or threatened abortion.
- A marked fall in prealbumin occurs in acute inflammation.
- *Increased serum hCG* is seen in trophoblastic neoplasms, toxemia, germ cell tumors, and breast cancer.
- *Decreased serum hCG* levels are observed in ectopic pregnancy and spontaneous abortion.

Interfering Factors

- False-negative urine tests and falsely low levels of hCG may be due to a dilute urine (low specific gravity) or a specimen obtained too early in pregnancy.
- False-positive urine tests are associated with proteinuria, hematuria, urinary tract infection, presence of excess pituitary gonadotropin, and certain drugs such as glucocorticosteroids, antiparkinsonism drugs, anticonvulsants, hypnotics, phenothiazines, and methadone.
- A positive test can be obtained 1–2 weeks after complete abortion.

Procedure

- Serum (5 mL) is obtained by venipuncture in a red-top tube.
- An early morning specimen is collected in a clean container for urine pregnancy test. This specimen usually contains the greatest concentration of hCG. However, specimens collected at any time may be used, but specific gravity must be at least 1.005. See specimen collection guidelines in Chapter 2.
- A 24-hour urine specimen is collected for quantitative hCG studies. See specimen collection guidelines in Chapter 2.
- Grossly bloody urine specimens are not acceptable; in this instance, a catheterized specimen should be obtained or a serum pregnancy test is ordered.

Nursing Interventions
▶Pretest

- Assess patient knowledge base before explaining test purpose and procedure.
- Ask female patient when she had last menstrual period.

▶Intratest

- Accurate test results depend on proper collection, preservation, and labeling. Be sure to include urine test start, completion, and collection times.

⟩*Posttest*
- Evaluate patient outcome. Provide counseling and support as appropriate for positive or negative outcomes.

PREGNANEDIOL

Timed Urine, Hormone

This test measures ovarian and placental function, specifically the principal metabolite of the hormone progesterone.

Indications
- Evaluate precocious puberty in girls.
- Assess amenorrhea and other menstrual disorders.
- Diagnose placental failure and fetal death.

Reference Values

Normal
- This test is difficult to standardize; it varies with age, gender, and weeks of pregnancy.

  Men (urine): <1.9 mg/24 hours or <5.9 μmol/day

  Women (urine):

      Follicular phase: <2.6 mg/24 hours or <8.1 μmol/day

      Pregnancy third trimester: 70–100 mg/24 hours or 218–312 μmol/day

      Postmenopausal phase: <1.4 mg/24 hours or <4.2 μmol/day

  Children: <1.1 mg/24 hours or <3 μmol/day

Clinical Implications
- *Increased pregnanediol levels* are associated with luteal ovarian cysts, arrhenoblastoma of ovary, hyperadrenocorticism, pregnancy, malignant neoplasm of trophoblast.
- *Decreased pregnanediol levels* are associated with amenorrhea, threatened abortion (if <50 mg/24 hours or 156 μmol/day, abortion is imminent), fetal death, toxemia, neoplasm of ovary, ovarian tumor, and hydatidiform mole.

Interfering Factors
- Improper specimen collection affects outcome.
- *Decreased values* with estrogen therapy, progesterone therapy, and oral contraceptives.

Procedure

- Collect urine in a clean container for 24-hour refrigeration; preservative may be required. Protect from light. See timed specimen collection guidelines in Chapter 2.
- Record date of last menstrual period.

Nursing Interventions

▶ Pretest

- Assess patient compliance. Obtain accurate menstrual history.
- Evaluate patient knowledge base before explaining test purpose and procedure.

▶ Intratest

- Accurate test results depend on proper collection, preservation, and labeling. Be sure to include test start and completion times.

▶ Posttest

- Evaluate patient outcome. Provide counseling and support as appropriate for menstrual disorders and pregnancy outcomes.

PRETRANSFUSION AND PRETRANSPLANT TESTS; IMMUNOHEMATOLOGY TESTS: OVERVIEW

Blood, Blood Banking

These tests are performed to select blood components that will have acceptable survival when transfused, to prevent possible transplant and transfusion reactions and infections, to identify potential problems such as hemolytic disease of newborns and the need for intrauterine transfusion, and to determine parentage. Immunohematology testing identifies highly reactive antigens on blood cells and their antibodies, possibly present in serum. All donated blood, as it is processed, must undergo several measurements for blood cell antigens and for infectious disease. These include donor blood tests for ABO groups, Rh type, antibody screen, hepatitis B surface antigen H (HBsAg), hepatitis B core antigen, hepatitis C virus (anti-HCV) (syphilis VDRL), human immunodeficiency virus (HIV-1 and HIV-2), human T-cell lymphocytic virus (HTLV-1 and HTLV-2), and human immunodeficiency virus antigen (HIV-1-Ag).

Required testing for whole-blood or red blood cell recipients include the following: ABO group, Rh type, antibody screen, crossmatch for compatibility between donor's cells and recipient's serum. Even though no crossmatch is needed for plasma administration, compatible ABO typing should be performed. Routinely, no crossmatch is needed for platelet administration; compatible ABO and Rh typing should be performed. If a patient becomes refractory, HLA-matched platelets may be administered. Granulocytes should be tested for HLA compatibility.

Histocompatibility locus A (HLA)—These antigens are found in blood cells and most tissues of the body. Because of previous transfusions or pregnancy, some patients develop antibodies against these antigens and, if given incompatible blood, may have a transfusion reaction. Other donated blood testing and processing considerations regarding autologous and directed donations, cytomegalovirus tests, and blood product irradiation are presented in the following list:

- *Autologous donations*—Blood recipient and donor are the same person and blood products donated by patients for their own use. Many patients opt to donate their own blood before scheduled surgery because of the concern over transfusion-transmitted diseases.
- *Allogenic*—Blood donor and blood recipient are not the same person; donations are blood products donated by one individual for use by other individuals.
- *Directed donations*—Recipients choose the donors who will donate blood for their transfusions. Laws in several states declare that this request must be honored in nonemergency situations. Standards and testing procedures must be identical to those required for an allogenic blood donor. (Autologous donors do not need to adhere to the same criteria as do allogeneic blood donors.) The following list addresses some general guidelines for autologous blood donors: There is no age limit, if healthy; no weight requirements. The volume of blood collected must comply with established weight provisions. Pregnant women can donate. Hematocrit should be 33% or more. If less than 33%, the patient's physician must approve the phlebotomy, usually in consultation with the blood bank medical director; and, normally, phlebotomy can be done at 3-day intervals; the final phlebotomy can be done at least 72 hours before the time of the scheduled surgery. Iron supplements may be prescribed to maintain adequate hemoglobin levels.
- *Cytomegalovirus testing*—Cytomegalovirus (CMV) testing is done for those patients at risk for transfusion-associated CMV infections. These types of CMV infections were first seen as a mononucleosis syndrome after cardiopulmonary bypass surgery and were thought to be related to the use of fresh blood during the

surgery. Clinical symptoms of transfusion-transmitted CMV infections include pneumonitis, hepatitis, retinitis, or disseminated infection. They generally occur in immunosuppressed patients such as premature infants weighing less than 1200 g at birth, bone marrow and organ transplant patients, and certain immunocompromised oncology patients. Therefore, to prevent these infections, CMV antibody testing is done. Patients at risk should receive CMV-seronegative blood and blood products. CMV in blood is associated with leukocytes. Leukocyte reduction with highly efficient leukocyte-reduction filters also appears to be an effective way of reducing CMV infection.

- *Irradiation of blood products*—Sometimes, blood products are irradiated before transfusion for certain immunosuppressed patients. Graft-versus-host disease (GVHD) is a rare complication that follows transfusion of severely immunosuppressed patients. GVHD occurs if donor lymphocytes from blood or blood products engraft and multiply in a severely immunodeficient recipient. The engrafted lymphocytes react against host (recipient) tissues. Clinical symptoms include skin rash, fever, diarrhea, hepatitis, bone marrow suppression, and infection, which frequently lead to death. GVHD can be prevented by irradiating blood products with a minimum dose (cesium 137) of 2500 rads in the center of the container and a minimum dose of 1500 rads delivered to all other parts of the component. This dose renders the T lymphocytes in a unit of blood incapable of replication. It does not affect platelets or granulocytes. Irradiation does affect the red cell membrane, causing it to "leak" potassium. All irradiated red cells are given a 28-day "outdate" or may keep their original "outdate" of less than 28 days.

- *Leukocyte reduction of blood products*—Leukocytes in blood products have long been known to be associated with nonhemolytic febrile transfusion reactions, possibly more due to cytokines produced by the leukocytes than due to the leukocytes themselves. Leukocyte reduction may reduce the number of these reactions. It may also decrease the possibility of alloimmunization to the HLAs on the leukocytes. Removing leukocytes very effectively reduces the danger of transfusion-transmitted CMV infection.

Indications

- Required of blood, organ, and tissue donors and potential recipients to prevent possible transfusion and transplant reactions and infection.

- Before surgery that may require transfusion, crossmatch to detect antibodies to *recipient's* serum that damage *donor* cells (major crossmatch), or detect antibodies in *donor's* cells that may affect RBCs of *recipient* (minor crossmatch).
- Detect and prevent hemolytic newborn disease and Rh typing when woman has had abortion or miscarriage.
- Determine the need for intrauterine transfusion and candidate for RhIG (Rh immunoglobulin).
- Determine parentage.

PRIONS

Blood

Recent research suggests that prions ("proteinaceous infectious particles") are bacteria that do not contain DNA or RNA and that occur in both inherited and infectious disease. No immune response to prions has been detected.

Indications
- Diagnose prion brain disease, such as Creutzfeldt-Jakob disease and spongiform encephalitis ("mad cow disease").

Reference Values

Normal
- Structural form, named PrPc (prion protein cellular), is found in lymphocytes and in CNS neurons.

Clinical Implications
- Abnormal finding of PrPc protein (disease-causing form) is pathogenic, which affects the cerebral cortex and cerebellum.
- Gerstmann-Sträussler-Scheinker (GSS) syndrome, a cause of hereditary dementia, occurs because of a mutation in the prion gene.
- Prion infectious disease may be transfusion related.

Procedure
- Brain biopsy samples are examined for evidence of the infectious prion or mutated gene in chromosome 20.

Nursing Interventions

▶ Pretest

- Explain the test purpose and procedure sensitively, as patients are often very sick and the infectious disease is usually fatal.
- Obtain from the patient or family any history of encephalopathy or dementia (hereditary) and related signs and symptoms. Behavioral changes include ataxia, peripheral sensory changes, and dementia.

▶ Posttest

- Interpret test results and explain supportive care and treatment.
- Monitor for encephalitis or dementia.
- Provide comfort, support, and special counseling regarding the progression of the disease. Death occurs about 12 months after the appearance of the first signs.

Proctoscopy—Anoscopy, Sigmoidoscopy, Proctosigmoidoscopy

Endoscopic GI Imaging

These examinations are used to view, diagnose, and treat disorders of the anal canal, rectum, and sigmoid colon linings with proctosigmoidoscopes (rigid or flexible), anoscopes, or proctoscopes.

Indications

- Routine (every 3–5 years) for cancer screening for individuals older than 50 years.
- Evaluate anal and perineal conditions such as hemorrhoids, abscesses and fistulae, structures and stenoses, rectal prolapse, fissures, and contractures.
- Assess anal pruritus, passage of blood or mucus in the stool, changes in bowel habits, lower abdominal or perineal pain, and unexplained anemia.
- Confirm or rule out inflammatory bowel disease, polyps, cancer, and benign tumors.

Reference Values

Normal

Normal-appearing anal canal, rectum, and sigmoid colon mucosa.

Clinical Implications

- Alterations in mucosa or changes in the vascular pattern, such as edematous, red, or denuded mucosa, granularity, friability, ulcers, thickened areas, pseudomembranes, or spontaneous bleeding.
- Inflammatory bowel processes such as chronic ulcerative colitis, Crohn's disease, acute or chronic proctitis, or pseudomembranous colitis, or antibiotic-associated colitis.
- Cysts, polyps, ulcers (adenomatous, familial, or diminutive), fistulae, strictures, infections, abscesses, hemorrhoids, and stenoses.
- Carcinomas or benign tumors such adenocarcinoma, carcinoids, and lipomas.

Procedure

- Digital examination of the anus and rectum is done before the procedure.
- For rigid proctoscopy, the patient assumes a knee-to-chest position. When the flexible proctoscope is used, the patient must be in the left lateral position, with the buttock over the edge of the table. The proctoscope or sigmoidoscope is then carefully inserted into the rectum.
- Specimens can be obtained and polyps can be removed during the procedure. Biopsy of the anal canal may require an anesthetic to be given to the patient.
- The patient may feel a very strong urge to defecate and may experience a feeling of bloating or cramping. These sensations are normal.
- The actual examination usually takes less than 10 minutes.

Nursing Interventions

◗ Pretest

- Explain test purpose and the procedure that the patient will experience. Special sensitivity to cultural, social, sexual, and modesty issues is needed.
- There is no need for the patient to fast. However, a restricted diet such as clear liquids the evening before the test may be prescribed.
- Laxatives and enemas may be administered the night before the examination. Enemas or a rectal laxative suppository may be administered the morning of the procedure.

◗ Intratest

- Position patient properly and drape adequately so that exposure is minimized.
- Explain that patient may experience gas pains, cramping, and urge to defecate as scope is advanced; slow, deep breathing and

abdominal muscle relaxation may reduce these sensations. (Sometimes sedatives, tranquilizers, or analgesics may be given prior to the examination.)

- Coach the patient in performing slow, deep breathing and abdominal muscle relaxation.
- Place specimens in appropriate preservatives, label correctly, and route to lab in a timely manner.

⋫Posttest

- Interpret test outcomes and counsel appropriately.
- Expect small amounts of blood in the stool if a biopsy or polypectomy was done. Instruct the patient to watch for signs of bowel perforation and to contact the physician immediately if perforation is suspected (see Clinical Alert).

CLINICAL ALERT

- Patients with acute symptoms, particularly those individuals with suspected ulcerative or granulomatous colitis, should be examined without any preparation (without enemas, laxatives, or suppositories).
- Perforation of the intestinal wall can be an infrequent complication of these tests.
- Symptoms of bowel perforation (an infrequent event) include rectal bleeding or hemorrhage, abdominal distention, and pain, fever, and malaise.
- Notify the physician immediately of any instances of decreased blood pressure, diaphoresis, or bradycardia.

PROGESTERONE

Blood, Hormone

Progesterone is a female sex hormone involved in the preparation of the uterus for pregnancy. This test is performed to confirm ovulation, evaluate function of the corpus luteum, and assess risk for early miscarriage.

Indications

- Study fertility.
- Assess ovarian production of progesterone. It is the single best test to determine whether ovulation has occurred.
- Monitor course of assisted reproduction.

Reference Values

Normal

	NG/ML	SI UNITS (NMOL/L)
Male (M)	<1.0	<3.2
Female (F)		
Follicular phase	0.1–0.7	0.5–2.3
Luteal phase (*increases* with increasing age)	2–25	6.4–79.5
First trimester	10–44	32.6–140
Second trimester	19.5–82.5	62.0–262
Third trimester	65–290	206–728

Clinical Implications

- *Increases* in congenital adrenal hyperplasia, lipid ovarian tumor, molar pregnancy (hydatidiform mole), and chorionepithelioma of ovary.
- *Decreases* in threatened abortion, galactorrhea-amenorrhea syndrome, hypogonadism, toxemia, miscarriage, and fetal death.

Interfering Factors

- *Decreases* are associated with exercise, after meals, and with some drugs.

Procedure

- Serum (5 mL) is obtained by venipuncture in a red-top tube.

Nursing Interventions

▶*Pretest*

- Explain purpose and procedure.

▶*Posttest*

- Evaluate patient outcomes, and in collaboration with physician, counsel appropriately about fertility, pregnancy, and fetal status.

PROLACTIN (HPRL)

Blood, Pituitary, Hormone

This test measures the amount of this pituitary hormone (essential for initiating and maintaining lactation), in presence of amenorrhea, galactorrhea (milky discharge from breasts), infertility, and in men with impotence.

Indications
- Diagnose and manage prolactin-secreting pituitary tumors.
- Evaluate galactorrhea and amenorrhea.
- Monitor the effectiveness of surgery, chemotherapy, and radiation treatment of prolactin-secreting tumors.

Reference Values

Normal
Nonpregnant women: 0–23 ng/mL or 0–23 μg/L
Pregnant women: 34–386 ng/mL by third trimester or 34–386 μg/L
Men: 0–20 ng/mL or 0–20 μg/L
Critical value: 200 ng/mL or 200 μg/mL indicates a prolactin-secreting tumor in a nonlactating woman.

Clinical Implications
- *Increased* in galactorrhea, amenorrhea, polycystic ovary syndrome, pituitary tumors (prolactinomas), sexual precocity of children, primary hypothyroidism, renal failure, anorexia nervosa, liver failure, and insulin-induced hypoglycemia. It can be increased with any large pituitary tumor or with pituitary stalk compression.
- *Decreased* in seizures, hypopituitarism, pituitary apoplexy (eg, Sheehan's syndrome), idiopathic hypogonadotropic hypogonadism, malnutrition, and polycystic ovaries.

Interfering Factors
- Many drugs may increase (estrogens, antidepressants, antipsychotics, antihypertensives) or decrease (dopaminergic drugs) values.
- Increases in newborns, pregnancy, postpartum period, stress, exercise, drugs, nipple stimulation, and lactation.

> **CLINICAL ALERT**
>
> - Normal prolactin levels do not rule out pituitary tumor.

Procedure
- A 12-hour fasting (5 mL) serum is obtained by venipuncture in a red-top tube. Draw specimen between 8:00 and 10:00 AM, 3–4 hours

after awakening. In the newborn, cord blood or capillary may be used.
- Avoid stress, excitement, or stimulation.

Nursing Interventions
▶ *Pretest*
- Explain purpose, procedure, and fasting.

▶ *Posttest*
- Evaluate patient outcome, and in collaboration with physician, counsel appropriately about meaning of increases.
- Explain the need for further testing for increased prolactin.

PROSTATE ULTRASOUND—PROSTATE SONOGRAPHY, TRANSRECTAL SONOGRAPHY OF THE PROSTATE

Ultrasound, GU Imaging

This noninvasive procedure images the prostate and surrounding tissues.

Indications
- Evaluate an abnormality detected on digital exam or by deviations in serum levels of prostate-specific antigen (PSA).
- Aid in staging of biopsy-proven prostate carcinoma.
- Evaluate infertility related to prostate pathology.
- Provide guidance for biopsy or other interventional procedures.

Reference Values

Normal
Normal size, volume, shape, and consistency of prostate gland.

Clinical Implications
- Prostate enlargement (glandular hypertrophy), presence of space-occupying lesions: tumors, abscesses, cysts, and prostatitis.

Interfering Factors
- Fecal material in rectum will obscure visualization of prostate.

Procedure
- Typically, the patient is required to administer an enema the night before and the morning of the procedure.

- Patient is asked to lie on an exam table on his or her left side with knees bent toward chest. A draped and lubricated rectal transducer is inserted into rectum. Water may be introduced to sheath surrounding transducer head. Patient may feel slight pressure. The transducer handle is rotated to produce images in a variety of planes.
- The procedure takes approximately 15–30 minutes.

Nursing Interventions
▸*Pretest*
- Explain purpose and procedure. Assure patient that no radiation is employed and that test is painless.

▸*Posttest*
- Evaluate patient outcomes; provide support and counseling (in collaboration with physician) about prostate abnormalities.

PROTEIN

Blood and Urine (Timed and Random)

Total Protein, SPE (Serum Protein Electrophoresis) Albumin, Alpha-1 Globulin, Alpha-2 Globulin, Beta Globulin, Gamma Globulin, IFE (Immunofixation Electrophoresis), Protein in Urine (Proteinuria)

These tests are used to determine total protein, albumin, and alpha-1, alpha-2, and beta and gamma globulins in the blood or urine.

Indications
- Investigate and monitor chronic inflammatory and lymphoproliferative disorders (Waldenström's macroglobulinemia, multiple myeloma), as well as patients with recurrent infections who are suspected of having immunodeficient disease.
- Identify dysproteinemia, hypogammaglobulinemia, acute and chronic inflammatory disorders, nephrotic syndrome, liver disease, gastrointestinal loss, and polyclonal and monoclonal gammopathies.
- Use as an index of nutrition and osmotic pressure in edematous and malnourished patients.
- Assess immune function.
- Work up for liver disease and diagnosis of nephrotic syndrome.

• Obtain urinary protein to assess severity of renal disease and for the differential diagnosis of nephrotic syndrome.

Reference Values

Normal

In an electric field, serum proteins are separated according to their size, shape, and electric charge at pH 8.6.

Total protein: 6.0–8.0 g/dL or 60–80 g/L

Albumin: 3.5–5.0 g/dL or 35–50 g/L

Alpha-1 globulin: 0.1–0.3 g/dL or 1–3 g/L

Alpha-2 globulin: 0.6–1.0 g/dL or 6–10 g/L

Beta globulin: 0.7–1.1 g/dL or 7–11 g/L

Gamma globulin: 0.8–1.6 g/dL or 8–16 g/L

24-hour urine: 10–140 mg/24 hours or 10–140 mg/day

Clinical Implications

• *Total protein increases* (hyperproteinemia/sum of circulating serum proteins) because of hemoconcentration as a result of dehydration with body fluid loss (vomiting, diarrhea, and poor kidney function), as well as in liver disease, multiple myeloma, Waldenström's macroglobulinemia, tropical disease, sarcoidosis, collagen disorders, chronic infections, and inflammatory states.

• *Total protein decreases* (hypoproteinemia) with insufficient nutritional intake (starvation, malabsorption), severe liver disease, alcoholism, prolonged immobilization (trauma, orthopedic surgery), hypothyroidism, and other chronic diseases (Crohn's disease, colitis).

• *Albumin increases* with intravenous infusions, dehydration; generally not found.

• *Albumin decreases* in poor nutrition states (inadequate iron intake), increased albumin loss (eg, nephrotic syndrome, third-degree burns), decreased synthesis states such as liver diseases, alcoholism, malabsorption syndromes, Crohn's disease, prolonged immobilization, and malignancy.

• *Alpha-1 globulin increases* with acute and chronic infections, febrile reactions, pregnancy.

• *Alpha-1 globulin decreases* are common when there is an alpha-1 antitrypsin deficiency and nephrosis.

• *Alpha-2 globulin increases* are found in biliary cirrhosis, obstructive jaundice, diabetic synonephrosis, multiple myeloma, and ulcerative colitis.

• *Alpha-2 globulin decreases* in acute hemolytic anemia.

- *Beta globulin increases* in certain liver and renal disorders; monoclonal gammopathies (eg, multiple myeloma).
- *Beta globulin decreases* in nephrosis, immunoglobulin A deficiency.
- *Gamma globulin increases* in Waldenström's macroglobulinemia (IgM), multiple myeloma (IgG, IgA), autoimmune and collagen disorders (polyclonal), liver diseases, and some leukemias.
- *Gamma globulin decreases* in hypogammaglobulinemia, nephrotic syndrome, immunosuppressive drug therapy, agammaglobulinemia, and advancing age.

The most frequently seen abnormalities on IFE include the following:

- A monoclonal protein in the serum or urine suggests a neoplastic process; a polyclonal increase in immunoglobulins is seen in chronic liver disease, connective tissue disease, and infection(s).
- In multiple myeloma, approximately 99% of patients have a monoclonal protein in the serum or urine. Waldenström's macroglobulinemia is always characterized by the presence of a serum monoclonal IgM protein.
- A monoclonal light chain (kappa or lambda) in the urine is referred to as a Bence Jones protein and is found in roughly 75% of patients with multiple myeloma and 80% of patients with Waldenström's macroglobulinuria.

Clinical Implications: Urine Protein

- *Increased* urine protein levels occur in renal diseases with glomerular damage (nephritis, glomerulonephritis, nephrosis, renal vein thrombosis, malignant hypertension, SLE).
- Proteinuria results from diminished tubular reabsorption (renal tubular acidosis, pyelonephritis, Wilson's disease, Fanconi's syndrome).
- Proteinuria results from increased serum protein levels, multiple myeloma, and Waldenström's macroglobulinemia; also present in congestive heart failure and toxemia.
- *Increases* may occur in nonrenal diseases and conditions such as fever, acute infections, traumas, leukemia, toxemia of pregnancy, diabetes, vascular disease (hypertension), and poisoning from turpentine, phosphorus, mercury, sulfosalicylic acid, lead, phenol, or opiates.

Interfering Factors: Serum Testing

- Gross hemolysis and prolonged specimen storage may decrease albumin fractions and increase total protein.
- The albumin band may appear split in patients receiving penicillin.

- X-ray contrast agents produce an uninterpretable pattern.
- If plasma is collected instead of serum, fibrinogen (present in plasma) can migrate between the beta and gamma fractions, causing a "bridging" effect. The plasma can be treated with thrombin to remove the interference of fibrinogen, and the same sample is retested.
- Prolonged bed rest and pregnancy lowers total protein levels.

Interfering Factors: Urine Testing

- Orthostatic proteinuria results from prolonged standing or physical exertion and is unrelated to renal damage.
- *Increases* with strenuous exercise, severe emotional stress, cold baths, and high-fat diet.
- Drugs can cause false-negative and false-positive results (cephalosporins, sulfonamides, penicillin, gentamicin, tolbutamide, acetazolamide, and contrast agents).
- Alkaline urine can give false-positive results with reagent dipstick.
- Very dilute urine can give falsely low protein value.
- False or accidental proteinuria may be present because of a mixture of pus and red blood cells in urinary tract infections or from menstruation.
- Increased protein occurs in pregnancy, newborn infants, women during the premenstrual state, and after consuming large amounts of protein and alcohol.
- *Decreased* urine protein with a high-fiber diet.

Procedure

- Serum (5 mL) is obtained by venipuncture in a red-top tube.
- If it is possible for a 24-hour urine to be collected, make appropriate arrangements because it is preferable to a random urine sample. Approximately 25 mL of urine from the 24-hour urine collection should be submitted for protein electrophoresis testing.
- Collect urine in a clean container and test as soon as possible. See specimen collection guidelines in Chapter 2.
- For the best assessment of a suspected monoclonal gammopathy, both serum and urine samples should be submitted simultaneously. Urine protein electrophoresis is required to diagnose Bence Jones protein.
- A confirmatory IFE on either serum or urine can be performed on the sample or samples submitted for the SPE or urine electrophoresis.

- Submit 25 mL from a 24-hour urine collection if a urine electrophoresis is to be performed simultaneously.

Nursing Interventions

▶Pretest
- Explain test purpose and specimen collection procedure.
- If a 24-hour urine is to be collected, give the patient specific instructions and a 24-hour collection container (see Chapter 2).

▶Posttest
- Evaluate patient outcome. Provide counseling and support for renal disease as appropriate and in collaboration with the physician.

CLINICAL ALERT

Proteinuria:
- Urine: >3000 mg/24 hours or >3000 mg/day indicates nephrotic syndrome.

PULMONARY FUNCTION TESTS (PFTs), SPIROMETRY, LUNG VOLUMES, DIFFUSION CAPACITY

Special Lung Study

Pulmonary function tests (PFTs) are used to evaluate the nature and extent of pulmonary disease and to identify the underlying ventilatory impairment.

Indications
- Assess the ventilatory status of patients complaining of chronic cough, shortness of breath, or chest pain (cardiac involvement ruled out).
- Evaluate the respiratory system preoperatively for patients with a history of smoking, occupational exposure, respiratory infections, or a familial history of lung diseases, undergoing abdominal or thoracic surgery.
- Monitor the course of bronchodilators, inhaled or oral steroids, or pulmonary side effects of antiarrhythmics (eg, amiodarone) and antineoplastics (eg, bleomycin).

- Monitor the effects of exposure to particulate matter in the workplace.

Reference Values

Normal
- Normal airway flow rates, lung volumes, and gas exchange.

Clinical Implications

Spirometry
- *Decreases in airway flow rates* are consistent with an obstructive ventilatory impairment, typically seen in patients with asthma, chronic bronchitis, emphysema, and cystic fibrosis.
- *Decreases in volume of air exhaled* are consistent with advanced obstructive ventilatory impairment and restrictive ventilatory impairment seen in interstitial pulmonary fibrosis, obesity, sarcoidosis, and thoracic cage deformities.

Lung Volumes
- *Increases in the functional residual capacity, residual volume, and total lung capacity* are consistent with air trapping or overdistension and commonly seen in patients with obstructive ventilatory impairments such as asthma, emphysema, and cystic fibrosis.
- *Decreases in these volumes* are consistent with restrictive ventilatory impairments, such as pulmonary interstitial fibrosis, lung resection, obesity, and asbestosis.

Diffusion Capacity
- A *decrease* in the diffusing capacity is consistent with gas-exchange defects, as seen in emphysema, anemia, and space-occupying lesions.

Interfering Factors
- Inhaled bronchodilators, caffeine intake, and smoking may affect results.
- Because the spirometry test is dependent on patient effort, any acute illness, nausea, GI disturbance, migraine headache, abdominal or chest pain, and recent respiratory infection may affect the results. Other interfering factors include inability to hold breath or anything that will not permit an airtight seal, such as nasogastric tubes, tracheal stoma, and perforated eardrum, or if a patient is on continuous oxygen and cannot be taken off for a few minutes.
- Elevated carboxyhemoglobin levels, which are seen in smokers, can cause a decrease in the diffusing capacity owing to the "back pressure" of carbon monoxide.

Procedure

- Patient's demographic data (eg, age, height, weight, sex, and race) are recorded, and via regression equations, the predicted values are determined.

Spirometry Procedure

- In a seated or standing position, the patient is instructed to inhale maximally and then exhale forcibly, rapidly, and completely into a spirometer through a specially designed mouthpiece.
- A minimum of three forced expiratory maneuvers are performed, with an appropriate rest period between each effort.
- Total test time is 15–20 minutes.

Lung Volume Procedure

- This is a two-part test:

  Part I—In a seated position, with nose clips on, the patient begins by breathing normally, inspiring maximally, and then exhaling slowly and fully. From the resultant tracing, several lung volumes and capacities are determined.

  Part II—In a seated position, the patient breathes either helium (approximately 10%) or oxygen (100%), depending on the method used, for several minutes via the pulmonary function analyzer.

- After completion of the test, several lung volumes or capacities (eg, functional residual capacity, residual volume, and total lung capacity) are determined.
- Test time is approximately 30 minutes.

Diffusion Capacity Procedure

- In seated position, with nose clips attached, the patient is instructed to exhale maximally and then inspire maximally a diffusion gas mixture through a mouthpiece and filter combination attached to the pulmonary function analyzer. Following a 10- to 15-second breath-hold, the patient is instructed to exhale and a sample of alveolar gas is captured for analysis.
- Test time is about 15–20 minutes.

Nursing Interventions
▶*Pretest*

- Assess for interfering factors and contraindications to testing, for example, chest pain, nausea, vomiting, or any other symptoms that could preclude a maximal effort during test procedure. Also, bronchodilators should be withheld for 4–6 hours and antihistamines for 48 hours if tolerated.

- Explain purpose and procedure, emphasizing that this is a noninvasive test requiring cooperation and effort. Combined tests take approximately 60–90 minutes. The patient should be encouraged not to smoke.

▶ Intratest

- The patient may experience lightheadedness, shortness of breath, or slight chest discomfort. These symptoms are transitory, and an appropriate rest period between maneuvers is generally all that is needed to alleviate these symptoms.

▶ Posttest

- Assess complaints of slight fatigue or chest discomfort related to the use of respiratory muscles during deep inspirations, followed by forced expirations. This is an expected outcome. Provide for rest as necessary.
- Evaluate other patient outcomes and counsel appropriately.
- Resume any pretest medications, as prescribed, that were held for procedure.

PULSE OXIMETRY

Noninvasive and Continuous Blood O_2 Test

A pulse oximeter is used to monitor a patient's arterial blood oxygen (Spo_2) saturation.

Indications

- Determine need for O_2 supplementation.
- Monitor adequacy of O_2 supply.

Reference Values

Normal

Spo_2: 94%–98% or 0.94–0.98
Critical value: <75% or <0.75

Clinical Implications

- *Decreases* occur in hypoxemia, pneumonia, pulmonary emboli, CNS depression, CHF, and cirrhosis and with inadequate tissue oxygenation.
- *Increases* with oxygen therapy.

Interfering Factors

The following factors affect oxygen saturation values:

- Movement
- Edema
- Low perfusion
- Hypothermia
- Dark skin
- IV contrast agents
- Venous pulsation
- Artificial nails and nail polish
- Outside light
- Abnormal hemoglobin
- Anemia
- Electronic noise
- Increased carboxyhemoglobin

Procedure

- The pulse oximeter sensor is applied to index, middle, or ring finger, using a special clip or adhesive. Other types are used on the forehead, nose, ear lobe, and toe or foot in infants and neonates.
- The site is checked every 8 hours and changed every 4 hours.
- The pulse oximeter displays SpO_2 and pulse rate values. Alarms sound, indicating high or low values.

Nursing Interventions

▸*Pretest*

- Explain purpose and placement of pulse oximeter sensor and how long sensor will be needed.

▸*Intratest*

- Check and change the sensor as required.

▸*Posttest*

- Counsel patient regarding meaning of values.

RADIOACTIVE IODINE (RAI) UPTAKE TEST (THYROID UPTAKE)

Nuclear Medicine Imaging, Endocrine Imaging

This test measures the ability of the thyroid to concentrate, retain, or receive radioactive iodine and is more useful in diagnosing hyperthyroidism than hypothyroidism.

Indications

- Evaluate hyperthyroid and hypothyroid conditions and assist in staging thyroiditis.

- Check thyroid response to medication for pituitary or hypothalamic dysfunction and effectiveness of radioiodine therapy.
- Include as part of a complete thyroid workup for symptomatic patients (eg, swollen neck, neck pain, jittery, sluggish, ultrasensitive to cold, goiter).

Reference Values

Normal

- 1%–13% or 0.01–0.13 absorbed by thyroid gland after 2 hours.
- 5%–20% or 0.05–0.20 absorbed by thyroid gland after 6 hours.
- 15%–40% or 0.15–0.40 absorbed by thyroid gland after 24 hours.

Clinical Implications

- *Increased uptake* (eg, 20% or 0.20 in 1 hour, 25% or 0.25 in 6 hours, 45% or 0.45 in 24 hours) suggests hyperthyroidism but is not diagnostic for the disorder.
- *Decreased uptake* (eg, 0% or 0.0 in 2 hours, 3% or 0.03 in 6 hours, 10% or 0.10 in 24 hours) may be caused by hypothyroidism but is not diagnostic for this disorder.
- *Decreased uptake* is observed in patients with rapid diuresis, renal failure, or malabsorption, even though the gland is functioning normally.
- *Increased uptake* is observed in renal failure, even though the gland is functioning normally.

Interfering Factors

- Many chemicals, drugs, and foods may interfere with the test by *lowering* the uptake:
  - Iodized foods and iodine-containing drugs such as Lugol's solution, expectorants, cough medicines, saturated solutions of potassium iodide, SSK, and vitamin preparations that contain minerals (1–3 weeks' duration for the effect of these substances in the body).
  - X-ray contrast agents such as iodopyracet (Diodrast), sodium diatrizoate (Hypaque), Renografin (diatrizoate meglumine and diatrizoate sodium), Lipiodol, Ethiodol (ethiodized oil), iophendylate (Pantopaque), iopanoic acid (Telepaque); 1 week to a year or more in duration. Consult with the nuclear medicine laboratory for specific times.
  - Antithyroid drugs such as propylthiouracil and related compounds (2–10 days' duration).

◦ Thyroid medications such as Cytomel (liothyronine sodium), desiccated thyroid, thyroxine synthroid (1–2 weeks' duration).
◦ Miscellaneous drugs—thiocyanate, perchlorate, nitrates, sulfonamides, Orinase (tolbutamide), corticosteroids, PAS, isoniazid, phenylbutazone (Butazolidin), thiopental (Pentothal), antihistamines, ACTH, aminosalicylic acid, amphenone, cobalt, coumarin anticoagulants. Consult with the diagnostic department for duration times, which may vary.

• Many compounds and conditions interfere by *enhancing* the uptake:

◦ Estrogen
◦ Barbiturates
◦ TSH
◦ Lithium carbonate
◦ Lithium

◦ Phenothiazines (1 week)
◦ Pregnancy
◦ Renal failure
◦ Cirrhosis
◦ Iodine-deficient diets

CLINICAL ALERT

• This test is contraindicated in pregnant or lactating women, in children, in infants, and in those individuals with iodine allergies.
• Whenever possible, this test should be performed before any other nuclear medicine procedures are done, before any iodine-based medications are given, and before any x-ray studies using iodine contrast agents.

Procedure

• Test is usually done in conjunction with a thyroid scan and assessment of thyroid hormone blood levels. A fasting state is preferred. A complete history and listing of all medications is a must for this test. The history should include nonprescription medications, vitamins, minerals, herbals, and patient dietary habits.
• A tasteless capsule of radioiodine is administered orally. (It can be administered intravenously if a quick test is desired.) The patient is usually instructed not to eat for 1 hour after the administration of radioiodine.
• After 2, 6, and 24 hours, the amount of radioactivity is counted and measured in the thyroid gland. There is no pain or discomfort involved.

- The patient will have to return to the laboratory at the designated time; the exact time of measurement is crucial in determining uptake.

Nursing Interventions
▶*Pretest*
- Explain purpose, procedure, fasting, and thyroid-uptake scan times. Reassure the patient regarding the safety of radiopharmaceutical.
- Advise that iodine intake is restricted for at least 1 week before testing, including foods such as seafood, kelp and kelp tablets, fish liver oils, some vegetables, and iodized salt and medications such as thyroid hormones, Lugol's solution, steroids, cough medications, vitamin and mineral preparations, nutritional supplements, and saturated solutions of potassium iodine (SSKI). Stress compliance with various procedural steps.
- Assess for iodine allergy and consult with physician regarding this information.

▶*Intratest*
- Stress that compliance with the restricted diet is necessary. Provide support.

▶*Posttest*
- Instruct the patient to resume medications and normal diet as ordered.
- Evaluate patient outcomes and counsel appropriately about further tests and possible treatment.
- Document any problems that may have occurred with the patient during the procedure.

RADIONUCLIDE CYSTOGRAM, VESICOURETERIC REFLUX (BLADDER AND URETERS) IMAGING

Nuclear Medicine, Genitourinary Imaging

This procedure, requiring catheterization, is usually done on pediatric patients to assess abnormal bladder filling and possible reflux into the ureters.

Indications
- Evaluate patients with suspected urine reflux from the bladder into the ureters and upper renal collecting system.

Reference Values

Normal

Normal bladder and ureter scan: Normal bladder filling without any reflux into the ureters.

Clinical Implications

- Any reflux is abnormal.
- Abnormal vesicoureteric reflux may be either congenital (immature development of the urinary tract) or caused by infection.

Procedure

- The patient is placed in a supine position. A special urinary catheter kit is used and a urinary catheter is inserted into the urethra.
- A urinary catheter kit with warmed sterile saline is prepared. An absorbent plastic backed pad is placed under the patient to absorb any leakage of radioactive material. If a urinary catheter is contraindicated for the patient, an alternative indirect renogram method may be used.
- Imaging begins during administration of the radiopharmaceutical technetium-99m (^{99m}Tc) pentetate. Saline is administered until the bladder is full or the patient needs to void. The patient is asked to void through the catheter.
- After imaging is complete, the catheter is removed.

Nursing Interventions

▸*Pretest*

- Explain the purpose and procedure of the bladder and ureter imaging.

▸*Intratest*

- Allow parents to accompany small children to the nuclear medicine department to reduce fears.

▸*Posttest*

- Counsel regarding outcome and need for further testing and treatment, and monitor appropriately.
- Special handling of patient's urine (gloves and handwashing before and after gloves are removed) is necessary for 24 hours after completion.
- Instruct family members of pediatric patients about disposal of urine and diapers.

RED BLOOD CELL (RBC) SURVIVAL AND SEQUESTRATION TIME TEST[*]

Blood and Stool Specimens

Nuclear Medicine Imaging of Organs

This blood test has its greatest use in the evaluation of known or suspected hemolytic anemia. Imaging of the heart, liver, and spleen is often done as part of the RBC sequestration test. Red blood cell survival is usually ordered in conjunction with blood volume determination and radionuclide iron uptake and clearance tests. When stool specimens are collected for 3 days, the test is often referred to as the gastrointestinal blood loss test.

Indications
- Determine how long the patient's RBCs stay in circulation.
- Assess for an obscure cause for anemia.
- Identify accessory spleens.
- Determine abnormal red cell production or destruction.
- Monitor effectiveness of therapy for hemolytic anemia.

Reference Values

Normal

Normal half-life ^{51}Cr-labeled red blood cell survival: approximately 25–35 days.
Chromium-51 (^{51}CR) in stool: <3 mL/24 hours.
Spleen-to-liver ratio is 1:1.
Spleen-to-precardium ratio is 2:1.

Clinical Implications
- Shortened red blood cell survival may be the result of blood loss, hemolysis, or removal of red blood cells by the spleen, as in:
  - Chronic granulocytic anemia
  - Pernicious anemia
  - Megaloblastic anemia of pregnancy
  - Hemolytic anemia
  - Hemoglobin C disease

---

[*]The publisher has decided to include this test for purposes of completeness, although it is rarely used today in many parts of the country.

- Sickle cell anemia
- Hereditary spherocytosis
- Uremia
- Prolonged red blood cell survival time may be the result of an abnormality in the red blood cell production as in thalassemia minor.
- If hemolytic anemia is diagnosed, further studies are needed to establish whether red blood cells have intrinsic abnormalities or whether anemia results from immunologic effects of the patient's plasma.
- Results will be normal in:
  - Hemoglobin C trait
  - Sickle cell trait

Procedure
- First, a venous blood sample of 20 mL is obtained.
- After 10–30 minutes, the blood is reinjected after being tagged with a radionuclide (^{51}Cr).
- Blood samples are usually obtained on the first day, again at 24, 48, 72, and 96 hours, and then at weekly intervals for 2–3 weeks. Time may be shortened depending on the outcome of the test.
- As part of this procedure, a radioactive detector may be used over the spleen, sternum, and liver to assess the relative concentration of radioactivity in these areas. This external counting helps determine if the spleen is taking part in excessive sequestration of red blood cells as a causative factor in anemia.
- A 72-hour stool collection may be ordered to detect gastrointestinal blood loss.

Nursing Interventions
▶*Pretest*
- Explain the purpose and procedure of the RBC survival time test. Emphasize that this test requires a minimum of 2 weeks of the patient's time, with trips to the diagnostic facility for venipunctures.
- If stool collection is required, advise the patient on the importance of saving all stool and that stool be free of urine contamination. Refer to Chapter 2 regarding specimen collection procedures.

CLINICAL ALERT
- The test is usually contraindicated in an actively bleeding patient.
- Record and report signs of active bleeding.
- Transfusions should not be given when the test is in progress.

▶ Intratest

- Reassure patient that test is proceeding normally and there are no potential problems related to transmission of blood-borne disease.
- Be certain that the patient returns to the laboratory at specific time for blood collection.

▶ Posttest

- Monitor injection site for extravasation or infiltration of radiopharmaceutical agent.
- Observe and treat mild reactions: pruritus, rashes, and flushing 2–24 hours after injection; sometimes nausea and vomiting may occur.
- Interpret test outcome and monitor appropriately for anemia.

Note: Radioactive iron is not presently available from the manufacturer. No date for its reintroduction has been given.

RENIN (ANGIOTENSIN); PLASMA RENIN ANGIOTENSIN (PRA)

Blood

Renin, an enzyme produced in the liver, converts angiotensinogen to angiotensin I, which is subsequently converted to angiotensin II, a potent vasoconstrictor. Renin and aldosterone help maintain a balance of potassium and sodium blood levels.

Indications

- Evaluate cause of hypertension.
- Differentiate primary versus secondary aldosteronism.
- Investigate renin-producing tumors of the kidney.

Reference Values

Normal

Normal sodium diet:
   Supine: 0.2–1.6 ng angiotensin I (AI)/mL/hour or 0.2–1.6 μg AI/hour/L
   Standing: 0.7–3.3 ng AI/mL/hour or 0.7–3.3 μg AI/hour/L
Low-sodium diet:
   Supine: Renin levels increase 2 times normal.
   Standing: Renin levels increase 6 times normal.

Renin direct:

    Supine: 12–79 mU/L or 12–79 mU/L

    Standing: 13–114 mU/L or 13–114 mU/L

Procedure

- Obtain a 5-mL venous blood sample in a lavender-top tube.
- Record posture and dietary status of patient at the time of blood drawing.
- A 24-hour urine sodium should be collected concurrently to aid in diagnosis.

Clinical Implications

- *Increased renin levels* occur in secondary aldosteronism with malignant hypertension, renovascular hypertension, reduced plasma volume due to low-sodium diet, diuretics, Addison's disease, hemorrhage, chronic renal failure, salt-losing status owing to GI disease, renin-producing tumors of kidney, Bartter's syndrome, and pheochromocytoma.
- *Decreased renin levels* are found in primary aldosteronism, unilateral renal artery stenosis, administration of salt-retaining steroids, congenital adrenal hyperplasia with 17-hydroxylase deficiency, and Liddle's syndrome.

Interfering Factors

- Levels vary in healthy persons and increase under influences that tend to shrink the intravascular fluid volume.
- Random specimens may be difficult to interpret unless dietary and salt intake of patient is regulated.
- Values are higher when the patient is in an upright position, when the test is performed early in the day, when the patient is on a low-sodium diet, during pregnancy, and with drugs such as diuretics and antihypertensives and foods such as licorice.
- Recently administered radioisotopes interfere with test results.
- Indomethacin and salicylates decrease renin levels.

Nursing Interventions

▶*Pretest*

- Explain test purpose and procedure.
- A regular diet that contains 180 mEq/L (180 mmol/L) of sodium and 100 mEq/L (100 mmol/L) of potassium must be maintained for 3 days before the specimen is obtained. A 24-hour urine sodium and potassium should also be done to evaluate salt balance. The blood test should be performed at the end of the 24-hour urine test.

- Instruct the patient that it is necessary to be in a supine position for at least 2 hours before obtaining the specimen. The specimen is drawn with patient in the supine position.
- Ensure that antihypertensive drugs, cyclic progestogens, estrogens, diuretics, and licorice are terminated at least 2 weeks and preferably 4 weeks before a renin-aldosterone workup.
- If a standing specimen is ordered, the patient must be standing for 2 hours before testing, and blood should be drawn with the patient in the sitting position.
- Do not allow caffeine ingestion the morning before or during the test.

 ▶*Posttest*
- Interpret test results and counsel appropriately regarding hypertension, further testing, and possible treatment.

RENOGRAM; RENAL IMAGING (WITH LASIX/DIURETIC FUROSEMIDE OR CAPTOPRIL)

Nuclear Medicine, GU Imaging

This procedure is performed in both adult and pediatric patients to study the function of the kidneys and to detect renal parenchymal or vascular disease as well as defects in excretion.

Indications
- Use a Lasix renogram to differentiate dilated renal collecting systems from obstructions.
- Use a Captopril renogram to evaluate the hypertensive patient for renal artery stenosis.
- Assess for renal disease.
- Evaluate upper urinary tract obstruction.
- Assess renal transplant efficacy.
- Evaluate hydronephrosis, obstruction, renal trauma, urinary tract infections in children, and reduced renal function in premature neonate.

| Reference Values | |

Normal

Normal images: Equal blood flow in both the right and left kidneys. In 10 minutes, 50% or 0.50 of the radiopharmaceutical agent should be excreted.

Clinical Implications

- Abnormal distribution pattern may indicate hypertension, obstruction due to stones or tumors, renal failure, decreased renal function, diminished blood supply, ineffective renal transplant.
- In pediatric patients, findings of urinary tract infections in male neonates; the finding shifts to females after 3 months of age.

Interfering Factors

- Diuretics, ACE inhibitors, and beta-blockers are medications that may interfere with the renogram results.

Procedure

Routine Renogram

- An IV line is started to facilitate hydration and administration of radiopharmaceuticals.
- Patient is positioned with camera located posteriorly.
- The radiopharmaceutical ^{99m}Tc mertiatide (MAG-3) is administered and imaging begins, which lasts 30 minutes.
- The nuclear medicine physician determines if the study needs to continue with either furosemide (Lasix) or captopril (Capoten).
- A routine renogram takes about 75 minutes.

Lasix Renogram

- Lasix is injected in the IV catheter and imaging continues for 20 to 30 minutes.
- Procedure time is about 90 minutes.

Captopril Renogram

- Blood pressure measurement is taken.
- Captopril is administered to the patient.
- Blood pressure measurements are taken every 15 minutes for a total of 60 minutes.
- Saline is administered for hydration.
- The renogram is repeated.
- Captopril renogram takes about 160 minutes.

CLINICAL ALERT

- A renogram may be performed in pregnant women when it is imperative that renal function must be ascertained.

Nursing Interventions

▶ *Pretest*

- Explain the purpose, procedure, and risks and benefits.
- Ensure that the patient is well hydrated with 2–3 glasses of water (unless contraindicated) in the preceding 2 hours before undergoing the scan (10-mL water/kg body weight).

▶ *Intratest*

- If patient is not adequately hydrated, fluids are given intravenously.
- Monitor the patient for side effects of medications, including blood pressure measurements at 15-minute intervals. Hypotension is the most likely drug side effect with captopril.

▶ *Posttest*

- Encourage fluids and frequent bladder emptying to promote excretion of radioactivity.
- Monitor injection site for extravasation or infiltration of the radiopharmaceutical agent.
- Observe and treat mild reactions (per order): pruritus, rashes, and flushing 2–24 hours after injection; sometimes nausea and vomiting may occur.
- Interpret test outcome and counsel and monitor appropriately.

> **CLINICAL ALERT**
>
> - The test should be performed before the intravenous pyelogram.
> - Severe impairment of renal function or massive enlargement of the renal collecting system may impair drainage even without true obstruction.

RETICULOCYTE COUNT

Blood, Anemia, Hematology

This test measures immature nonnucleated red blood cells and is done in the differential diagnosis of anemia. Reticulum is present in newly released blood cells for 1–2 days before the cell reaches its full mature state.

Indications

- Differentiate anemias due to bone marrow failure in aplastic anemia from those due to hemorrhage or red blood cell destruction.

- Monitor effectiveness of treatment in pernicious anemia (treatment with vitamin B_{12} or transfusion) and recovery of bone marrow function.
- Determine radiation effects on patients and exposed workers.

Reference Values

Normal

Men: 0.5%–1.5% (expressed as % of total erythrocytes) or 0.005–0.015

Women: 0.5%–2.5% or 0.005–0.025

Infants: 2%–5% or 0.02–0.05

Children: 0.5%–4% or 0.005–0.04

Reticulocyte index (RI) = 1.0 or 1% increase in RBC production above normal or corrected reticulocyte count (CRC)

Clinical Implications

- *Reticulocytes increase* (reticulocytosis) in hemolytic anemias, hemoglobinopathies, sickle cell anemias, 3–4 days after hemorrhage, increased RBC destruction, and treatment of anemias and malaria.
- *Reticulocytes decrease* in iron deficiency and aplastic anemia, untreated pernicious anemia, chronic infection, radiation therapy and exposure, marrow tumors, endocrine disorders, myelodysplastic syndromes, and alcoholism.

Interfering Factors

- Specimen older than 24 hours affects outcome.
- Recent transfusion decreases values.

Procedure

- A 5-mL blood sample is obtained by venipuncture in a lavender-top tube. Place the specimen in a biohazard bag.
- A blood smear is prepared after mixing blood with a supravital stain and examined microscopically.

Nursing Interventions

▶*Pretest*

- Explain purpose and procedure of testing.

▶*Posttest*

- Evaluate patient outcome and counsel regarding possible repeat testing.
- Recently approved treatment for myelodysplastic syndromes include demethylating agents, e.g., azacitidine and decitabine.

RETINAL IMAGING

Eye

This imaging technique, scanning laser ophthalmoscope (SLO), is used to evaluate the retina.

Indications
- Evaluate for retinal diseases (eg, macular degeneration).
- Assess for the effects of systemic disease (eg, diabetes or hypertension) on the retina.
- Monitor eye disease progression.

Reference Values

Normal
- Retinal scan: Healthy eye and retina with no disease noted.

Clinical Implications
- Abnormal results show evidence of bleeding in the eye, most often associated with diabetes, hypertension, or macular degeneration.

Procedure
- Through digitally imaging the back of the eye, SLO technology uses different colored lasers to scan a picture of the retina onto a computer screen (Optomap). This exam allows for a more thorough exam of the retina than by the routine ophthalmoscope exam.
- SLO is recommended for all patients during routine eye exams to more accurately follow the health of the eyes.
- Procedure time is approximately 25 minutes.

Nursing Interventions
▸*Pretest*
- Explain the purpose of the eye test and procedure.
- If the patient uses contact lenses, these may be worn during the procedure.
- Generally, there is minimal or no discomfort during the procedure. However, some individuals' eyes may be sensitive to the flashing light of the lasers.

▶*Posttest*
* Interpret test results and counsel the patient appropriately.
* Refer the patient to the appropriate medical specialist if problems related to medical diagnosis, such as bleeding in the eye related to diabetes or hypertension, are identified.
* The patient may be instructed to return a year later for repeat tests to evaluate disease progression.

RETINAL NERVE FIBER ANALYSIS

Eye

This procedure, by use of microscopic laser technology, measures the thickness of the retinal nerve fiber of the eye.

Indications
* Evaluate for glaucoma.
* Assess for vision loss.

Reference Values

Normal
* No abnormalities of retinal nerve fiber.
* Normal thickness of retinal nerve layer.

Clinical Implications
* Abnormal appearance of the optic nerve is associated with changes in the eye that occur in glaucoma. Changes may be associated with vision loss.

Procedure
* Instruct the patient to sit upright in the examining chair.
* Place the patient's forehead and chin in cuplike holders and check one eye at a time. Twenty sectional images are obtained in less than 1 second and then analyzed to determine the thickness of the nerve layer.
* Inform the patient that the procedure may take approximately 30 minutes.

Nursing Interventions

▶*Pretest*
- Explain the test purpose and procedure.
- Inform the patient that contact lenses may be left in place.

▶*Posttest*
- Evaluate outcomes, counsel the patient appropriately, and explain if there is a need for further testing and possible treatment of abnormal outcomes.

RETROGRADE PYELOGRAM

X-Ray and Endoscopic Upper Urinary Tract Invasive Imaging With Contrast

This invasive x-ray examination of the upper urinary tract visualizes the proximal ureter and renal anatomy.

Indications
- Evaluate poorly functioning renal tissue, urinary tract in the presence of calculi or obstruction, and poorly perfused renal tissue.
- Done when IVU reveals kidney nonvisualization.

Reference Values

Normal
Normal contour and size of kidneys, patent ureters.

Clinical Implications
- Abnormal findings: Obstruction of urinary tract, tumors, calculi, congenital abnormalities, and reflux.

Interfering Factors
- Retained feces, barium, or intestinal gas will obscure visualization of urinary tract.
- Metallic objects that overlie area of exam will interfere with organ visualization.
- Severe obesity adversely affects image quality.

Procedure

- Sedation and local anesthesia are required.
- A catheter is introduced into the ureter up to the level of the renal pelvis through a cystoscope.
- Contrast media is injected, and x-ray films are taken.
- The total exam time is generally less than 1 hour.

Nursing Interventions

▶*Pretest*

- Assess for test contraindications, eg, pregnancy or history of allergy to iodine.
- Explain exam purpose and procedure. No food is allowed for approximately 8 hours before the study. Some labs also have fluid restrictions for patients undergoing retrograde pyelography.
- Instruct the patient to remove certain jewelry and metallic objects from abdominal area.
- Note that a bowel prep may be necessary, consisting of cleansing enemas and/or laxatives. Check protocol at laboratory performing the study.

▶*Intratest*

- Encourage patient to follow breathing and positional instructions.

▶*Posttest*

- Check vital signs for at least 24 hours. Monitor for signs of iodine-contrast allergy.
- Provide the patient with plenty of fluids, food, and rest after study.
- Record urine output and appearance for at least 24 hours. Hematuria and dysuria are common for several days after exam.
- Administer analgesics, if necessary.
- Evaluate patient outcomes; provide support and counseling.

RH TYPING, BLOOD TYPE

Blood, Pretransfusion

This test is used to determine whether an individual is Rh positive or Rh negative. TABLE 3.4 reviews the Rh nomenclature.

Indications

- Rh-positive blood administered to an Rh-negative person may sensitize the person to form anti-D (Rh_1).

TABLE 3.4 COMPARISON OF TERMS USED IN RH SYSTEM NOMENCLATURES

WEINER	FISHER-RACE
Rh_1	D
Rh_2	C
Rh_3	E
Rh_4	c
Rh_5	e
Rh_6	f(ce)
Rh_{12}	G

- Rh_1(D)-positive blood administered to a recipient having serum anti-D (Rh_1) could be fatal.
- Identify RhIG (Rh immunoglobulin) candidates.
- Rh typing must also be done for patients who have had abortions or miscarriages.

Reference Values

Normal

	INCIDENCE
White	85% Rh positive (have the Rh antigen)
	15% Rh negative (lack the Rh antigen)
African American	90% Rh positive (have the Rh antigen)
	10% Rh negative (lack the Rh antigen)

Clinical Implications

- The significance of Rh antigens is based on their capacity to immunize the patient as a result of receiving a transfusion or becoming pregnant.
- Antibodies for Rh_2(C) are frequently found, together with anti-Rh_1(D) antibodies, in the Rh-negative, pregnant woman whose fetus or child is type Rh positive and possesses both antigens.
- With exceedingly rare exceptions, Rh antibodies do not form unless preceded by antigenic stimulation, as occurs with pregnancy and abortions; blood transfusions; and deliberate immunization, most commonly of repeated IV injections of blood for the purpose of harvesting a given Rh antibody.

Procedure

- Obtain a 7-mL blood specimen via venipuncture.

Nursing Interventions

▶ *Pretest*

- Explain purpose and procedure of Rh typing.
- See Chapter 1 guidelines for safe, effective, informed *pretest* care.

▶ *Posttest*

- Interpret test outcome, inform, and counsel regarding Rh type. Women of childbearing age may need special consideration.

RH DISEASE TEST, RH ANTIBODY TITER TEST, D_0 ANTIGEN

Blood of Rh-Negative Pregnant Woman

This test is performed to determine the Rh antibody level in an Rh-negative or pregnant woman whose partner is Rh positive.

Indications

- Check the presence before and after delivery in Rh-negative women.
- Detect fetal maternal bleed.
- Predict need for amniocentesis.
- Prevent hemolytic disease of the newborn.
- Monitor Rh or other antibody formation in cases of potential mother-baby blood incompatibility.

Reference Values

Normal

- Negative is zero, ie, no antibody D_0 antigen detected; low ratio 1:16.
- No ABO incompatibility between mother and fetus.
- Not Rh immunized.

Clinical Implications

- Some institutions have established a critical titer for anti-D below which hemolytic disease of the newborn (HDN) is considered unlikely. No further investigations are undertaken unless the critical titer level is reached.

Procedure

- Obtain a 10-mL venous blood sample from the mother, using a yellow-top (ACD) and clotted-blood tube.

Nursing Interventions

▸*Pretest*
- Explain the test purpose and procedure.
- Follow Chapter 1 guidelines for safe, effective, informed *pretest* care.

▸*Posttest*
- Interpret test outcome and counsel appropriately.
- Follow Chapter 1 guidelines for safe, effective, informed *posttest* care.

ROSETTE TEST, FETAL RED CELLS (FETAL-MATERNAL BLOOD)

Blood, Maternal, at Time of Delivery of Baby

This qualitative test detects Rh-positive fetal cells in the Rh-negative maternal circulation.

Indications
- Detect the presence of Rh-positive fetal cells in the Rh-negative mother's circulation.

Reference Values

Normal
Negative for fetal blood loss; no Rh positive; and no rosetting fetal RBCs detected in maternal blood.

Clinical Implications
- When the test sample contains few or no Rh-D–positive fetal cells, rosetting or agglutination is absent, and the fetomaternal bleed (fetal blood loss) is less than 30 mL, one dose of parenteral Rh-immune globulin (RhIG) will prevent immunization.
- If the fetal blood loss into the maternal circulation exceeds 30 mL, a quantitative or semiquantitative test (ie, Kleihauer-Betke test) must be performed to calculate the amount of Rh-immune globulin to administer.

Procedure
- A 7-mL venous blood EDTA sample is obtained from the mother shortly after delivery.

- This test is performed and examined for rosettes or mixed-field agglutinates. Following manufacturer's guidelines, the presence of rosettes above a predetermined number indicates a fetal bleed that exceeds 30 mL of the whole blood.

Nursing Interventions

▶*Pretest*
- Explain testing purpose, procedure, and timing (immediately after delivery).
- See Chapter 1 guidelines for safe, effective, informed *pretest* care.

▶*Intratest*
- Refer to Chapter 2 for venous blood specimen collection.

▶*Posttest*
- Interpret test outcome. Counsel regarding Rh-immune globulin administration and follow-up maternal testing.
- Follow Chapter 1 guidelines for safe, effective, informed *posttest* care.

RUBELLA/GERMAN MEASLES ANTIBODY TEST

Blood, Viral Infection

This test measures IgG and IgM antibody formation in response to rubella virus, the causative agent of German measles.

Indications
- Determine the patient's susceptibility to rubella virus.
- Determine the immune status of patient or health care worker.
- Confirm rubella infection.
- Identify potential carriers of rubella who may infect women of childbearing age.

Reference Values

Normal

Negative for IgG or IgM antibodies: Not immune to rubella virus.
Positive for rubella IgG antibody: Immune to rubella virus.
Positive for rubella IgM antibody: Indicates a current or recent infection with the rubella virus.

Clinical Implications

- A fourfold rise in titer between acute and convalescent samples indicates a recent infection. Once a person has been infected, the titer remains high for many years. This indicates immunity; repeat infections are rare. Immunization with rubella vaccine causes production of rubella antibodies.
- Positive tests indicate immunity.
- Negative tests and titers indicate no previous infection and no immunity.

Procedure

- Serum (5 mL) is obtained by venipuncture in a red-top tube.

Nursing Interventions

▶ Pretest

- Assess patient's knowledge of test. Explain reason for testing and blood test procedure.
- Advise pregnant women that rubella infection in first trimester of pregnancy is associated with miscarriage, stillbirth, and congenital abnormalities.

▶ Posttest

- Advise women of childbearing age if test is negative to obtain immunization before becoming pregnant.
- Vaccination during pregnancy is contraindicated.
- Advise patients with positive test that they are immune to further infection.

SALIVARY GLAND IMAGING

Nuclear Medicine Parotid Gland Imaging

This study is helpful in the evaluation of swelling or associated pain of the parotid or salivary glands.

Indications

- Detection of tumors or masses.
- Investigate blockage of the ducts.
- Diagnose Sjögren's syndrome.

Reference Values

Normal

No evidence of tumor-type activity or blockage of ducts.
Normal size, shape, and position of the glands.

Clinical Implications

- The reporting of a hot nodule amidst normal tissue that accumulates the radionuclide is associated with tumors of the ducts; Warthin's tumor, oncocytoma, and mucoepidermoid tumor.
- The reporting of a cold nodule amidst normal tissue that does not accumulate the radionuclide is associated with benign tumors, abscesses, or cysts, which are indicated by smooth, sharply defined outlines; adenocarcinomas are indicated by ragged, irregular outlines.
- Diffuse decreased activity occurs in obstruction, chronic sialadenitis, or Sjögren's syndrome.
- Diffuse increased activity occurs in acute parotitis.

Procedure

- The radionuclide ^{99m}Tc pertechnetate is injected intravenously.
- Imaging is performed immediately following the injection. There are three phases to imaging: blood flow, uptake or trapping mechanism, and secreting capability.
- If a secretory function test is being performed to detect blockage of the salivary duct, three-fourths of the way through the test, ask the patient to suck on a lemon slice. If the salivary duct is normal, this causes the gland to empty. This is not done in studies undertaken for tumor detection.
- Total test time is 45 to 60 minutes.

Nursing Interventions

▶ Pretest

- Explain the purpose, procedure, benefits, and risks.
- No pain or discomfort is involved.
- Lemon may be given to the patient to stimulate parotid secretion.

▶ Posttest

- Interpret test outcome and monitor appropriately.

SCHILLING, VITAMIN B$_{12}$ TEST*

Timed Urine Nuclear Medicine Procedure

This timed urine test evaluates the body's ability to absorb vitamin B$_{12}$ from the gastrointestinal tract and is based on the anticipated urinary excretion of an administered dose of radioactive vitamin B$_{12}$. It is an indirect test of intrinsic factor deficiency.

Indications
- Determine *cause* of vitamin B$_{12}$ deficiency.
- Diagnose pernicious anemia and malabsorption syndromes.

Reference Values

Normal
- Excretion of 10% or more of test dose of cobalt-tagged vitamin B$_{12}$ appears in urine within 24 hours.
- Less than 5% is abnormal and indicates failure to absorb vitamin B$_{12}$.

Clinical Implications
- An abnormal low value (eg, <7%) or borderline (7%–10%) is consistent with either the absence of intrinsic factor or defective absorption in the ileum.
- When the absorption of radioactive vitamin B$_{12}$ is low, the test must be repeated with intrinsic factor to rule out intestinal malabsorption (confirmatory Schilling test). If the urinary excretion rises to normal levels, it indicates a lack of intrinsic factor, suggesting the diagnosis of pernicious anemia. If the urinary excretion does not rise, malabsorption is considered the cause of the patient's anemia.

Procedure
- Patient must fast for 12 hours before the test and for 2 hours after. (Fasting is continued for 3 hours after vitamin B$_{12}$ doses are administered.)
- A small capsule of radioactive B$_{12}$ labeled with ^{57}Co is administered orally.

---

*The publisher has decided to include this test for purposes of completeness, although it is rarely used today in many parts of the country.

- Two hours later, an intramuscular injection of nonradioactive B$_{12}$ is given.
- Total urine is collected for 24–48 hours from time the patient receives the injection of vitamin B$_{12}$.

Interfering Factors

- The single most common source of error in performing the test is *incomplete collection of urine.* Some laboratories may require a 48-hour collection to allow for a small margin of error.
- Urinary excretion of B$_{12}$ is depressed in elderly patients, diabetic patients, patients with hypothyroidism, and those with enteritis.
- Renal insufficiency and benign prostatic hypertrophy may cause reduced excretions of radioactive vitamin B$_{12}$ and a 48- to 72-hour urine collection is advised because eventually all of the absorbed material will be excreted. Urine specific gravity and volume are checked.
- Fecal contamination of the urine may invalidate the test.

CLINICAL ALERT

- No laxatives are to be used during testing.
- Bone marrow aspiration should be done before the Schilling test, because the vitamin B$_{12}$ administration in the test will destroy the diagnostic characteristics of the bone marrow.

Nursing Interventions

▶ Pretest

- Explain the test purpose, procedure, and collection of 24-hour urine specimen. Record accurate weight.
- A random sample urine specimen is usually obtained before vitamin B$_{12}$ doses are administered.
- The patient is to fast from midnight. Water is permitted during the fasting period.
- Be certain that patient receives the nonradioactive vitamin B$_{12}$. If the intramuscular dose of vitamin B$_{12}$ is not given, radioactive vitamin B$_{12}$ will be found in the liver instead of the urine.

▶ Intratest

- Ensure the patient remains fasting for 3 hours after the oral vitamin B$_{12}$ has been given.
- Food and drink are permitted after the doses of vitamin B$_{12}$ are given. The patient is encouraged to drink as much as can be tolerated during the entire test.

- Assess for compliance with 24-hour urine. Be certain that none of the urine is discarded. The urine specimen can be tested for creatinine excretion as a check on adequacy of collection.

▶*Posttest*
- Evaluate patient outcomes; monitor and counsel appropriately. Explain that if outcomes are normal, further blood testing that is more specific will be required.

SCROTAL ULTRASOUND (SCROTAL SONOGRAM), TESTICULAR SONOGRAM (TESTICULAR ULTRASOUND)

Ultrasound Imaging of Testes

This noninvasive procedure images the testes and their surrounding structures.

Indications
- Identify and characterize testicular mass.
- Evaluate cause of testicular pain or potential changes resulting from testicular trauma.
- Evaluate structural causes of male infertility and identify location of undescended testes.

Reference Values

Normal
Normal location, size, and appearance of scrotal and testicular tissues.

Clinical Implications
- Presence of space-occupying lesions: tumors, abscesses, hematomas, hydrocele, gland enlargement or echo changes suggestive of inflammatory process, spermatocele, varicocele, infarct, undescended testes, and torsion as evidenced by lack of Doppler signal.

Procedure
- Penis is retracted and scrotum is supported on a rolled towel. After a coupling gel is applied to expose scrotum, a handheld transducer is gently moved across the skin.
- A Doppler ultrasound or color-flow Doppler evaluation may be done to assess the presence of torsion of the testes.
- Exam time is about 10–30 minutes.

Nursing Interventions

▶ Pretest
- Explain exam purpose and procedure. Assure patient that no radiation is employed and that test is painless.
- No preparation is required.

▶ Posttest
- Remove or instruct patient to remove any residual gel from skin.
- Evaluate patient outcomes; provide support and counseling.

Sedimentation Rate (SED Rate), Erythrocyte Sedimentation Rate (ESR)

Blood, Inflammation

This test measures the sedimentation rate or settling of RBCs and is used as a nonspecific measure of many diseases, especially inflammatory conditions.

Indications
- Diagnose inflammatory disease, rheumatic fever, rheumatoid arthritis, respiratory infections, and temporal arthritis.
- Monitor steroid treatment of inflammatory disease.

Reference Values

Normal
Same for standard and SI units.
Men: Aged <50: 0–14 mm/hour; 50–85 years: 0–19 mm/hour; >85 years: 0–29 mm/hour
Women: Aged <50: 0–19 mm/hour; 50–85 years: 0–29 mm/hour; >85 years: 0–41 mm/hour
Children: 0–10 mm/hour

Clinical Implications
- *Increased rate* is seen in inflammation, collagen and autoimmune disorders, infections, subacute bacterial endocarditis, cancers, toxemia, heavy metal poisoning, nephritis, anemia, gout, myocardial infarct, malignancy, and multiple myeloma.
- *Normal or no increase is seen* in polycythemias, sickle cell anemia, spherocytosis, congestive heart failure, hypofibrinogenemia, and pyruvate kinase deficiency.

- Variable deviations can be seen in acute disease, convalescence, unruptured acute appendicitis, angina pectoris, viral diseases and infectious mononucleosis, renal failure, allergy, and peptic ulcer.

Interfering Factors

- *Increased in* pregnancy (after 12 weeks), postpartum, menstruation, drugs (heparin and oral contraceptives), presence of cholesterol, globulins, fibrinogen, C-reactive protein, and anemia.
- *Decreased with* certain drugs (steroids, aspirin) and decreased fibrinogen level in newborns, and blood specimens allowed to stand before testing (>24 hours), high glucose, high albumin, high phospholipids, and high RBC and WBC counts.

Procedure

- A 4.0 mL of whole-blood specimen is obtained by venipuncture in a lavender-top tube.
- Do not allow blood sample to stand more than 24 hours, as rate can be falsely decreased.

Nursing Interventions

▸*Pretest*

- Explain purpose and procedure. Obtain appropriate medication history. Fasting is not necessary, but a fatty meal may cause plasma alterations.

▸*Posttest*

- Evaluate patient outcomes and counsel appropriately about inflammation, anemia, or collagen and autoimmune disorders, among others.
- Explain need for repeat testing to monitor progress and evaluate prescribed therapy.

SENTINEL NODE LOCATION BEFORE BIOPSY (BREAST, MELANOMA)

Prebiopsy Special Studies (Lymphoscintigraphy, Nuclear Medicine Imaging), Nuclear Gamma Radiation Probe, and/or Blue Dye

The concept of identifying and localizing the sentinel node or nodes before biopsy is that these nodes receive initial lymphatic drainage and are the first filter to remove metastatic cells; thus, if this node is free of disease, then the rest of the nodes in the patient will also be free of disease. Three methods are used: lymphoscintigraphy (preoperative), nuclear probe localization (intraoperative), and blue-dye injection (intraoperative).

Indications
Lymph Nuclear Medicine Imaging, Lymphoscintigraphy
- Detect metastasis.
- Map all sentinel nodes.
- Stage and monitor cancers (eg, melanoma, breast, head, neck, and skin).

Nuclear Gamma Probe
- Detect the most sentinel nodes.
- Provide auditory confirmation.

Blue Dye Staining
- Staining provides visual confirmation of nodes.
- Mapped tumor route urine will turn blue and skin will stain too.

CLINICAL ALERT

- Only when the sentinel node is positive is a complete nodal dissection performed.

Reference Values

Normal
- No evidence of tumor activity; no blocked lymphatic drainage.
- Sentinel node: Negative; symmetrical nodes.

Clinical Implications
- Abnormal findings reveal metastatic nodes and routes of spread.
- Asymmetry may indicate lymph flow obstruction.

Procedure
Lymph Nuclear Medicine Imaging (Lymphoscintigraphy)
- For the breast, the radiopharmaceutical (larger volume) is injected subcutaneously into the breast, adjacent to the suspected breast tumor. (For lymphedema, it is injected into the webs of fingers and toes.)

- For melanoma, 4–6 intradermal injections are made around the tumor or excision site, avoiding scar tissue.
- Immediate imaging is done with the patient in the position expected during surgery.

Nuclear Radiation (Gamma) Probe (Which Produces Sound)

- A previously administered radiopharmaceutical and gamma probe sound radiation detector permit node detection and are used to determine where the initial operative incisions can be made. Of the three procedures, the probe is the most sensitive.

Blue Dye (Not Externally Visible)

- The feet are injected in the web between the toes, and the hands are injected between the second and third fingers.

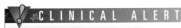
CLINICAL ALERT

- Allergic reaction to the dye may occur.

Nursing Interventions

▸ Pretest

- Explain the purpose of preoperative sentinel node identification procedure.
- Acknowledge the fear and anxiety that relate to test outcomes of metastatic disease.
- Inform the patient that if the sentinel node is positive, a complete nodal dissection is performed and surgery usually follows soon after.

▸ Intratest

- Usually, no sedation or analgesia are ordered.
- The site of lymph nodes is marked with indelible pen.
- Provide support, assist with positioning, and assure the patient that testing is proceeding as expected.

▸ Posttest

- Monitor injection site (breast, toes, fingers, or around tumor excision site). Check for signs of inflammation or bleeding.
- If surgery is planned, prepare according to established protocol.
- Administer pain medication related to prebiopsy procedures.

SEVERE ACUTE RESPIRATORY SYNDROME (SARS)

Blood, Sputum, Stool

This test is used to diagnose severe acute respiratory syndrome (SARS), which has been linked to a coronavirus (SARS-CoV). SARS is spread by person-to-person contact or contact with infected material.

Indications
• Assess for virus.
• Evaluate symptoms consistent with exposure.

Reference Values

Normal
• Negative for SARS-CoV antibody.

Clinical Implications
• Detection of the antibody to SARS-CoV in a convalescent-phase serum obtained more than 28 days after the onset of symptoms is evidence of the disease.

Procedure
• Collect a respiratory tract or blood or stool specimen.
• Respiratory specimens may be collected from nasopharyngeal aspirates or swabs or oropharyngeal swabs. Nasopharyngeal aspirates are collected by instilling 1.0–1.5 mL of nonbacteriostatic saline into one nostril and then subsequently aspirating, via a plastic catheter, into a sterile vial. Nasopharyngeal or oropharyngeal specimens can be obtained by inserting a swab into the nostril or posterior pharynx, respectively. (Do not use swabs with wooden sticks or calcium alginate, as they may contain substances that can interfere with the analysis.) The swabs should then be placed into sterile vials containing 2.0 mL of viral media. If the sample is to be shipped, it should be either packed in cold packs (4°C) for domestic travel or dry ice for international shipping.
• Obtain 5.0–10.0 mL of whole blood in a serum separator tube or in an EDTA tube. If collected in a serum separator tube, the blood is allowed to clot and is then centrifuged.
• Collect 10–50 mL of stool, place the specimen in a stool cup, and cap it securely. Place specimens in a biohazard bag.

Nursing Interventions

▶*Pretest*

- Explain the purpose and procedure of testing.
- Close contact (eg, living with or taking care of a person with SARS, or sharing eating or drinking utensils) or close conversation (<3 ft) may result in transmission of the disease.

▶*Posttest*

- Counsel, monitor, and treat the patient appropriately.
- Report evidence of SARS to local, state, and federal health departments as appropriate.

SEXUALLY TRANSMITTED DISEASE (STD) TESTING: OVERVIEW

Tissue, Blood, Vaginal Fluid, Rectal Swabs, Aspirates

Sexually transmitted diseases are caused by a variety of agents such as *Neisseria gonorrhoeae* (gonorrhea), herpes simplex virus (types 1 and 2; genital herpes), hepatitis B virus (hepatitis B), *Haemophilus*, chancroid/*Calymmatobacterium* (granuloma inguinale), *Chlamydia trachomatis* (serotypes L1, L2, and L3), *Chlamydia trachomatis* (serotypes D–K), *Molluscum contagiosum* virus, *Candida albicans*, *Phthirus pubis* (pubic or crab louse pediculous), *Sarcoptes scabiei* (scabies), *Treponema pallidum* (syphilis), *Trichomonas vaginalis* (trichomonas), *Gardnerella vaginalis*, *Mobiluncus curtisii*, *M. muliebris* (vaginitis), *Ureaplasma urealyticum*, human DNA papillomavirus (venereal warts), HIV (AIDS), and enteric organisms (*Giardia lamblia*, *Entamoeba histolytica*, *Cryptosporidium*, *Shigella*, *Campylobacter fetus*, and strongyloids/worms; gastrointestinal infections).

The diagnosis of sexually transmitted disease is made by isolating the causative organism from urine, semen, urethral, vaginal, cervical or oral swabs, prostatic secretions, tissue biopsy, and blood or stool specimens.

CLINICAL ALERT

- A consent for testing to diagnose sexually transmitted diseases (STDs) may be required.
- Tracing sexual partners is a very important part of diagnosis and treatment.

- Asymptomatic carriers are more common than generally realized.
- Even though diagnosed with one sexually transmitted disease, other types of sexually transmitted pathogens may be found in the same patient.
- The disease may recur because the patient becomes reinfected by a nontreated sexual partner.
- Precise diagnosis and vigorous treatment of STDs is especially important in pregnancy to prevent transmission of the disease to the newborn.

SICKLE CELL TESTS

Blood, Genetic

Hemoglobin S, Sickledex, Hb Electrophoresis, Sickle Cell Anemia

These blood tests are routinely done as a screening for sickle cell anemia or trait and to confirm these disorders. This test detects the presence of hemoglobin S (Hb S), an inherited recessive gene.

Indications
- Screen for sickle cell disease or trait.
- Include as part of workup following the detection of sickle-shaped cells on peripheral blood smear.
- Confirm sickle cell trait and diagnose sickle cell anemia.
- Evaluate hemolytic anemias.

Reference Values

Normal
Adults: Negative; no Hb S present.

Clinical Implications
- A positive test means that hemoglobin S is present and that great numbers of erythrocytes have assumed the typical sickle cell (crescent) shape.
- *Sickle cell trait:* Definite confirmation of sickle cell trait by hemoglobin electrophoresis reveals the following heterozygous (A/S)

pattern: Hb S, 20%–40%; HbA$_1$, 60%–80%; Hb F, small amount. This means that the patient has inherited a normal Hb gene from one parent and an Hb S gene from the other (heterozygous pattern). This patient does not have any clinical manifestations of the disease, but some of the children of this patient may inherit the disease if the patient's mate also has the recessive gene pattern.

- *Sickle cell anemia:* Definite confirmation of sickle cell anemia by hemoglobin electrophoresis reveals the following homozygous (S/S) pattern: Hb S, 80%–100%; Hb F, most of the rest; HbA$_1$, 0% or small amount. This means that an abnormal Hb S gene has been inherited from both parents (homozygous pattern). Such a pattern has all the clinical manifestations of the disease.

Interfering Factors

- False-positive results are due to other abnormal hemoglobins (D and G).
- False-negative results in patients with pernicious anemia and polycythemia.
- Infants younger than 3 months have false-negative results owing to a high amount of Hb F.

Procedure

- A 5- to 7-mL venous blood sample is obtained in a purple-top tube.
- Note any blood transfusions 3–4 months prior on a lab slip or computer screen.
- Hemoglobin electrophoresis is more specific and should be done in all positive Sickledex screens.

Nursing Interventions

▶ Pretest

- Explain purpose and procedure of sickle cell tests. Obtain signed, witnessed consent form if required for genetic testing.
- Provide genetic counseling and education.

▶ Posttest

- Evaluate patient outcome and counsel and monitor appropriately.
- Advise genetic counseling if outcomes reveal sickle cell trait or anemia.
- Prenatal testing can be performed to determine whether the fetus will have sickle cell disease, carry the trait, or be unaffected. In three of four cases, if both parents carry the gene, the prenatal test will reveal that the fetus will *not* have sickle cell disease.

SKIN TESTS

Special Skin Study

Allergy, Penicillin Allergy, Tuberculosis (TB), Blastomycosis, Coccidiomycosis, Histoplasmosis, and Toxoplasmosis; Trichophyton Anergy (Candida and Mumps)

Skin tests aid in diagnosis of previous infections and indicate status of immune system when antigens are injected intradermally and interpreted on the basis of delayed (24, 48, and 72 hours) skin reactions (delayed cutaneous hypersensitivity [DCH]).

Indications
- Screen high-risk groups.
- Confirm sensitivity to allergens and identify at-risk persons for penicillin—immediate or accelerated reactions, presence of IgE antibodies, no predictive value.
- Evaluate immune function.
- Determine susceptibility or resistance to specific infections.
- Control contacts of TB in a communicable stage.
- Perform a two-step TB skin test for noninfected new employees and new residents (of hospitals, nursing homes, homeless shelters, correctional institutions, and alcohol and drug treatment centers); the foreign born from countries with a high prevalence of the disease; and patients 55 years and older. The test is performed to reduce the likelihood that a "boosted" reaction will be interpreted as recent infection, not routine for contact case investigation.

Reference Values

Normal

Negative or nonsignificant for cutaneous hypersensitivity to allergens, tuberculosis, blastomycosis, coccidiomycosis, histoplasmosis, and toxoplasmosis, candida, mumps, and penicillin.

Clinical Implications
- *Positive* or significant reactions for *allergens: Exaggerated response to allergy extracts such as house dust and pollen.*
- *Positive* or significant reaction for *tuberculosis: Zone of induration 10 mm or more in diameter.*

- *Positive* or significant reaction to trichophyton read at 24–72 hours; zone of erythema and induration of 5 mm or more.
- *Positive* or significant reaction for *blastomycosis: Zone of erythema and induration by 5 mm or more in diameter.*
- *Positive* or significant reaction, read in 24–72 hours to *coccidioidomycosis: Zone of erythema and induration of 5 mm or more in diameter.*
- *Positive* or significant reaction, read at 24–72 hours to *histoplasmosis: Zone of erythema induration of 5 mm or more in diameter.*
- *Positive* or significant reaction read at 24–72 hours to *toxoplasmosis: Zone of erythema area over 10 mm in diameter.*
- *Positive* or significant reaction read at 24–72 hours to candida or mumps: *Zone of induration 5 mm or more.*
- Anergy (a defect in cell-mediated immunity associated with impaired or lack of response to injected antigens) has been correlated with malnutrition, immunosuppressive therapy, and increased risk of infection, disease, and death. (See DISPLAY 3.9.)

Interfering Factors Causing False-Negative Reactions

- Improper administration, interpretation, or use of outdated antigen.
- Test is applied too soon after exposure to the antigen (DCH takes 2–20 weeks to develop).

DISPLAY 3.9 **Skin Tests**

Skin Test	Reading Time	Positive Reaction
PPD	48–72 hours	**≥5 mm considered positive for:** Close contacts with an infected person. Persons with abnormal chest x-ray study indicating old healed TB. Persons with known or suspected HIV infection. **≥10 mm considered positive for:** Other medical risk factors. Foreign born from high-prevalence areas. Medically underserved, low-income populations, alcoholics and intravenous drug users, residents of long-term care facilities (including correctional facilities and nursing homes), staff in settings where disease would pose a hazard to large number of susceptible persons. **≥15 mm considered positive for:** Persons without risk factors for TB.

- Concurrent viral illnesses (eg, rubeola, influenza, mumps, and probably others) or recent administration of live attenuated virus vaccines (eg, measles).
- Anergy may be associated with immune-suppressing chronic illnesses; diabetes, uremia, sarcoidosis, metastatic carcinomas, Hodgkin's disease, acute lymphocytic leukemia, hypothyroidism, chronic hepatitis, and cirrhosis; some antineoplastic agents, radiation therapy, and corticosteroids (if possible, discontinue steroids at least 48 hours before DCH skin testing); congenital immune deficiencies, malnutrition, shock, severe burns, trauma, severe disseminated infections; miliary or cavitary TB, cocci granuloma, and other disseminated mycotic infections, gram-negative bacillary septicemia, and leukocytosis ($>15,000$ cells/mm^3).

Interfering Factors Causing False-Positive Reactions

- Improper interpretation: Patient sensitivity to minor ingredients in the antigen solutions such as the phenol or thimerosal preservatives and cross-reactions between similar antigens.

Procedure

- Perform all skin tests intradermally into the flexor surface of the arm.
- Use a separate sterile TB syringe for each antigen. Immediately after the antigen is drawn up, make the injection intradermally in the flexor surface of the forearm.
- A small bleb 6–10 mm in diameter will form if the injection is made at the correct depth. If a bleb does not form or if the antigen solution leaks from the site, repeat the injection.
- When applying more than one skin test, make the injections at least 5-cm apart.
- Perform any serologic blood tests before testing or wait for 48–96 hours.
- For two-step procedure, administer TB monitoring skin test (0.1 mL, 5 tuberculin units) for all persons noted for indications. Strictly enforce reading results in 48–72 hours. If *positive*, do not administer second PPD and refer for follow-up. If induration is present but does not classify as positive, retest *immediately* using other arm and read results in 48–72 hours. If *negative*, administer second PPD 1–2 weeks after first PPD, using same strength as first and using the same arm. Read results in 48–72 hours. If reaction at second test is negative (0 mm), no further testing is performed now. Make plans to administer one-step tubercular test yearly or every 3–6 months if high risk.

Interpreting Reactions

- Read all tests at 24, 48, and 72 hours. Reactions occurring before 24 hours indicate an immediate rather than a delayed hypersensitivity.
- Measure the diameter of the induration in two directions (at right angles) with a ruler and record each diameter in millimeters.
- Record test results in the health care record and include the millimeters of induration present and a picture of the arm showing the location of the tests.

CLINICAL ALERT

- In patients who are highly sensitive, or when higher than recommended doses are used, exaggerated local reactions may occur, including erythema, pain, blisters, necrosis, and scarring. Although systemic reactions are rare, a few cases of lymph node enlargement, fever, malaise, and fatigue have been reported.
- To prevent severe local reactions, never use second test strengths as the initial agent. Use diluted first strengths in patients with known or suspected hypersensitivity to the antigen.
- Have epinephrine and antihistamines on hand to treat severe allergic reactions that may occur.
- Health care workers in contact with suspected or confirmed TB must wear a properly fitted, high-efficiency, dust- or mist-proof mask.

Nursing Interventions

▶ *Pretest*

- Explain purpose and procedure of skin testing. Assess for allergy to candida or tetanus toxoid and eggs (mumps) when injecting two other skin antigens at the same time as PPD (done to detect false-negative TB results).

▶ *Intratest*

- For intradermal injection, cleanse skin with an alcohol swab (or inner aspect of the forearm) and allow to dry. Stretch skin taut. Inject substance under skin so that a discrete pale elevation of skin—a wheal, 6–10 mm in diameter—is formed.
- Document site of test for follow-up reading of results.

▶ *Posttest*

- Evaluate patient outcomes and counsel regarding outcomes, need for follow-up tests and treatment, and chest x-ray studies and sputum cultures in positive TB skin tests.

- Discuss initial and continued therapy and institute infection and case control as required.
- Read test results per specific skin test kit protocols. Examine in a good light. Base interpretation on induration, not erythema. Run your finger lightly over the area of normal skin to indurated zone. Measure the diameter of induration across the forearm (perpendicular to the long axis) and record in millimeters.

> ### CLINICAL ALERT FOR TB SKIN TESTING
>
> - Persons who meet any of the following high-risk criteria should receive preventive therapy regardless of age: *5 mm or more* (>5 mm) induration and infected with HIV or risk of HIV with unknown HIV status; close contact with recently diagnosed TB; or abnormal chest x-ray study showing fibrotic lesions likely to represent old healed TB; *10 mm or more* (>10 mm) induration and recent conversion initiation of 2-year period and younger than 35 years; or IV drug user who is HIV positive; or those with medical conditions at increased risk for TB (sclerosis, gastrectomy, intestinal bypass, body weight 10% or more below ideal), chronic renal failure, diabetes, immunosuppression, malignancies, and some blood disorders; *15 mm or more* (>15 mm) and recent conversion within a 2-year period and 35 years or older.
> - Penicillin scratch/skin testing: The inner volar surface of the forearm is usually used.
> - A nonbleeding scratch of 3–5 mm in length is made in the epidermis with a 20-gauge needle. If bleeding occurs, another site should be selected and another scratch should be made using less pressure. A small drop of the test solution is then applied and rubbed gently into the scratch using an applicator, toothpick, or the side of the needle. The scratch test site should be observed for the appearance of a wheal, erythema, or pruritus.
> - A positive reaction is signified by the appearance within 15 minutes of a pale wheal (usually with pseudopods) 5–15 mm or more in diameter. As soon as a positive response is elicited, or 15 minutes have elapsed, the solution should be wiped off the scratch.
> - If the scratch test is negative or equivocal (ie, a wheal of <5 mm in diameter with little or no erythema or itching appears), an intradermal test may be performed.
> - If significant reaction, treat and proceed to desensitization. Skin responses to penicillin testing will develop within 15 minutes.

SLEEP STUDY—CARDIORESPIRATORY, SLEEP DISORDERED BREATHING STUDY (SDB), SLEEP APNEA

Special Breathing Study

This test assesses cardiac and respiratory parameters during sleep. Specifically, the test is used to determine whether a patient has sleep apnea or sleep-disordered breathing (SDB). Typically, SDB tests are performed in a clinical setting; however, recent technological advances have made it possible to perform studies in the patient's home.

Indications

- Evaluate breathing patterns during sleep in which there are observed periods of apnea (cessation of breathing).
- Evaluate heart rate and rhythm during sleep.
- Determine if sleep apnea is a contributory factor to excessive daytime sleepiness.
- Perform preoperative evaluation for bariatric surgery.
- Assess overweight individuals who snore and are hypersomnolent.

Reference Values

Normal

- Apnea/Hypopnea Index (AHI): <5 per hour in the adult and <10 per hour in the older adult (60 years or older)
- Oxygen Desaturation Index (ODI): <5 per hour
- Apnea (A): <5 per hour
- Hypopnea (H): <5 per hour
- Heart rate will normally decrease during sleep; however, it should remain somewhat constant and the rhythm should be normal.

Clinical Implications

- Sleep-disordered breathing (SDB) can be divided into two major categories: obstructive sleep apnea (OSA) and central sleep apnea (CSA). An AHI of >5 is consistent with SDB, with values of >40 or 50 consistent with severe sleep apnea.
- Brady-tachyarrhythmia (most common in OSA) or any other dysrhythmia.

Interfering Factors

- Electrophysiologic artifacts, defective electrodes, diaphoresis, environmental noises, or inability to fall asleep will affect study results.

- Use of sleeping medications, alcohol, and caffeine interferes with test results.
- Elevating the head of the bed or using two or more pillows during the study should be discouraged unless the patient normally sleeps that way.

Procedure

- The SDB study is done during the patient's normal sleeping times.
- The patient is instructed to perform his or her normal daily activities on the day of the study.
- In clinical setting, the patient reports to the hospital 1 or 2 hours before normal sleep time. If this is a home study, patient will need to report at least 2 hours before sleep time to have electrodes applied.
- The preparation includes taping firmly in place ECG and impedance electrodes (chest), airflow thermistor (below nose), and pulse oximetry sensor (finger).
- During the study, continuous recordings of heart rate, chest wall movement, oral/nasal airflow, and oxygen saturation levels are made. Some systems will also monitor and record positional changes and snoring.
- A total study time of 6–8 hours is necessary to ensure adequate recording times for all stages of sleep.
- Recordings of the cardiorespiratory parameters are made on a paper-based or digital system and subsequently hand- or computer scored and edited.

Nursing Interventions
▸*Pretest*

- Explain purpose and procedure, emphasizing that this is a noninvasive study requiring them only to relax and fall asleep. Instruct the patient to adhere to normal sleep patterns before sleep studies so the patient comes to the test neither sleep deprived nor overrested.

▸*Intratest*

- Observe to ensure proper recording and check for loose electrodes.
- Provide a bedside commode as recording cables may not be long enough to reach the bathroom.
- Expect periods of apnea or hypopnea with decreases in oxygen saturation in these patients, although interventional discretion should be exercised.

▸*Posttest*

- Remove electrodes, record vital signs, and discharge.
- Assess for complaints and counsel appropriately.

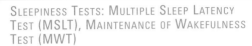

SLEEPINESS TESTS: MULTIPLE SLEEP LATENCY
TEST (MSLT), MAINTENANCE OF WAKEFULNESS
TEST (MWT)

*Special Study of Sleep Disorders (Includes EEG,
EOG, and EMG)*

The multiple sleep latency test (MSLT) is used as an objective measure of excessive daytime sleepiness and determines its severity. An alternative to this test is the maintenance of wakefulness test (MWT), which measures the ability of an individual to stay awake rather than to fall asleep.

Indications
- Diagnose narcolepsy or falling asleep at inappropriate times.
- Verify suspected narcolepsy.
- Evaluate effectiveness of drug therapy for daytime hypersomnolence.
- The MWT is useful to evaluate effectiveness of treatment in patients with excessive daytime sleepiness.

Interfering Factors
Caffeinated beverages can delay sleep, whereas sedatives (hypnotics) shorten sleep onset. Additionally, sleep deprivation may produce false-positive MSLT results. Daytime naps, environmental noise, lights, and temperature can have an side effect on the patient's ability to fall asleep.

Reference Values

Normal
MSLT: Mean sleep latency >10 minutes.
MWT: Mean sleep latency >35 minutes on the 40-minute test;
    >18 minutes on the 20-minute test.
No sleep onset REM periods (SOREMs).

Clinical Implications
MSLT
- An average sleep onset of 6–9 minutes is considered a "gray area" diagnostically, because these tests are performed in a laboratory setting and not in the patient's home environment. Re-evaluation may be necessary if the patient complains and symptoms persist.

- An average sleep onset of <5 minutes and two or more REM periods in the five to six naps is diagnostic for narcolepsy.

MWT
- Falling asleep before 25 minutes is associated with problems of maintaining vigilance.

Procedure
- Typically, the MSLT is administered the morning following a sleep study. Following the sleep study, the patient dresses, eats (avoiding caffeine), and reports back to the sleep laboratory.
- The electrodes are reapplied if necessary. The electrodes used include ECG, electroencephalogram (EEG), electro-oculogram (EOG), and chin electromyogram (EMG).
- The first nap begins 1.5 to 2 hours after morning awakening, with a minimum of four additional naps at 2-hour intervals throughout the day.
- The nap is terminated after 20 minutes, unless the patient falls asleep, in which case, the recording is continued for 15 minutes after sleep onset. (In the MWT, each trial [rather than nap] is either 20 or 40 minutes in length.)
- *Note:* The term "nap" indicates a short intentional or unintentional episode of subjective sleep taken during habitual wakefulness, whereas the term "falling asleep" or "sleep onset" is defined objectively by electroencephalographic (EEG) recordings (ie, stage 1 of NREM sleep).
- Between naps, the patient must remain awake and is encouraged to move around.
- Following the naps, all equipment is disconnected and the patient is discharged.

Nursing Interventions
▶Pretest
- Explain the test purpose and procedure. Remind the patient not to change daily routine on the day of testing.
- Reassure the patient that lead wires, monitors, and sensors will not interfere with sleep.
- Remind the patient that no alcohol or caffeinated beverages should be consumed the day of the test.
- Use standard sleep questionnaires or scales (eg, Epworth Scale, Stanford Scale).
- Follow the guidelines in Chapter 1 regarding safe, effective, informed *pretest* care.

▶*Posttest*
- Explain test outcome and possible need for follow-up testing.
- Follow the guidelines in Chapter 1 for safe, effective, informed *posttest* care.

SPUTUM CULTURE

Sputum, Infection

Sputum specimens are examined to identify organisms causing a respiratory illness. Pertinent symptoms include cough with sputum production, fever, chest pain, and shortness of breath.

Indications
- Diagnose disease of the lower respiratory tract.
- Determine antibiotic or drug sensitivity and course of treatment and evaluate effectiveness of therapy or medication.

Reference Values

Normal
- Negative culture for pathogenic organisms.

Clinical Implications
- Pathogens indicative of tuberculosis, fungal infections, and causing pneumonia, bronchitis, and bronchiectasis.
- Possible organisms are group A *Streptococcus*, *Streptococcus pneumoniae*, species of *Enterobacteriaceae*, Staphylococcus aureus, *Mycobacterium* sp., and *Legionella* sp.

Interfering Factors
- Antibiotics may cause false-negative cultures or may delay growth of organisms.
- Unsatisfactory sputum samples: contaminated specimens or "dry" specimens.

Procedure
- Instruct the patient to provide a deep-coughed specimen into a sterile container (1–3 mL is generally sufficient).

- If the patient is unable to expectorate a satisfactory specimen, ultrasonic nebulization, chest physiotherapy, nasotracheal or tracheal suctioning, or bronchoscopy can be used.
- The best sputum specimens are collected in the early morning.

Nursing Interventions
▶*Pretest*
- Explain the purpose, procedure, and all aspects of specimen collection.
- Instruct the patient not to touch inside of sputum container.

▶*Intratest*
- Patient should clear nose and throat and rinse mouth before expectorating, take several deep breaths, perform a series of short coughs, and then cough deeply and forcefully.
- Sputum specimens are usually not refrigerated but taken to the laboratory immediately.

▶*Posttest*
- Evaluate patient outcome and counsel appropriately about treatment and self-care for respiratory illness. Provide monitored care.

 STOOL ANALYSIS, ROUTINE FECAL STUDIES AND CULTURE

Stool

Fat, Meat Fibers, Occult Blood (Fecal Blood), Parasites, *Giardia* and *Cryptosporidium* Antigens, Stool Culture Leukocytes, APT Test for Swallowed Blood, Stool Electrolytes

Stool analysis determines the various properties of the feces for diagnostic purposes. Examination of fecal material for pathogenic organisms, electrolytes, occult blood, blood cells, and swallowed blood is also done.

 CLINICAL ALERT

- Stool analysis and all fecal studies must be done before administration of barium, antidiarrheal medications, antibiotics, bismuth, oil, enemas, or laxatives.

Indications

- Screen for colon cancer, asymptomatic ulcerative lesions of GI tract.
- Evaluate GI diseases in persons with diarrhea and constipation.
- Rule out in a stool culture the presence of enteric pathogens, such as *Salmonella, Shigella, Campylobacter, Yersinia, Escherichia coli* (pathogenic), and *Clostridium difficile*, and large numbers of *Staphylococcus* and *Pseudomonas.*
- Detect *Giardia lamblia*, most common intestinal parasite in the United States, and detect *Cryptosporidium* antigen in feces.
- Screen immunocompromised persons for parasitic infectious diseases.
- Use fat analysis as gold standard to diagnose malabsorption syndrome.
- Detect the presence or absence of fecal leukocytes before the isolation of a bacterial pathogen.
- Assess stool electrolytes to evaluate electrolyte imbalance in persons with diarrhea (stools must be liquid for electrolyte test).
- Use stool and serum osmolality to calculate osmotic gap and diagnose intestinal disaccharide deficiency.
- Differentiate swallowed blood syndrome from infant GI hemorrhage.

Reference Values

Normal

MACROSCOPIC EXAMINATION	OUTCOMES
Amount	100–200 g/day
Color	Brown
Odor	Varies with pH of stool and diet and depends on bacterial fermentation and putrefaction
Consistency	Plastic; not unusual to see seeds in a vegetable diet; visible undigested fiber, both small and dry in a high-meat diet
Size, shape	Formed, soft plastic; soft and bulky for a high-fiber diet; dry in a high-protein diet
Gross blood, mucus, pus, and parasites	None

MICROSCOPIC EXAMINATION	OUTCOMES
Fat	Colorless, neutral fat (18%), and fatty acid crystals and soaps
Undigested food, meat fibers, starch, trypsin	None to small amount
Eggs and segments of parasites	None
Culture	Negative for pathogens, bacteria, viruses, and yeasts
Giardia antigen	Negative
Leukocytes	Negative

CHEMICAL EXAMINATION	OUTCOMES
Water	Up to 75%
pH	Neutral to weakly alkaline (pH 6.5–7.5)
Occult blood	Negative
Urobilinogen	50–300 EU/100 g or 500–3000 EU/kg
Porphyrins	Coproporphyrins: <200 μg/24 hours or <305 nmol/day
	Uroporphyrins: <1000 μg/24 hours or <1.2 μmol/day
Nitrogen	<2.5 g/24 hours or <178 mmol/day
APT test for swallowed blood	Negative in adults, positive in newborns. Test result will indicate whether blood present in newborn feces or vomitus is of maternal or fetal origin
Trypsin	Positive in small amounts in adults; present in greater amounts in normal children
Osmolality, used with stool Na + K to calculate osmotic gaps	200–250 mOsm or 250 mg/dL; osmolality is $2\times$ sodium plus potassium
Sodium	5.8–9.8 mEq/24 hours or mmol/day
Chloride	2.5–3.9 mEq/24 hours or mmol/day
Potassium	15.7–20.7 mEq/24 hours or mmol/day
Lipids (fatty acids)	0–6 g/24 hours

Clinical Implications: Color

The color of feces changes in disease states: *Yellow to yellow green*—severe diarrhea; *black*—bleeding >100 mL of blood into upper GI tract; *tan or clay*—common bile duct blockage and pancreatic insufficiency; *pink, bright red to maroon*—bleeding from lower GI tract from tumors, fissures, inflammatory process, or hemorrhoids.

Interfering Factors: Color

- Stool darkens on standing.
- Color is influenced by diet: Green with spinach; black with cherries and high meat; light with high-milk and low-meat diets; red with beets.
- Color is also influenced by drugs: yellow green (sterilization of bowel by antibiotics); black (iron, bismuth, charcoal); green (indomethacin); light white (barium, antacids); brown (anthraquinone); red (tetracyclines in syrup); among many others.

Clinical Implications: Mucus

- Mucus is abnormal and appears in conditions of parasympathetic excitation. Translucent mucus on surface of formed stool in spastic constipation and emotionally disturbed patients. Bloody mucus clinging to stool (cancer of colon, inflammation of the rectal canal). Copious amounts of mucus of 3–4 L in 24 hours (villous adenomas) and mucus with pus and blood (enteritis, intestinal tuberculosis, shigellosis, salmonellosis, ulcerative colitis).

Interfering Factors: Mucus

- Dulcolax suppositories cause excess mucus.

Clinical Implications: Consistency

- Diarrhea mixed with mucus and red blood cells (cancer, amebiasis, cholera, typhus, typhoid); diarrhea mixed with mucus and white blood cells (ulcerative colitis, shigellosis, salmonellosis, enteritis, and intestinal TB).
- Altered size and shape indicate motility or abnormalities in colon wall as a narrow ribbonlike stool (spastic bowel, partial obstruction); small, round, hard stools (habitual constipation); and severe fecal retention (huge impacted masses with a small amount of liquid stool as overflow).

Clinical Implications: Cultures

- Presence of parasites, enteric disease-causing organisms, and viruses. Large numbers of *Candida albicans*, *Staphylococcus aureus*, and *Pseudomonas aeruginosa* are considered pathogenic in the presence of previous antibiotic therapy. Cryptosporidiosis is a cause of severe protractile diarrhea.

Clinical Implications: Electrolytes

- Electrolyte abnormalities occur in the following conditions:
  - Idiopathic proctocolitis: *Increased* sodium (Na^+) and chloride (Cl^-), *normal* potassium (K^+).
  - Ileostomy: *Increased* sodium (Na^+) and chloride (Cl^-), *low* potassium (K^+).
  - Cholera: *Increased* sodium (Na^+) and chloride (Cl^-).
- Chloride is greatly increased in stool in the following conditions: Congenital chloride diarrhea; acquired chloride diarrhea; secondary chloride diarrhea; idiopathic proctocolitis; and cholera.
- Stool osmolality of 500 mg/dL (500 mOsm) per day is suspicious for factitious disorders (eg, laxative abuse, ingestion of rat poison). Higher levels indicate high amounts of stool-reducing substances. The osmotic gap is increased in osmotic diarrhea caused by the following conditions: saline laxatives; sodium or magnesium citrate; and carbohydrates (lactulose or sorbitol candy).

Interfering Factors: Electrolytes

- Formed stools invalidate the results. Stools *must* be liquid for electrolyte tests.
- The stool cannot be contaminated with urine.
- Surreptitious addition of water to the stool specimen considerably lowers the osmolality. Stool osmolality *must* be <240 mOsm/kg to calculate the osmotic gap.

 CLINICAL ALERT

- *Giardia* antigen detection results should not be the only criterion to form diagnosis but rather correlate test results to patient's clinical symptoms. Test three consecutive stool specimens for the *Giardia* antigen before considering test results negative.

Clinical Implications: Occult Blood

- Positive test caused by cancer of colon and stomach; occurs in ulcerative colitis, ulcers, diaphragmatic hernia, and rectal carcinoma.

Interfering Factors: Blood in Stool

- Many foods and drugs may give false-positive outcomes. Drugs include salicylates, steroids, indomethacin, iron (large doses), Coumadin, vitamin C (ascorbic acid), bromides, colchicine, alcohol, and iodine, among others. Foods with hemoglobin and

myoglobin enzymes and peroxidase activity such as meat and some vegetables (horseradish, turnips).
- Other factors include bleeding hemorrhoids, hematuria, menstrual contaminants, and vigorous exercise (long-distance runners).

Clinical Implications: Fecal Fat, Fatty Acids, Meat Fibers

- *Increases in fecal fat and fatty acids* occur with lack of lipase, enteritis and pancreatic disease, surgical removal and resection of a part of intestine, and in malabsorption syndromes (Crohn's disease and sprue).
- *Increased meat fibers* in malabsorption syndrome, pancreatic dysfunction, and gastrocolic fistula (correlates with the amount of fat excreted).

Interfering Factors: Fat

- Increased neutral fat may occur with the use of rectal suppositories and oily perineal creams, castor and mineral oil; low-calorie dietetic mayonnaise; and high-fiber diet or Metamucil.

Clinical Implications: Leukocytes

- Large amounts of leukocytes (primarily neutrophils) accompany the following conditions:
  a. Chronic ulcerative colitis
  b. Chronic bacillary dysentery
  c. Localized abscesses
  d. Fistulas of the sigmoid rectum or anus
- Primarily neutrophilic leukocytes appear in the following conditions:
  a. Shigellosis
  b. Salmonellosis
  c. *Yersinia* infection
  d. Invasive *Escherichia coli* diarrhea
  e. Ulcerative colitis
- Primarily mononuclear leukocytes appear in typhoid.
- Absence of leukocytes is associated with the following conditions:
  a. Cholera
  b. Nonspecific diarrhea (eg, drug or food induced)
  c. Viral diarrhea
  d. Amebic colitis
  e. Noninvasive *E. coli* diarrhea
  f. Toxigenic bacteria (eg, *Staphylococcus*, *Clostridium*)
  g. Parasites (eg, *Giardia*, *Entamoeba*)

Clinical Implications: APT Test for Swallowed Blood

- Fetal hemoglobin, which is pink in color, is present in gastric hemorrhage of the newborn.

- Adult hemoglobin, which is brownish in color, is present in swallowed blood syndrome in the infant.

Interfering Factors: APT Test for Swallowed Blood

- The test is invalid with black, tarry stools because the blood has already been converted to hematin.
- The test is invalid if there is insufficient blood present; grossly visible blood must be present in the specimen.
- Vomitus with pH < 3.9 produces an invalid test result.
- The presence of maternal thalassemia major produces a false-positive test result because of increased maternal hemoglobin F.

CLINICAL ALERT

- The blood in the newborn's stool is the result of blood swallowed during delivery or may be from a fissure of the mother's nipple in breast-fed infants. This condition must be differentiated from GI hemorrhage of the newborn. The test is based on the fact that the infant's blood contains largely fetal hemoglobin, which is alkali resistant. This blood can be differentiated from the mother's blood using laboratory methods.

Procedure for Random Collection and Transport of Stool Specimens

- Observe standard universal precautions when procuring and handling specimens.
- Collect feces in a dry, clean, urine-free container that has a properly fitting cover.
- The specimen should be uncontaminated with urine or other bodily secretions such as menstrual blood. Stool can be collected from the diaper of an infant or incontinent adult. Samples can be collected from temporary ostomy bags.
- While wearing gloves, collect the entire stool specimen and transfer it to a container with a clean tongue blade or similar object. A 2.5-cm (walnut size) or 64.7-mg (1-oz) sample of liquid stool may be sufficient for some tests.
- For best results, cover specimens and deliver to laboratory immediately after collection.

Procedure for Stool Culture

- Often parasite testing and stool culture are ordered together. In this case, the specimen is divided in half and one portion is refrigerated for culture and one portion is kept at room temperature for ova and parasites. A diarrheal stool will give good results. Stool passed into toilet bowl must *not* be used for cultures.

- For individuals who develop diarrhea of unknown etiology, obtain *two* stool cultures, one for enteric pathogens (culture and sensitivity) and a second specimen (50 mL of liquid stool) for *C. difficile* culture and toxin.
- Use a wooden spatula and transfer at least 1 in (2.54 cm) or walnut-sized portion of fecal material to specimen container. Place in a biohazard bag.
- Collect stool specimens before antibiotic therapy is initiated and as early in the course of the disease as possible.
- If mucus or blood is present, it definitely should be included with the specimen, because pathogens are more likely to be found in these substances.

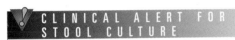

CLINICAL ALERT FOR
STOOL CULTURE

- At least three specimens, collected every other day or within a 10-day time frame, are needed to make a positive stool culture diagnosis.

Procedure for Ova and Parasites

- Observe standard precautions. Collect feces in a dry, clean, urine-free container.
- Warm stools are best for detecting ova and parasites. Do *not* refrigerate specimens for ova and parasites.
- Special vials that contain 10% formalin and polyvinyl alcohol (PVA) fixative may be used for collecting stool samples to test for ova and parasites. In this case, specimen storage temperature is not critical.
- Because of the cyclic life cycle of parasites, three separate random stool specimens for analysis are recommended.
- Place the specimen in a biohazard bag.

Procedure for Occult Blood

- Obtain a random stool specimen. Follow testing method (or instruct patient to do so), as given in manufacturer's directions exactly, or results are not reliable. Use a portion from the center of formed stool. A liquid stool may give false-negative results with filter paper methods. Time the reaction exactly.

Procedure for Fat and Meat Fibers

- Collect a 24- or 72-hour specimen following specimen collection guidelines in Chapter 2. If a 72-hour specimen is ordered, each individual stool specimen is collected properly, identified, and labeled and sent immediately to the laboratory.
- Specimens for fat testing should be obtained with mineral oil; bismuth or magnesium compounds cannot be used.
- If testing for meat fibers is ordered, specimens obtained with a warm saline enema or Fleet Phospho-Soda are acceptable.

Procedure for Leukocytes

- Collect a random stool specimen. Mucus or liquid stool specimens can be used.

Procedure for APT for Swallowed Blood

- Collect a random sample from a newborn infant; observe universal precautions.
- The following are acceptable specimens:
  a. Blood-stained diaper
  b. Grossly bloody stool
  c. Bloody vomitus or gastric aspiration
- Place specimen or specimens in a biohazard bag and deliver to the laboratory as soon as possible.
- In the laboratory, the blood is dissolved and treated with NaOH for alkali denaturation. Fetal hemoglobin is alkali resistant, and the solution of blood remains pink. Swallowed blood of maternal origin contains adult hemoglobin, which is converted to brownish hematin when the alkali is added.

Nursing Interventions

♦ Pretest

- Explain purpose and diet requirements, procedure for stool collection, interfering factors, and need to follow appropriate procedure.

- Supply the appropriate specimen collection container. Withhold antibiotic therapy until after specimen collection for leukocytes.
- Note that barium procedure and laxatives should be avoided for 1 week before specimen collection.
- Do not collect specimen while hemorrhoids are bleeding, while blood is present in the urine, or during menstrual period, until 3 days after menses have stopped.

▶Intratest
- Provide privacy during stool collection.
- Observe standard precautions when collecting stool specimen.
- Provide assistance with specimen collection for patients who require help, ie, disabled, children, and confused.
- Follow the manufacturer's directions for prepackaged specimen containers.
- Stress compliance with specimen collection procedure.

▶Posttest
- Evaluate patient compliance and outcomes and counsel the patient appropriately. Explain the need for repeat or further testing, if ordered.
- Report blood in stool immediately and document it in the medical record.

STRESS TEST, EXERCISE TESTING, GRADED EXERCISE TOLERANCE TEST, SUBMAXIMAL EFFORT

Special Cardiac and Respiratory Study

Exercise stress testing is used to evaluate the cardiac and respiratory response to graded exercise. It may be used to delineate cardiac versus respiratory limitation to exercise and subsequent management of the patient.

Indications
- Diagnose ischemic heart disease and investigate angina, dysrhythmias, inordinate BP elevation, valve competence, and pacemaker function.
- Measure functional capacity for work, sports, or participation in rehabilitation programs; predict potential response to medical or surgical treatment; and set limits for an exercise program.
- Evaluate upper limits of physiologically responsive pacemakers.

Reference Values

Normal

- Negative: No significant symptoms, arrhythmias, or other ECG changes at 85% (this is considered a submaximal test level) of the maximum predicted heart rate.
- Normal response to graded exercise: Increase in systolic BP (diastolic levels remain near normal) and heart rate; less than a 4% (absolute) decrease in oxygen saturation levels.

Interfering Factors

- False-positive results may reflect left ventricular hypertrophy, digitalis toxicity, ST-segment abnormality at rest, hypertension, valvular heart disease, left-bundle branch block, anemia, hypoxia, vasoregulatory asthenia, Lown-Ganong-Levine syndrome (ie, ventricular pre-excitation), panic or anxiety attack, and Wolff-Parkinson-White syndrome.

Procedure

- Electrode sites are prepared, electrodes are secured, and a baseline ECG tracing is recorded. Additionally, the baseline HR, BP, and oxygen saturation (via pulse oximetry) are recorded.
- The patient walks a motor-driven treadmill or pedals an ergometer, and as work rate is increased, the ECG, HR, BP, and oxygen saturation are continuously monitored.
- The test is terminated if ECG abnormalities, fatigue, weakness, abnormal blood pressure changes, or other intolerable symptoms occur during the test.
- Recovery-stage assessments are usually recorded in the testing area until the patient is stable.

Nursing Interventions

▶*Pretest*

- Explain the test purpose and procedure and demonstrate the equipment.
- Advise patient to abstain from stressful exercise or stress testing for the prior 12 hours. No food, coffee, or smoking is allowed within 2 hours of the test. Water may be taken.
- Certain medications (beta-adrenergic blocking agents) are withheld, dosages reduced, tapered gradually, or discontinued before testing.
- Instruct the patient to report symptoms and sensations.
- Walking shoes or tennis shoes, shorts, loose trousers or slacks, bra, and a front-button blouse are suggested attire.

▶ *Intratest*
- Be alert to signs of anxiety, pain, hypotension, fatigue, or dysrhythmias and other signs and symptoms that may indicate a need to abort the test.
- Provide feedback and reassurance.

▶ *Posttest*
- The patient should not be discharged from the test area until stable. No excessive exercise is permitted for the remainder of the day. Report significant signs or symptoms (eg, arrhythmia, angina) at once.

CLINICAL ALERT

- Patients with unstable angina, congestive heart failure, or severe myocardial dysfunction are at greater risk during stress testing.

SYPHILIS DETECTION TESTS

Blood, Bacterial Infection

VDRL, RPR, FTA-ABS, FP-PA

These tests are performed to diagnose syphilis, a venereal disease caused by *Treponema pallidum.* VDRL (Venereal Disease Research Laboratory) and rapid plasma reagin (RPR) are nontreponemal (nonspecific) tests that determine the presence of regain; fluorescent treponema antibody (FTA-ABS) test and treponema pallidum partiate agglutinate (TP-PA) are treponemal (specific) tests that determine the presence of antibodies to *Treponema pallidum.* VDRL and RPR, an ERT (automated reagin test), are used as screening tests. The more complex FTA-ABS and TP-PA tests are used to confirm syphilis and are not used for screening.

Indications
- Evaluate bacterial infection with *Treponema pallidum.*
- Screen for and confirm syphilis.
- Monitor treatment.

Reference Values

Normal
- Nonreactive: Negative for syphilis.

Clinical Implications
- Positive for infection with *Treponema pallidum* when both the screening and confirmatory tests are reactive.

Interfering Factors
- False-positive reactions: Biologic false-positive (BFP) reactions can occur in nontreponemal tests in patients who abuse drugs, or who have diseases such as lupus erythematosus, mononucleosis, malaria, leprosy, or viral pneumonia; or who have been recently immunized; or rarely during pregnancy.
- False-negative reactions: Nontreponemal tests may give negative results early in the disease or during inactive or late stages of disease, or when the patient has a faulty immunodefective mechanism.

Procedure
- Serum (5 mL) is obtained by venipuncture in a red-top tube. Place the specimen in a biohazard bag.
- Fasting is usually not required.

Nursing Interventions

▶Pretest
- Assess patient's knowledge of test and clinical history. Assess for interfering factors.
- Explain purpose and blood test procedure. Advise patient to avoid alcohol ingestion for at least 24 hours before blood draw because alcohol decreases reaction intensity in tests that detect reagin.

▶Posttest
- Evaluate patient outcomes and counsel appropriately.
- If result is a biologic false positive, assess patient's understanding that he or she does not have syphilis.

CLINICAL ALERT

- Sexual partners of patients with primary, secondary, or early latent syphilis should be evaluated for signs and symptoms of syphilis and should undergo a blood test for syphilis.
- After treatment, patients with early syphilis should be tested at 3-month intervals for 1 year.

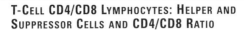

T-Cell CD4/CD8 Lymphocytes: Helper and Suppressor Cells and CD4/CD8 Ratio

Blood for Altered Immunity

T-cell subset analysis is a surface marker for the T-helper cells and T-suppressor cells and is used in the clinical assessment of two major disease states (lymphoproliferative leukemia and lymphoma) and in immunodeficient states (HIV and organ transplant).

Indications

- Monitor CD4 counts.
- Monitor effectiveness of therapy through repeat testing of CD4 levels.
- Assess immune deficiencies.
- Assess transplant patients for threat of organ rejection or host infection.
- HIV-positive patients should be tested every 3–6 months to monitor their level of CD4 T lymphocytes.

Reference Values

Normal

	Percent	Absolute Counts (Cells/μL)	SI Units (10^9/L)
Total T cells (CD3)	60–80	3500 ± 600	3.5 ± 0.60
Helper T cells (CD4)	30–60	1700 ± 300	1.7 ± 0.30
Suppressor T cells (CD8)	20–40	1600 ± 150	1.6 ± 0.15
Total B cells	5–20	200 ± 100	0.2 ± 0.10
Helper/suppressor ratio	>1.0		

Clinical Implications

- When the CD4 count falls below 500/mm^3, the patient can be diagnosed with AIDS and can receive AZT (zidovudine or azidothymidine) or other antiretroviral drug.

- When the CD4 count is less than 200/mm^3, prophylaxis against *Pneumocystis carinii* pneumonia is recommended.

Procedure
- Obtain a 7-mL venous blood sample using a lavender-top tube.

Nursing Interventions

▸*Pretest*
- Explain the test purpose and procedure.

▸*Posttest*
- Evaluate patient outcomes and counsel appropriately.

TESTICULAR/SCROTAL IMAGING

Nuclear Medicine, Genitourinary (GU) Imaging

This procedure is performed on an emergency basis in the evaluation of acute, painful testicular swelling. It is also used in the differential diagnoses of torsion or acute epididymitis and in the evaluation of injury, trauma, tumors, and masses.

Indications
- Differentiate inflammation from ischemia in patients with pain.
- Done on an urgent basis when torsion is suspected.
- In pediatric patients, done to diagnose acute and latent testicular torsion, epididymitis, or testicular hydrocele and to evaluate testicular masses such as abscesses and tumors.

Reference Values

Normal
Normal blood flow to scrotal structures.

Clinical Implications
- Abnormal concentrations reveal tumors, hematomas, infection, and torsion (with reduced blood flow and acute epididymitis); in the neonatal patient, torsion is primarily due to developmental anomalies.
- In the patient with "hot" areas, infection is likely; if "cold" areas are present, then ischemia is likely.
- Imaging is most specific soon after the onset of pain, before abscess is a clinical consideration.

Procedure

- The patient lies on his back under the gamma camera and the penis is gently taped back onto the lower abdominal wall. In pediatric patients, for proper positioning, towels are used to support the scrotum. Lead shielding is often placed in the perineal area, with the scrotum under one layer of lead foil to reduce any background radioactivity.
- The radionuclide (^{99m}Tc pertechnetate) is injected intravenously.
- Imaging is performed in two phases: First, as a dynamic blood flow study of the scrotum, and, second, as an assessment of distribution of radiopharmaceutical in the scrotum.
- Total examining time is 30–45 minutes.

Nursing Interventions

▸*Pretest*
- Explain the purpose and procedure of the test.
- If the patient is a child, a parent (preferably the father) should accompany him.

▸*Intratest*
- Provide privacy during the procedure to lessen embarrassment.

▸*Posttest*
- Interpret test outcome and counsel appropriately.
- Monitor injection site for extravasation or infiltration of the radiopharmaceutical agent.
- Observe and treat mild reactions: pruritus, rashes, and flushing 2–24 hours after injection; sometimes nausea and vomiting may occur.

TESTOSTERONE—TOTAL AND FREE

Blood, Hormone

These tests measure testosterone hormone production in both men (secreted by testes and adrenals) and women (secreted by ovaries and adrenals).

Indications

- Evaluate hypogonadism in men and masculinization in women.
- Investigate male precocious puberty.
- Assess testicular function, pituitary gonadotropin function, and impotency.

- Diagnose hypopituitarism.
- Detect ovarian and adrenal tumors in women with symptoms of hirsutism, anovulation, amenorrhea, and polycystic ovaries.
- Use as a part of fertility workup.

Reference Values

Normal

TESTOSTERONE—TOTAL

Men: 270–1070 ng/dL or 9–38 nmol/L
Women: 15–70 ng/dL or 0.5–2.4 nmol/L
Children: 2–20 ng/dL or 0.07–0.70 nmol/L

TESTOSTERONE—FREE

Men: 50–210 pg/mL or 174–729 pmol/L (diminished in normal, elderly man)
Women: 1–8.5 pg/mL or 3.5–29.5 pmol/L

Clinical Implications

- *Decreased testosterone totals in men* with hypogonadism (pituitary failure), Klinefelter's syndrome, hypopituitarism, orchidectomy, hepatic cirrhosis, and delayed puberty.
- *Increased testosterone totals in men* with hyperthyroidism, syndromes of androgen resistance, adrenal tumors, and precocious puberty and adrenal hyperplasia in boys.
- *Increased testosterone totals in women* with adrenal neoplasms, ovarian tumors (virilizing), trophoblastic disease in pregnancy, hirsutism, and hilar cell tumor.
- *Decreased free testosterone in men* with hypogonadism and increase of sex hormone-binding globulin, especially in elderly men.
- *Increased free testosterone in women* with hirsutism, polycystic ovaries, and masculinization.

Interfering Factors

- Levels affected by radiopharmaceutical administration approximately 24 hours before testing.
- Levels are high in morning, decrease to 50% in men and 30% in women by midafternoon.
- Alcoholism in men decreases levels.
- Estrogen therapy in men increases levels.
- Many drugs, including androgens and steroids, decrease levels.

Procedure

- Obtain a 5-mL serum sample by venipuncture in a red-top tube. Blood should be drawn at 7:00 AM for highest levels.

Nursing Interventions

▶*Pretest*

- Explain purpose and procedure of the test.
- Do not administer any radiopharmaceutical within 1 week of test.

▶*Posttest*

- Evaluate outcomes, monitor, and counsel appropriately.

THERAPEUTIC DRUG MANAGEMENT (TDM)

Blood, Urine, Saliva, Drug Therapy

Therapeutic drug management (TDM) is a reliable and practical approach to managing adequate and nontoxic individual patient drug therapy. Determination of drug levels is especially important when the potential for drug toxicity is significant or when an inadequate or undesirable response follows the use of a standard dose. It provides an easier and more rapid estimation of dosage requirements than does observation of the drug effects themselves. For some drugs, monitoring is routinely useful (digoxin); for others, it can be helpful in certain situations (antibiotics). The plasma level of drugs needed to control the patient's symptoms is called the therapeutic concentration and is usually maintained by a combination of drug dosage and interval. At steady state, drug levels are the same after every dose. Steady state is reached at 3–5 half doses, and the rate of drug administration is equal to the rate of drug elimination. Monitoring at intervals minimizes the possibility of the development of dose-related side effects. If single drug therapy is not effective, therapeutic monitoring allows the clinician to select supplementary medication and monitor its effect upon the primary drug. Common classes of monitored drugs include antibiotics, cardiac therapeutics, anticonvulsants, antipsychotics, and antiasthma, among others.

Definitions

- **Therapeutic values** refer to the desirable range of drug concentrations in the serum or blood. When the drug concentration is

within the therapeutic range, the desired pharmacologic response is likely to occur.
- **Peak drug level** is the highest drug concentration occurring within a dosing interval.
- **Trough drug level** occurs just before administration of the next dose of drug (used for most drugs).
- **Toxic (panic or critical) values** are drug concentrations above the therapeutic range associated with an increasing risk of toxicity or undesirable effects.
- **Half-life** is the time required for a 50% decrease in the serum concentration relative to the initial concentration of the drug.

Indications

- Select or adjust drug dosage, level, or interval and modify therapy.
- When noncompliance (nonadherence) is suspected and patient motivation to maintain medication is poor.
- When physiologic status is altered by factors such as age, weight, menstrual cycle, body water, and stress.
- With coadministered (multiple) drugs, which may cause either synergistic or antagonistic drug reaction.
- When pathology is present that influences drug absorption and elimination, such as cardiovascular dysfunction, liver clearance (caffeine, phenobarbital), renal clearance (urinary output and pH, digoxin); gastrointestinal and poor absorption; and altered plasma protein binding (or change in blood proteins that carry drug).
- Some drugs have a very small safety range (therapeutic window or concentration). Factors that affect concentration include genetic variability, absorption, metabolism, route of excretion, drug tolerance, tissue storage, site of action, disease processes, and drug toxicity.

Reference Values

(See Table 3.5.)

Procedure

- Blood, urine, or saliva specimens may be tested. Most often, a venous sample of blood is obtained. Serum or plasma can be used, depending on the drug being tested and laboratory protocols (see Chapter 2).
- Record sampling time.
- Serum separation tubes may not be used for drug monitoring because small amounts of the drug adhere to the separator gel barrier.

(text continues on page 549)

TABLE 3.5 BLOOD PLASMA CONCENTRATIONS OF COMMONLY MONITORED DRUGS

DRUG	THERAPEUTIC LEVEL	TOXIC/CRITICAL LEVEL
Acetaminophen (Tylenol)	10–30 μg/mL (SI: 66–199 μmol/L)	>200 μg/mL (SI: >1324 μmol/L)
Acetylsalicylic acid (aspirin)	100–300 μg/mL (SI: 0.72–2.17 mmol/L)	>300 μg/mL (SI: >2.17 mmol/L)
Alcohol	Driving while intoxicated: 100 mg/dL or 21.7 μmol/L	>200 mg/dL (SI: >43.4 mmol/L)
Amikacin	Infections: 25–30 μg/mL (SI: 42.7–51.2 μmol/L)	Peak: >35 μg/mL (SI: >60 μmol/L)
	Serious infections: 20–25 μg/mL (SI: 34.2–42.7 μmol/L)	Trough: >10 μg/mL (SI: >17.1 μmol/L)
	Urinary tract infections: 15–30 μg/mL (SI: 25.6–51.2 μmol/L)	
	Trough: Life-threatening infections: 4–8 μg/mL (SI: 6.8–13.7 μmol/L)	
	Serious infections: 1–4 μg/mL (SI: 1.7–6.8 μmol/L)	
Amiodarone (Cordarone)	0.5–2.5 μg/mL (SI: 1–4 μmol/L)	>3.5 μg/mL (SI: 6 μmol/L)
Amitriptyline (Elavil)	100–250 ng/mL (SI: 360–900 nmol/L)	>500 ng/mL (SI: 1805 nmol/L)
Caffeine	5–15 μg/mL (SI: 26–77 μmol/L)	>30 μg/mL (SI: 155 μmol/L)
Carbamazepine (Tegretol)	6–12 μg/mL (SI: 25–51 μmol/L)	>15 μg/mL (SI: 64 μmol/L)
Chloramphenicol (Chloromycetin)	15–20 μg/mL (SI: 46–62 μmol/L)	>40 μg/mL (SI: 124 μmol/L)

(table continues on page 542)

TABLE 3.5 (continued)

DRUG	THERAPEUTIC LEVEL	TOXIC/CRITICAL LEVEL
Chlordiazepoxide (Librium)	0.1–3 µg/mL (SI: 0–10 µmol/L)	>23 µg/mL (SI: >77 µmol/L)
Clonazepam (Klonopin)	20–80 ng/mL (SI: 63–254 nmol/L)	>80 ng/mL (SI: >254 nmol/L)
Clorazepate (Tranxene)	0.12–1 µg/mL (SI: 0.36–3.01 µmol/L)	Not defined
Cyclosporine	100–400 ng/mL (SI: 83–333 nmol/L)	Not well defined—nephrotoxicity may occur at any level
Desipramine (Norpramin)	50–300 ng/mL (SI: 188–1126 nmol/L)	Possible toxicity: (>300 ng/mL; SI: >1126 nmol/L)
Diazepam (Valium)	0.2–1.5 µg/mL (SI: 0.7–5.3 µmol/L)	Check with your laboratory (SI: 0.7–5.3 µmol/L)
Digitoxin (Crystodigin)	20–35 ng/mL (SI: 26–46 nmol/L)	>45 ng/mL (SI: 59 nmol/L)
Digoxin (Lanoxin)	CHF: 0.8–2.0 ng/mL (SI: 1.0–2.6 nmol/L); arrhythmias: 1.5–2.5 ng/mL (SI: 1.9–3.2 nmol/L)	>2.0 ng/mL (SI: >2.6 nmol/L) Fatal: >3.5 ng/mL (SI: >4.5 nmol/L)
Disopyramide (Norpace)	Atrial arrhythmias: 2.8–3.2 µg/mL or 8.3–9.4 µmol/L Ventricular arrhythmias: 3.3–7.5 µg/mL or 9.7–22.0 µmol/L	>7 µg/mL (SI: >20.7 µmol/L)
Doxepin (Sinequan)	30–150 ng/mL (SI: 107–537 nmol/L)	>500 ng/mL (SI: >1790 nmol/L)

Ethchlorvynol (Placidyl)	2–9 µg/mL (SI: 14–55 µmol/L)	>20 µg/mL (SI: >138 µmol/L)
Ethosuximide (Zarontin)	40–100 µg/mL (SI: 280–710 µmol/L)	>150 µg/mL (SI: >1062 µmol/L)
Fenoprofen (Nalfon)	20–65 µg/mL (SI: 82–268 µmol/L)	Not available
Flecainide (Tambocor)	0.2–1.0 µg/mL or 0.4–2.0 µmol/L	21.3 µg/mL fatal or 43.2 µmol/L
Fluoxetine (Prozac)	100–800 ng/mL (SI: 289–2314 nmol/L)	>2000 ng/mL (SI: >6.5 µmol/L)
Gentamicin (Garamycin)	Peak: Serious infections: 6–8 µg/mL (SI: 12–17 µmol/L) Life-threatening infections: 8–10 µg/mL (SI: 17–21 µmol/L) Urinary tract infection: 4–6 µg/mL (SI: 8–12 µmol/L) Synergy against gram-positive organisms: 3–5 µg/mL (SI: 6.3–10.4 µmol/L) Trough: Serious infections: 0.5–1 µg/mL Life-threatening infections: 1–2 µg/mL (SI: 2.1–4.2 µmol/L)	Check with your laboratory
Haloperidol (Haldol)	5–15 µg/mL (SI: 10–30 nmol/L)	>42 ng/mL (SI: >84 nmol/L)
Ibuprofen (Motrin, Advil)	10 µg/mL or 48 µmol/L antipyretic effect	>200 µg/mL (SI: >970 µmol/L) may be associated with severe toxicity

(table continues on page 544)

TABLE 3.5 (continued)

DRUG	THERAPEUTIC LEVEL	TOXIC/CRITICAL LEVEL
Imipramine (Tofranil) (desipramine is an active metabolite of imipramine)	Imipramine: 150–200 ng/mL (SI: 530–890 nmol/L) Desipramine: 150–300 ng/mL (SI: 560–1125 nmol/L) (Utility of serum monitoring is controversial)	>300 ng/mL (SI: >1070 nmol/L)
Isoniazid	1–7 µg/mL (SI: 7–51 µmol/L)	20–710 µg/mL (SI: 146–5176 µmol/L)
Kanamycin (Kantrex)	Peak: 25–35 µg/mL (SI: 52–72 µmol/L) Trough: 4–8 µg/mL (SI: 8–16 µmol/L)	Peak: >35 µg/mL (SI: >72 µmol/L) Trough: >10 µg/mL (SI: >21 µmol/L)
Lidocaine (Xylocaine)	1.5–5.0 µg/mL (SI: 6–21 µmol/L)	Potentially toxic: >6 µg/mL (SI: >26 µmol/L) Toxic: >9 µg/mL (SI: >38 µmol/L)
Lithium (Eskalith)	Acute mania: 0.6–1.2 mEq/L (SI: 0.6–1.2 mmol/L) Maintenance level: 0.8–1 mEq/L (SI: 0.8–1 mmol/L)	>2 mEq/L (SI: >2 mmol/L)
Meperidine (Demerol)	70–500 ng/mL (SI: 283–2020 nmol/L)	>1000 ng/mL (SI: >4043 nmol/L)
Methotrexate	Variable	Toxic: Low-dose therapy, >91 ng/mL (SI: >200 nmol/L); high-dose therapy: > 454 ng/mL (SI: >1000 nmol/L)

Mexiletine (Mexitil)	0.5–2 µg/mL (SI: 2.8–11.2 µmol/L)	Potentially toxic >2 µg/mL (SI: >11 µmol/L) associated with seizures
Nitroprusside	Nitroprusside is converted to cyanide ions in the bloodstream. It decomposes to prussic acid, which is converted to thiocyanate. Monitor thiocyanate levels if the infusion is longer than 4 days' duration or more than 4 µg/kg/minute	
Thiocyanate	6–29 µg/mL (SI: 103–500 µmol/L)	Toxic: 35–100 µg/mL (SI: 602–1721 µmol/L) Fatal: >200 µg/mL (SI: >3443 µmol/L)
Cyanide	Normal: <0.2 µg/mL (SI: <4.6 µmol/L) Normal smoker: <0.4 µg/mL (SI: <9.3 µmol/L)	Toxic: >2 µg/mL (SI: >46 µmol/L) Potentially lethal: >3 µg/mL (SI: >70 µmol/L)
Nortriptyline (Pamelor)	50–150 ng/mL (SI: 190–570 nmol/L)	>500 ng/mL (SI: >1900 nmol/L)
Oxazepam (Serax)	0.2–1.4 ug/mL (SI: 0.7–4.9 µmol/L)	Check with your laboratory
Pentobarbital (Nembutal)	Hypnotic: 1–5 µg/mL (SI: 4–22 µmol/L) Coma: 10–50 µg/mL (SI: 88–221 µmol/L)	>10 µg/mL (SI: >44 µmol/L)
Phenobarbital	Infants/children: 15–30 µg/mL (SI: 65–129 µmol/L) Adults: 20–40 µg/mL (SI: 86–182 µmol/L)	>40 µg/mL (SI: >172 µmol/L) Toxic concentration: Slowness, ataxia, nystagmus: 35–80 µg/mL (SI: 151–345 µmol/L); coma with reflexes:

(table continues on page 546)

TABLE 3.5 (continued)

DRUG	THERAPEUTIC LEVEL	TOXIC/CRITICAL LEVEL
		65–117 µg/mL (SI: 280–504 µmol/L); coma without reflexes: >100 µg/mL (SI: >431 µmol/L)
Phenytoin (total) (Dilantin)	Children/adults: 10–20 µg/mL (SI: 40–79 µmol/L) Neonates: 8–15 µg/mL (SI: 31–59 µmol/L)	Toxic: 30–50 µg/mL (SI: 11–198 µmol/L) Lethal: >100 µg/mL (SI: >400 µmol/L)
Phenytoin (free)	1–2.5 µg/mL (SI: 4–10 µmol/L)	Toxic: 30–50 µg/mL (SI: 120–200 µmol/L) Lethal: >100 µg/mL (SI: >400 µmol/L)
Procainamide	4–10 µg/mL (SI: 17–42 µmol/L)	>14 µg/mL (SI: >59.5 µmol/L)
N-Acetylprocainamide (NAPA)	15–25 µg/mL (SI: 60–100 µmol/L)	Check with your laboratory
Combined	10–30 µg/mL (SI: 39–120 µmol/L)	Check with your laboratory
Propoxyphene (Darvon)	0.1–0.4 µg/mL (SI: 0.3–1.2 µmol/L)	>0.5 µg/mL (SI: >1.5 µmol/L)
Propranolol (Inderal)	50–100 ng/mL (SI: 190–390 nmol/L)	
Protriptyline (Vivactil)	70–250 ng/mL (SI: 266–950 nmol/L)	>500 ng/mL (SI: >1900 nmol/L)
Quinidine	2–5 µg/mL (SI: 6.2–15.4 µmol/L)	>7.0 µg/mL (SI: >22 µmol/L)
Theophylline	8–20 µg/mL (SI: 44–1114 µmol/L)	>20 µg/mL (SI: >111 µmol/L)
Aminophylline bronchodilator		
Thioridazine (Mellaril)	1.0–1.5 µg/mL (SI: 2.7–4.1 µmol/L)	>10 µg/mL (SI: >27 µmol/L)

Tobramycin (Nebcin)	Peak: Serious infections: 6–8 µg/mL (SI: 12–17 µmol/L)	>12 µg/mL (SI: ≥26 µmol/L)
	Life-threatening infections: 8–10 µg/mL (SI: 17–21 µmol/L)	
	Urinary tract infection: 4–6 µg/mL (SI: 8–12 µmol/L)	>12 µg/mL (SI: ≥26 µmol/L)
	Synergy against gram organisms: 3–5 µg/mL (SI: 6–11 µmol/L)	>5 µg/mL (SI: ≥11 µmol/L)
	Trough: Serious infections: 0.5–1 µg/mL (SI: 1–2 µmol/L)	>4 µg/mL (SI: >16 µmol/L) (SI: 4–8 µmol/L)
	Life-threatening infections 1–2 µg/mL (SI: 2–4 µmol/L)	
Tocainide (Tonocard)	5–12 µg/mL (SI: 22–52 µmol/L)	>15 µg/mL (SI: ≥52 µmol/L)
Trazodone (Desyrel)	0.5–2.5 µg/mL (SI: 2–10 µmol/L)	Potentially toxic: >2.5 µg/mL (SI: >10.0 µmol/L)
		Toxic: >4 µg/mL (SI: >8 µmol/L)
Valproic acid (Depakene)	50–100 µg/mL (SI: 350–690 µmol/L) Seizure control may improve at levels of >100 µg/mL, but toxicity may occur at levels of 100–150 µg/mL (SI: 693–1040 µmol/L).	>200 µg/mL (SI: >1390 µmol/L)
Verapamil (Calan, Isoptin, Covera)	50–200 ng/mL (SI: 100–410 nmol/L)	>400 ng/mL (SI: >410 nmol/L)

(table continues on page 548)

TABLE 3.5 (continued)

DRUG	THERAPEUTIC LEVEL	TOXIC/CRITICAL LEVEL
Warfarin	2–5 µg/mL (SI: 6.5–16.2 µmol/L) Warfarin levels are not useful for monitoring degree of anticoagulation. They may be useful if a patient with unexplained coagulopathy is using the drug surreptitiously or if it is unclear whether clinical resistance is due to lack of drug intake	
Volatile Drug Screen		
Methanol		>50 mg/dL (SI: >15.6 mmol/L)
Ethanol		>300 mg/dL (SI: >65 mmol/L) >400 mg/dL severe toxicity (SI: >86.8 mmol/L)
Isopropanol		>1000 mg/L (SI: >16.6 mmol/L)

- The time the specimen is drawn is extremely important with respect to the peak and the trough.
- Urine and saliva specimens may also be tested for marijuana, cocaine, phenylcyclohexylpiperidine (PCP; Angel dust), amphetamines, and morphine.

Nursing Interventions
▶*Pretest*
- Explain therapeutic drug management purpose and procedure.

▶*Posttest*
- Verify drug test results; distinguish between therapeutic and critical values. Therapeutic values within the normal range denote appropriate usage and interval. A toxic or critical value denotes a serious condition and requires quick action.
- Counsel and monitor appropriately for adverse or toxic drug effects.

THIRTY-DAY CARDIAC EVENT MONITOR
Special Noninvasive (ECG) Heart Procedure

This test is used to monitor and record heart rate and rhythm for 30 consecutive days. This type of presymptom monitor increases the likelihood of detecting a cardiac arrhythmia from 10%–20%, as is typically seen with Holter monitoring, to 90%.

Indications
- Document cardiac arrhythmias in patients who complain of syncopal episodes, palpitations, chest pain, lightheadedness, or shortness of breath.
- Diagnose a serious cardiac arrhythmia (eg, ventricular tachycardia, sinus arrest).
- Record transient symptomatic arrhythmias.

Reference Values

Normal
Normal cardiac rhythms and heart rates.

Clinical Implications
- Abnormal findings include inappropriate heart rates, that is, bradycardia, tachycardia, or bradycardia-tachycardia syndrome.
- Cardiac arrhythmias, for example, atrial fibrillation, atrial flutter, premature ventricular contractions, ventricular arrhythmias.

Interfering Factors

- Inability to place and secure leads properly.
- Unable to keep a diary, perceive arrhythmia, depress the event button, replace battery, or download over a telephone.
- Significant changes in normal routines or activities.

Procedure

- Explain the monitoring procedure to the patient.
- Instruct the patient on proper two-channel electrode application (which remain in place for 30 days), including site preparation and lead placement, connection of leads to the monitor, battery replacement, event marking, and downloading over the telephone.
- Instruct the patient to depress the event button on "feeling" a cardiac symptom, for example, palpitation or a "racing" sensation.
- Approximately eight events can be retained before it must be downloaded via telephone.

Nursing Interventions

▸Pretest

- Explain monitoring purpose and procedure to patient. Provide written instructions and diagram.
- Demonstrate proper skin site preparation and lead placement, the downloading and subsequent memory clearance of recordings, and the handling, battery replacement, and care of monitor.
- Emphasize the importance of depressing the event button whenever symptoms are felt and to record activity at that time.
- Encourage patient to continue normal daily activities and that the monitor needs to be used for the entire 30-day period.

▸Posttest

- Explain proper procedure for discontinuing monitor recording and returning monitor (through a preaddressed, postage-paid box, in some instances).
- Evaluate patient outcomes and monitor and counsel appropriately.

THORACOSCOPY

Endoscopic Imaging of Chest Cavity, Interventional Procedure

Thoracoscopy is the examination of the thoracic cavity with an endoscope.

Indications

- Evaluate and examine tumor growth, effusions, empyema, inflammatory processes, and pneumothorax.
- Perform laser procedure and biopsies of pleura, mediastinal nodes, and lungs.
- Visualize the parietal and visceral pleura, pleural spaces, thoracic walls, mediastinum, and pericardium.
- Perform laser procedures; assess tumor growth, pleural effusion, empyema, inflammatory processes, and conditions predisposing to pneumothorax.

Reference Values

Normal

Thoracic cavity tissues, parietal and visceral pleura, pleural spaces, thoracic walls, mediastinum, and pericardium: Normal and free of disease.

Clinical Implications

- Abnormal findings include carcinoma (metastatic or primary), empyema, effusions, conditions predisposing to pneumothorax or ulcers, inflammatory processes, and diseases such as tuberculosis, coccidioidomycosis, and histoplasmosis.

Procedure

- A thoracoscopy is considered an operative procedure. The patient's state of health, particular positioning needed, and the procedure itself determine the need for either local or general anesthesia. Chest tubes are usually placed and connected to negative suction and sometimes to gravity drainage. Lung expansion and tube placement are confirmed by x-ray postoperatively.
- The lung is collapsed (intentional pneumothorax) for visualization of the chest cavity.
- The patient should be fasting at least 8 hours preoperatively.
- Start an IV line if ordered and administer preoperative medications.
- Skin preparation and correct positioning are done in the operating room.

Nursing Interventions

▸Pretest

- Explain thoracoscopy test purpose and procedure and describe what the patient will experience.

▶*Posttest*
- Monitor vital signs, respiratory status, lung sounds, and arterial blood gases (if ordered); report abnormalities promptly. Check chest tube patency, drainage, bubbling, and fluctuation of fluid level in drainage tubing and record. Report abnormalities promptly.
- Administer pain medication as needed; monitor respiratory status closely. Assist the patient to cough and deep breathe frequently. Encourage ambulation and leg exercises frequently.

> ## CLINICAL ALERT
>
> - Watch for signs of increasing respiratory problems or hemorrhage. Report promptly and take appropriate action.
> - *Do not clamp chest tubes unless specifically ordered.* Clamping the chest tubes may produce a tension pneumothorax.
> - Sudden sharp pain, together with dyspnea, uneven chest wall movement, tachycardia, anxiety, and cyanosis may signal development of a pneumothorax—notify physician immediately and document completely and carefully.

THYROID FUNCTION TESTS

Blood, Endocrine

T_4 Free (Thyroxine), T_4 Total, T_3 (Triiodothyronine) Uptake, T_3 Total, Free Thyroxine Index (FTI) (T_7), Thyroid-Stimulating Hormone (TSH) (Thyrotropin)

These tests are indirect and direct measurements of thyroid status and function.

Indications
- Determine thyroid function and rule out hypothyroidism and hyperthyroidism.
- Evaluate thyroid replacement therapy.

Reference Values

Normal

T_4 Free (FT_4): 0.7–2.0 ng/dL or 9–26 pmol/L

T_4 Total:
    Adults: 5.4–11.5 µg/dL or 69.5–148.0 nmol/L
    Children: 6.4–13.3 µg/dL or 82.4–171.2 nmol/L
T_3 Uptake: 25%–35% (arbitrary units); 0.8–1.30 (ratio between patient specimen and standard control).
T_3 Total (triiodothyronine):
    Adults: 80–200 ng/dL or 1.23–3.07 nmol/L
    Adolescents: 100–220 ng/dL or 1.53–3.37 nmol/L
    Children: 125–250 ng/dL or 1.92–3.83 nmol/L
Free thyroxine index (FTI) T_7: 1.2–4.5 (index); Calculation: T_4 total $\times T_3$ Uptake (%)/100. (Check with laboratory for normal values).
TSH (thyrotropin):
    Adults: 0.2–5.4 mIU/L or 0.2–5.4 mIU/L
    Children: 0.7–6.4 µIU/mL or 0.7–6.4 µIU/mL

Clinical Implications: Free T_4

• *Increased FT_4 levels are associated with*
  a. Graves' disease (hyperthyroidism).
  b. Hypothyroidism treated with thyroxine.
  c. Euthyroid sick syndrome.
• *Decreased FT_4 levels are associated with*
  a. Primary hypothyroidism.
  b. Secondary hypothyroidism (pituitary).
  c. Tertiary hypothyroidism (hypothalamic).
  d. Hypothyroidism treated with triiodothyronine.

Interfering Factors: Free T_4

• Values are increased in infants at birth. This value rises even higher after 2–3 days of life.
• Many drugs, eg, heparin, will falsely elevate its levels.

Clinical Implications: T_4 Total

• T_4 total increases in hyperthyroidism, thyrotoxicosis (Hashimoto's disease), acute thyroiditis (first stage), and liver disease (hepatitis), D-thyroxine therapy, and neonates.
• T_4 total decreases in hypothyroidism, hypoproteinemia, and triiodothyronine treatment.

CLINICAL ALERT

• T_4 values are higher in neonates owing to their elevated thyroxine-binding globulin (TBG). Values rise abruptly in the first few hours after birth and decline gradually until the age of 5 years.

Interfering Factors

- T_4 total increases with the use of certain drugs (estrogen, birth control pills, TSH, thyroid extract, D-thyroxine, anticonvulsants, heroin, and methadone), pregnancy, and iodine contrast medium.
- Values decrease with salicylates and anticoagulants.

Clinical Implications: T_3UP or T_3U

- This test is an indirect measurement of the unsaturated thyroxine-binding globulin (TBG) in the blood (inversely proportional).
- T_3 uptake (T_3UP) is useful only when the T_4 test is performed.
- *Decreased T_3UP levels* are found in hypothyroidism and other situations in which TBG is elevated, such as pregnancy or estrogen therapy.
- *Increased T_3UP levels* are found in hyperthyroidism and in situations in which TBG is decreased.

Interfering Factors: T_3UP

- *Decreased T_3UP levels* occur in normal pregnancy, with estrogens, antiovulatory drugs, methadone, and heparin.
- *Increased T_3UP levels* occur with drugs such as dicoumarol, heparin, steroids, phenytoin, and large amounts of salicylates.

Clinical Implications: Total T_3

- *Increased T_3 values* are associated with:
  Hyperthyroidism
  T_3 thyrotoxicosis
  Daily dosage of 25 μg or more of T_3
  Acute thyroiditis
  TBG elevation from any cause
  Daily dosage of 300 μg or more of T_4
- *Decreased T_3 levels* are associated with:
  Hypothyroidism (however, some clinically hypothyroid disease patients will have normal levels)
  Starvation and state of nutrition
  Acute illness
  TBG decrease from any cause

Interfering Factors: Total T_3

- Values are increased in pregnancy and with the use of drugs such as estrogens and antiovulatory compounds, methadone, and heroin.
- Values are decreased with the use of drugs such as anabolic steroids, androgens, large doses of salicylates, and phenytoin.

Clinical Implications: FTI/T$_7$
- *FTI increases* in hyperthyroidism.
- *FTI decreases* in hypothyroidism.

Clinical Implications: TSH
- *TSH increases* in adults and neonates with primary hypothyroidism, Hashimoto's thyroiditis, TSH antibodies, thyrotoxicosis, thyrotropin-producing tumors, and hypothyroid disease patients not receiving sufficient replacement hormone.
- *TSH decreases* in hyperthyroidism, secondary pituitary or hypothalamic hypothyroidism, euthyroid sick patients, treated Graves' disease, and overreplacement of thyroid hormone in the treatment of hypothyroidism.

Interfering Factors: TSH
- *Decreases* during treatment with T$_3$, aspirin, corticosteroids, and heparin and during first-trimester pregnancy.
- *Increases* during treatment with lithium, potassium iodide TSH injection, and dopamine.
- Values are normally high in neonatal cord blood. The TSH level returns to normal in 1–2 weeks.

Procedures for T$_4$ Free, T$_4$ Total, T$_3$ Uptake, T$_3$ Total, TSH
- Blood (10 mL) is obtained by venipuncture in a red-top tube.
- To get a valid T$_4$ Total, thyroid treatment should be discontinued 1 month before testing.

Procedure for FTI (T$_7$)
- A calculation is made, based on results of T$_3$ uptake and T$_4$ total:

$$FTI = T_4 \text{ total} \times T_3 \text{ uptake } (\%)/100.$$

- The free thyroxine (Free T$_4$) index permits meaningful interpretation by balancing out most nonthyroidal factors. Actual measurement of the free T$_4$ gives a more accurate picture of the thyroid status when the TBG is abnormal in pregnant women or those persons who are being treated with estrogen, androgens, phenytoin, or salicylates.

Nursing Interventions
▶*Pretest*
- Explain purpose, procedure, and interfering factors of thyroid function tests.

▶*Posttest*
- Ask the patient to resume normal activities.
- Interpret test results and counsel as appropriate.

THYROID SCAN

Nuclear Medicine Endocrine Imaging

This procedure measures the uptake of the thyroid and evaluates the size, shape, and function of thyroid tissue.

Indications
- Establish thyroid origin of neck masses and evaluate functional activity of thyroid nodules.
- Monitor effectiveness of thyroid therapies (medication, radiation, or surgery).
- Differentiate type of hyperthyroidism: Graves' disease or Plummer's disease.
- Pediatric indications include evaluation of neonatal hypothyroidism or thyrocarcinoma (lower incidence than adults).

Reference Values

Normal
- Normal or evenly distributed concentration of radioactive iodine; normal size, position, shape, site, weight, and function of thyroid; absence of nodules.

Clinical Implications
- *Decreased uptake:* Hypothyroidism, cancer of the thyroid, and prolonged Hashimoto's disease.
- *Increased uptake:* Hyperthyroidism, Graves' disease, and autonomous nodules.
- Cold nodules or lesions occur in malignant nodules, colloid nodules, adenomas, cysts, and inflammatory areas (eg, thyroid).
- Benign adenomas may appear as nodules on increased uptake of iodine (hot nodules) or may appear as nodules on decreased uptake of iodine (cold nodules).

Interfering Factors
- Ingested iodine medications, foods containing iodine, and contrast iodinated agents (eg, used in IVP, cardiac catheterization, CT scans with intravenous injections, myelogram, kidney studies, and other arteriograms). These agents may interfere with test results for approximately 2 months.

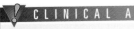

CLINICAL ALERT

- Test is contraindicated when allergy to iodine or shellfish is present.
- Contraindicated in pregnant or lactating women.

Procedure
- The patient ingests a capsule containing radioactive iodine (^{123}I).
- The uptake quantification and scan are performed 4 to 6 hours and 24 hours after ^{123}I administration.
- The thyroid gland and neck area are imaged.
- Imaging time is 45 minutes.

Nursing Interventions
▶ Pretest
- Explain the thyroid imaging purpose and procedure.
- Advise that iodine intake is restricted for at least 1 week before the procedure, because of the thyroid gland's response to small amounts of iodine.
- Assess for iodine allergy and consult with physician regarding these data.

▶ Intratest
- Provide support; reassure the patient that the test is proceeding normally.
- Allow a parent to accompany a child.

▶ Posttest
- Evaluate patient test outcome; monitor and counsel as necessary.
- Observe and treat mild reactions (per orders): pruritus, rashes, flushing 2–24 hours after injection; sometimes nausea and vomiting may occur.
- If iodine has been administered, observe the patient for signs and symptoms of allergic reactions.

THYROID SONOGRAM—THYROID ULTRASOUND, THYROID ECHOGRAM, NECK ULTRASOUND

Ultrasound Imaging of Endocrine Gland and Neck

This noninvasive procedure is used to visualize and determine the size of the thyroid gland.

Indications

- Identify and characterize masses (cysts and solids) and infectious processes.
- Estimate gland weight before administering radioiodine drugs for Graves' disease to monitor therapeutic outcomes.
- Use as guide during biopsy or cyst aspiration.

Reference Values

Normal

- Normal size and anatomy of thyroid and surrounding structures, including muscles and blood vessels.
- Normal homogenous thyroid pattern.

Clinical Implications

- An abnormal pattern may consist of a *cystic*, *complex*, or solid echo pattern.
- Gland enlargement and presence of space-occupying lesions: Cysts, solid masses such as adenomas or nodules, hematomas, and abscesses. Also, it may reveal parathyroid lesions or changes in lymph nodes.
- Certain congenital deformities.

Interfering Factors

- Very small lesions (1 cm) may escape detection. Lesions >4 cm in diameter give a mixed echogram that is difficult to correlate with a specific disease.
- Sonography cannot differentiate benign from malignant lesions.
- Parathyroid lesions or other extrathyroid masses may not be differentiated from intrathyroid lesions.

Procedure

- Patient lies on his or her back and a pillow is placed under the shoulders for comfort.
- A coupling medium, generally gel, is applied to exposed hyperextended neck in order to promote transmission of sound. An ultrasound transducer is slowly moved across the skin.
- Thyroid biopsy may be performed with ultrasound guidance.
- Exam time is about 30 minutes.

Nursing Interventions

♦Pretest

- Explain the test purpose and procedure.

▶*Posttest*
• Evaluate patient outcomes; provide support and counseling (in collaboration with the physician) about thyroid disease.

TORCH TEST

Blood, Mixed Infections

TORCH is the acronym for toxoplasma, rubella, cytomegalovirus, and herpes simplex virus (antibodies) and identifies agents frequently implicated in congenital infections of the newborn and confirmed by the demonstration of specific IgM-associated antibodies in the infant's blood.

Indications
• Evaluate and differentiate possible congenital infection with one or more of the TORCH agents.
• Test both the mother and the newborn for exposure.

Reference Values

Normal
Negative for antibodies to toxoplasma, rubella, cytomegalovirus, and herpes simplex virus.

Clinical Implications
• Presence of IgG antibodies suggests transfer of antibodies from mother to newborn.
• The presence of IgM antibodies suggests congenital infection.

Interfering Factors
• TORCH screen is not always useful because antibody production may not occur in detectable amounts early in the infection.
• TORCH is more useful in excluding a possible infection than proving etiology.

Procedure
• Obtain a 3-mL venous or cord blood sample following specimen collection guidelines in Chapter 2. Use a red-top tube. Place the specimen in a biohazard bag.

Nursing Interventions
▶*Pretest*
• Explain the test purpose and procedure.

▶*Posttest*
• Evaluate patient outcomes; monitor and counsel appropriately for intrauterine and congenital infections.

Total Blood Plasma Volume, Red Cell Volume*

Radionuclide Laboratory Study, Venous Blood Samples

The purpose of these tests is to determine circulating blood volume.

Indications
• Evaluate gastrointestinal and uterine bleeding.
• Aid in the diagnosis of hypovolemic shock.
• Screen patients suspected of having polycythemia vera (eg, elevated RBC volume and normal plasma volume).
• Determine the required blood component for replacement therapy, as in persons undergoing surgery.
• Increased or decreased volume of red blood cell mass.
• Plasma volume establishes a vascular baseline, to determine changes in plasma volume before and after surgery.
• Evaluate fluid and blood replacement in gastrointestinal bleeding and in burn and trauma cases.
• ^{51}Cr red blood cell volume study determines the percentage of the circulating blood composed of red blood cells.
• Performed in connection with red blood cell survival, gastrointestinal blood loss, or ferrokinetic studies.

Reference Values

Normal
Total blood volume: 55–80 mL/kg (0.055–0.080 L/kg) in men and women
Red blood cell volume (RBCV): 20–35 mL/kg (0.020–0.035 L/kg) (greater in men than in women)
Plasma volume (PV): 30–45 mL/kg (0.030–0.045 L/kg) in men and women

---

*The publisher has decided to include this test for purposes of completeness, although it is rarely used today in many parts of the country.

Clinical Implications

- Normal total blood volume with decreased red blood cell content indicates the need for a transfusion of packed red blood cells.
- Polycythemia vera may be differentiated from secondary polycythemia.
- Increased total blood volume due to an increased red blood cell mass suggests polycythemia vera; elevated RBC volume and normal plasma volume.
- Normal or decreased total blood volume due to a decreased plasma volume suggests secondary polycythemia. The red blood cell volume is most often normal.

Procedure

- Obtain venous blood samples, one from each arm, at different time intervals. Document time and the arm that is used for each sample. One sample is mixed with a radionuclide.
- After 15–30 minutes, the blood with the radiopharmaceutical (eg, ^{131}I or ^{125}I) is reinjected.
- About 15 minutes later, another venous blood sample is obtained for counting and red blood cell mass determination in the laboratory.

 CLINICAL ALERT

- If intravenous blood component therapy is ordered for the same day, the blood volume determination should be done before the intravenous line is started.
- Test is contraindicated in the presence of active bleeding and edema.

Nursing Interventions

▶ *Pretest*

- Explain the purpose, procedure, and benefits and risks of volume tests.
- Measure and weigh the patient and record measurements just before the test, if possible.

▶ *Intratest*

- Explain that the blood injected is the patient's *own* blood and that it is not possible for a blood-borne disease to occur.

▶ *Posttest*

- Monitor blood draw and radiopharmaceutical agent injection sites for extravasation and infiltration.

- Observe and treat mild reactions: pruritus, rashes, and flushing 2–24 hours after injection; sometimes nausea and vomiting may occur.
- Interpret test outcome, monitor appropriately, and counsel about follow-up tests and appropriate treatment.

TOXOPLASMOSIS (TPM) ANTIBODY TESTS

Blood, Parasitic Infection

This test is used to diagnose toxoplasmosis by detecting antibodies to the protozoan parasite *Toxoplasma gondii*. TPM may be acquired by ingesting inadequately cooked meat, and congenital TPM may cause fetal death.

Indications
- Evaluate *Toxoplasma* infection in patients with enlarged lymph glands and other infectious mononucleosis-like symptoms.
- Assess pregnant women who may be asymptomatically infected.
- Diagnose congenital toxoplasmosis.
- Evaluate immunocompromised patients in whom the disease may become very serious or fatal.

Reference Values

Normal
Negative for antibodies to *Toxoplasma gondii*.

Clinical Implications
- Any titer in a newborn is abnormal.
- Titer 1:16–1:64 indicates past exposure. Titer 1:256 indicates recent exposure or current infection. Titer 1:1024 indicates significant exposure and may reflect active disease, and titer of 1:16 or less occurs with ocular toxoplasmosis; rising titers are of greatest significance.

Interfering Factors
- False-positive results in patients with high rheumatoid factor levels.
- False-negative results in immunocompromised patients because of their impaired ability to produce antibody.
- Newborns may have antibody received from their mothers and should be retested.

Procedure

- Serum sample (5 mL in adults) is obtained by venipuncture following specimen collection guidelines in Chapter 2. Use a red-top tube. Place specimen in a biohazard bag.

Nursing Interventions

▶*Pretest*

- Explain purpose and blood test procedure.
- Inform pregnant women that parasite can be passed to fetus, causing neurologic and eye problems, and may lead to fetal death.

▶*Posttest*

- Advise patient if results are not significant that the test may be repeated to check for rising titer.
- Diagnosis of congenital toxoplasmosis may require additional test procedures, such as demonstration of the parasite in cerebral spinal fluid and detection of nonmaternal antibodies in the serum.

TRANSDERMAL TESTING

Skin

Transdermal iontophoresis is a noninvasive method for extracting certain substances (eg, sweat) using patches or collection devices on intact skin.

Indications

- Diagnose cystic fibrosis as an alternative to blood sampling.
- Predict and compare blood concentrations with transdermal results.
- Monitor drug therapy (eg, lithium) for bipolar disease.
- Use to detect abnormally high concentrations of electrolytes (eg, sodium) and glucose.

Reference Values

Normal

- Sweat sodium: <70 mEq/L or <70 mmol/L
- Sweat chloride: <40 mEq/L or <40 mmol/L
  - Borderline: 40–60 mEq/L or 40–60 mmol/L
  - >60 mEq/L or >60 mmol/L is consistent with cystic fibrosis

- Electrolytes (sodium, potassium, calcium, magnesium) and glucose within expected ranges.
- Drugs (eg, cocaine and caffeine) within expected range.

Clinical Implications

- Abnormally increased values in cystic fibrosis.
- Abnormal glucose metabolism.
- Therapeutic range of prescribed medications (eg, lithium levels).

Interfering Factors

- Dehydration and edema, especially in areas of collection sites, may interfere with test results.

Procedure

- Sweat-inducing techniques are performed using applied electrodes and collection devices (eg, patches, gauze pads, or other means).
- A slight current is delivered.
- Content of electrically collected sweat is chemically analyzed.
- Electrodes are removed and then cleaned.
- Testing time varies.

Nursing Interventions

▶Pretest

- Explain the test purpose and procedure. A slight stinging sensation is usually experienced.
- Explain that no fasting is required.

▶Posttest

- After collection patches are removed, carefully wash and dry the skin to prevent irritation caused by collection devices.
- Inform the patient that he or she may resume normal activities.
- Interpret test results and counsel and monitor patient as appropriate. Provide genetic counseling when positive sweat test indicates cystic fibrosis.

CLINICAL ALERT

- Cystic fibrosis is transmitted as an autosomal recessive trait. The Caucasian carrier rate is 1 in 20, whereas the African-American carrier rate is 1 in 60 to 1 in 100.

TRANSESOPHAGEAL ECHOCARDIOGRAPHY (TEE)
Ultrasound Endoscopic Cardiac Imaging

This test permits optimal ultrasonic visualization of the heart when traditional transthoracic (noninvasive) echocardiography fails or proves inconclusive.

Indications
- When a transthoracic echocardiogram has been unsatisfactory, as in the presence of obesity, trauma to the chest wall, and chronic obstructive pulmonary disease.
- When results of traditional transthoracic echocardiography do not agree or correlate with other clinical findings.

Reference Values

Normal
Normal position, size, and function of heart valves and heart chambers.

Clinical Implications
- Heart valve diseases
- Pericardial effusion
- Congenital heart disease
- Aortic dissection
- Left ventricular dysfunction
- Endocarditis
- Intracardiac tumors or thrombi

Procedure
- A topical anesthetic is applied to the pharynx. A bite block is inserted into the mouth.
- The patient assumes a lateral decubitus position while the lubricated endoscopic instrument is inserted to a depth of 30–50 cm. The patient is asked to swallow to facilitate advancement of the device.
- Manipulation of the ultrasound transducer provides a number of image planes.
- Various images of heart anatomy can be displayed by rotating the top of the instrument and by varying the depth of insertion into the esophagus.

- *Note:* A variety of medications may be used during this procedure. Generally, these drugs are intended to sedate and anesthetize, reduce secretions, and serve as an ultrasound contrast agent.

Nursing Interventions
▶*Pretest*
- Explain the procedure and its purpose, as well as its benefits and risks.
- Ensure the patient is on NPO status for at least 4–8 hours before the procedure to reduce the risk of aspiration.

▶*Intratest*
- Provide support; assure the patient that the test is proceeding normally.

▶*Posttest*
- Evaluate posttest outcomes. Explain possible follow-up procedures and treatments to the patient.

TRANSPLANT TESTING/ORGAN AND TISSUE
Blood

Blood testing is done before and after procuring organs and tissues for donation and grafting. This testing is done for both the donor and the recipient. Tissue donation takes place after cardiac as well as brain death. Types of donors include living donors and brain-dead donors. Organs that can be donated include lungs, heart, liver, kidney, pancreas, and small intestine. Examples of tissues that can be donated include corneas, dura mater of the brain, skin, bone, cartilage, tendons, ligaments, and peripheral blood progenitor cells.

Indications
- Match donor and recipient.
- Identify compatible blood and histocompatibility antigens or human leukocyte antigen (HLA) types.
- Prevent rejection and immune reactions.
- Prevent transmission of infections and genetic diseases.
- Identify immunologic risk factors.
- Identify HLAs to be avoided and irrelevant antigens.
- For some, evaluate kidney or liver function.

Reference Values

Normal

- Normal blood; no evidence of exposure to or presence of infectious disease; no exposure to drugs, biological hazards, toxic substances, or high levels of metal; acceptable levels of percent reactive antibodies (PRAs).

Clinical Implications

- Abnormal values indicate no match or a poor match and unacceptable levels of sensitization regarding PRAs.
- Blood positive for previously mentioned factors. This varies for each disease, organ, or tissue.

Procedure

- Venous blood specimens are obtained. See TABLE 3.6.

 CLINICAL ALERT

- Success of transplants depends on ability to deter immune reaction and rejection.
- Victims of poisoning are eligible to be organ and tissue donors.
- Proper informed consent must be obtained from family for organ or tissue donation. These are surgical procedures.
- A federal procurement organization covers a donor network in the United States.

Nursing Interventions

▶*Pretest*

- Obtain a health history that includes past and present infections, malignancies, neurodegenerative disease, recipient of human pituitary gland hormones, or high-risk behavior (eg, drug abuse).

▶*Posttest*

- Interpret test outcomes and check for signs of transplant rejection. Posttransplant rejections occur more frequently in the presence of cytokines, ALA, complement, infection with bacteria, viruses or fungi, toxoplasmosis disease, accelerated vascular disease, and metabolic diseases (eg, diabetes).
- Counsel the patient about possible aggressive treatment with antirejection drugs.

(text continues on page 569)

TABLE 3.6 LABORATORY TESTS PERFORMED ON THE DONOR AND RECIPIENT FOR ORGAN AND TISSUE TRANSPLANT*

TESTS OF DONOR AND RECIPIENT†	LUNG (PORTION) D	R	LIVER (PORTION) D	R	KIDNEY D	R	PANCREAS D	R
Blood type	X	X	X	X	X	X	X	X
HLA typing					X		X	
Bilirubin	X		X	X				X
BUN	X		X		X			
WBC	X		X					
CBC		X			X	X		X
Platelets				X				X
Hgb/Hct	X		X					
PT/PTT						X	X	X
Electrolytes	X	X			X			
Calcium	X						X	
Magnesium	X			X			X	X
Phosphorous				X	X			X
Creatinine	X	X	X		X	X		
Serum amylase								X
Albumin				X				X
Total protein				X				
ALT				X	X			X
AST				X				X
Hepatitis A		X						
Hepatitis B	X		X	X	X	X	X	X
Hepatitis C	X			X	X			X
Liver panel		X		X	X			
Epstein-Barr virus	X	X		X	X			X
Anti-HIV-1 and -2	X	X		X	X	X	X	X
Anti-HTLV-1					X		X	
PRA		X						
VDRL/RPR	X		X	X			X	
CMV	X	X	X	X	X	X		X
VZV	X	X		X	X			
Measles/rubella	X	X						

TABLE 3.6 (continued)

TESTS OF DONOR AND RECIPIENT†	LUNG (PORTION)		LIVER (PORTION)		KIDNEY		PANCREAS	
	D	R	D	R	D	R	D	R
Mycology smear (fungus/yeast)	X	X						
Bronchoscopy‡	X							

D, donor; R, recipient; HLA, human leukocyte antigen; BUN, blood urea nitrogen; WBC, white blood cells; Hgb/Hct, hemoglobin/hematocrit; PT/PTT, prothrombin time/partial thromboplastin time; ALT, alanine aminotransferase; AST, aspartate aminotransferase; HIV, human immunodeficiency virus; HTLV-1, human T-cell lymphotropic virus type 1; PRA, percent reactive antibodies; VDRL/RPR, Venereal Disease Research Laboratory/rapid plasma reagin test; CMV, cytomegalovirus; VZV, varicella-zoster virus (chickenpox); mycology smear, yeast and fungi; ALT, albumin, alkaline phosphatase; AST, direct and fetal protein, total protein.

*Pretransplant testing is continually changing and can vary from one institution to another; therefore, check with your transplant department and/or the laboratory.

†*Note:* Female organ recipients of childbearing age will undergo a STAT pregnancy test.

‡Although bronchoscopy is technically a procedure, it is listed as part of the donor workup for a lung transplant.

TUBERCULOSIS (TB) TESTS: QUANTIFERON TB TEST (QFT), TUBERCULIN SKIN TESTING (TST)

Blood, Skin

These tests diagnose TB-infected persons who are at increased risk for TB development and who will benefit from treatment. The QuantiFERON TB test (QFT) is used to detect latent TB. The QFT measures interferon-gamma (IFN-γ), a component of cell-mediated immune activity to TB response. Tuberculin skin testing (TST) screens for new or latent TB infection in high-risk groups. The TST measures lymphocyte response to TB in persons sensitized to the TB antigen. This test measures a delayed hypersensitivity response (48–72 hours).

Reference Values

Normal

- QuantiFERON TB test (QFT):
  Negative: <0.35 IU/mL of IFN-γ
  Positive: ≥0.35 IU/mL of IFN-γ

- Tuberculin skin testing (TST): Negative is nonsignificant for cutaneous hypersensitivity (area of induration <10 mm)

Clinical Implications

- For the QuantiFERON TB test:
  A positive test result indicates that TB infection is likely.
  A negative test result indicates that TB infection is unlikely but cannot be excluded.
- For tuberculin skin testing (TST): Positive is significant reaction: Area of induration >10 mm.

Procedure

- For TST, perform intradermal injection into the flexor surface using PPD (protein derivative of tuberculin) (0.1 mL, 5 TU)
- For QFT, obtain a venous whole-blood specimen using a green-topped tube. Process within 12–48 hours after collection. Do not refrigerate or freeze.

Nursing Intervention

▶*Pretest*

- Explain the reason for testing (eg, pre-employment screening, resident of nursing homes, known or suspected HIV, unexplained weight loss, close contact with recently diagnosed person with TB, symptoms such as coughing up blood, or fever).
- Obtain a recent history of signs and symptoms.

▶*Posttest*

- For TST, read, interpret, and record skin reaction and the arm used.
- Evaluate test outcome and counsel patient regarding the need for further follow-up (eg, x-rays, sputum cultures) in positive tests.
- Educate the patient regarding prevention and therapy (eg, medications).

TUMOR MARKERS

Blood, Urine, Cancer

Tumor cells differ from normal cells in many ways. Laboratory tests, such as tumor markers, are potential methods for diagnosis and monitoring of patients with tumors. Tumor markers include genetic markers (abnormal chromosomes or oncogenes [genes that function abnormally]), oncogene receptors, enzymes, hormones, hormone receptors, oncofetal antigens, glycoproteins, tumor antigens on cell surfaces, and substances produced in response to tumor growth (eg, cell-reactive protein, circulating complexes, prostate-specific antigen).

Tumor markers are used and developed to obtain greater sensitivity and specificity in determining tumor activity. Because tumor markers lack specificity and are not pathognomonic for one type of neoplasm, diagnosis still derives from a comprehensive patient medical history, physical examination, and other diagnostic procedures (TABLE 3.7).

Tumor marker tests measure the presence of substances produced or secreted by malignant tumor cells that are found in the serum of patients with specific types of carcinomas. Tumor markers are generally classified into two major categories:

- Normal cell products synthesized in excess by tumor cells (cell-surface protein, secreting products, and associated antigens).
- "Ectopic" proteins produced normally by one type of cell (ie, pituitary, ACTH production) but synthesized in other neoplastic cells (ACTH production of small-cell lung carcinoma).

Indications

- Detect malignancy to pinpoint the tissue of origin.
- Assess extent of tumor or disease, tumor staging, and estimate progress or prognosis.
- Obtain greater sensitivity and specificity about tumor activity through the use of *selective* tumor markers.
- Evaluate tumor burden, change, and clinical course.
- Monitor effect of therapy and disease recurrence.

Cell Surface Glycoproteins and Mucins

Reference Values

Normal

- CA 125 (ovarian cancer, glycoprotein antigen, and serum carbohydrate antigen): <34 U/mL (or <34 arb units/L)
- CA 19-9 (mucin, modified form of Lewis antigen, carbohydrate antigen, pancreatic-hepatobiliary cancer): <70 U/mL (or <70 arb units/L)
- CA 50 (antibody, detects protein in those lacking Lewis gene and in gastrointestinal and pancreatic cancers): <17 U/mL (or <17 arb units/L)
- CA 15-3 (glycoprotein antigen, found in breast milk globules [CA 27-29, similar to CA 15-3, metastatic breast cancer, breast-cystic fluid protein, BCFP], used in conjunction with CEA): <30 U/mL (or <30 arb units/L)

(text continues on page 574)

TABLE 3.7 Characteristics of Selected Tumor Markers

Type of Marker	Characteristics	Examples
Cell surface glycoproteins mucins	Found on normal and tumor cells. Requires increased production or damage to tissue to produce increased levels. Based upon the specific monoclonal cell line that produces an antibody against the cancer antigen. Cleared by liver	CA 125 (ovarian, endometrial), CA 19-9 (colorectal, pancreatic), CA 50, CA 27.29 (breast), CA 15-3, CA 549 (breast, ovarian), CA 21, and CA 29
Oncofetal antigens	Produced by specific cells during fetal life and in only trace amounts by adults. With activation of cells normally producing these markers, levels increase, although almost near to fetal levels. Levels also increase with benign proliferation of cells in organs normally manufacturing these proteins	Alpha-fetoprotein (AFP; liver, germ cell), CEA (colorectal, GI, pancreatic, lung, breast, tissue), polypeptide antigen (TPA; breast, ovarian, bladder), hCG (liver, germ cell)
Normal cell and enzyme production	Produced by normal cells and in excessive amounts by tumors of these cells. Typically produced by a limited number of cell types represents the largest group of tumor markers	Monoclonal immunoglobulin, hormones, enzymes (PSA: prostate; alkaline phosphatase: bone sarcoma, liver, leukemia)
Hormones	Excessive hormone can be produced by the endocrine tissue (normotopic) and by nonendocrine tissue (ectopic syndrome). An elevation of a certain hormone (ACTH)	CA 242 and CA 50 (pancreatic, colorectal); CA 72-4 (GI, ovarian); ACTH (small-cell lung cancer); antidiuretic hormone (lung, adrenal cortex, pancreas, duodenum);

		by the pituitary is normotopic, but by small-cell lung cancer is ectopic	calcitonin (medullary thyroid); gastrin (glucagoma); hCG (testicular, nonseminoma); prolactin (pituitary adenoma, renal, lung)
Genetic markers	Usually present in tumor cells and not typically found in circulation (may be identified by PCR). Often due to mutations, so differ from form found in normal cells. Some are specific to tumor type, and some relate to prognosis	Oncogenic, chromosomal translocations, chromosomal mutations
Markers of host response tumor or altered cell metabolism	Nonspecific markers of tissue injury; when used with enzymes may indicate organ involved (which may be site of primary tumor or metastasis)	Acute phase reactant proteins to tumor necrosis factor A, acidic glycoprotein, tissue enzymes (alkaline phosphatase, LDH), products of metabolism (uric acid, polyamines)
Cellular marker related to prognosis	Found only within cells, not in circulation. Can be used only when tissue is sampled (biopsy, cytology for some tumors). Often labile and requires rapid transport to laboratory and immediate freezing	Steroid hormone receptors, DNA ploidy, S-phase analysis (% of cells synthesizing DNA, cathepsin D)
Urine tests	Tests for bladder tumors and transitional cell carcinoma (TCC) of the urinary tract. Higher levels are associated with suspected recurrence	NMP (nuclear matrix protein) (urinary tract cancer); BTA (bladder tumor analytes) (bladder tumors)

Clinical Implications: CA 125

- *Increased in cancer: Epithelial ovarian, fallopian tube, endometrium, endocervix, liver, pancreas.*
- *Lesser increases: Colon, breast, lung, and gastrointestinal.* Progressive decline in positive therapy response—a rise after successful therapy may predict recurrent tumor. *Noncancer: Increased* in pregnancy, advanced stage of endometriosis, pelvic inflammatory disease, cirrhosis, severe liver necrosis and hepatitis, peritonitis and ascites, other GI and pancreas diseases, Meigs' syndrome, pleural effusion, and pulmonary disease.

Interfering Factors: CA 125

- False-positive results in pregnancy and normal menstruation.
- Falsely elevated levels with liver diseases and ascites.

Clinical Implications: CA 19

- *Increased in cancer: Primarily pancreatic and hepatobiliary. Mild elevation in gastric, colorectal, and lung cancers.*
- *Noncancer increases: Pancreatitis, cholecystitis, cirrhosis, gallstones, and cystic fibrosis (minimal elevations).*
- Falsely elevated levels with obstructive jaundice.

Clinical Implications: CA 50

- *Increased in cancer: Gastrointestinal and pancreatic.*
- *Noncancer increases: None identified.*

Clinical Implications: CA 15-3 (27, 29):

- *Increased in cancer: Metastatic breast is greatly elevated. Limited volume in primary or small tumor burden of breast cancer because levels are not as high. Increased* in pancreas, lung, colorectal, ovarian, and liver cancers.
- *Noncancer increases:* Benign breast or ovarian disease.
- *Levels decreased* with therapy and *increased* rise after therapy suggests progressive disease.
- Falsely elevated levels with liver disease.

🖎 Oncofetal Antigens

Reference Values

Normal

- *Carcinoembryonic antigen* (CEA, cell surface glycoprotein): <5.0 ng/mL (<5.0 µg/L)

- *Alpha-fetoprotein* (AFP, a glycoprotein produced by fetal liver, yolk sac, and smaller amounts in fetal GI tract and kidney): <15 ng/mL or <15 µg/L
- *Human chorionic gonadotropin* (hCG, produced by placenta syncytiotrophoblast): <5 IU/L or <5 mIU/mL

Clinical Implications

- *Carcinoembryonic (CEA): Increased in cancer:* Primarily colon cancer (especially metastatic or recurrence). Others include lung, metastatic breast, pancreas, prostate, ovary, uterus, bladder, limbs, neuroblastoma, leukemia, thyroid, and osteogenic carcinoma. *Noncancer: Increased* in inflammatory bowel disease, active ulcerative colitis, pancreatitis, bronchitis, pulmonary emphysema, pulmonary and rectal infections, polyps, chronic renal failure, cirrhosis, peptic ulcers, fibrocystic breast disease, and smoking. Most levels decline with remission of disease.

Interfering Factors

- Falsely elevated with liver disease.

Clinical Implications

- *Alpha-fetoprotein (AFP): Increased in cancer:* Primary hepatocellular cancer, embryonal cell (nonseminomatous germ cell), testicular tumors, yolk sac ovarian tumors, teratocarcinoma, gastric, pancreatic, renal, lung, colon, and breast can cross-react with LH, increases with gonadal failure. *Noncancer increases:* Fetal distress and death, neural tube defects, viral hepatitis, primary biliary cirrhosis, partial hepatectomy, ataxia-telangiectasia, Wiskott-Aldrich syndrome, multiple pregnancy, and abortion.

Interfering Factors

- Falsely elevated with liver injury.

Clinical Implications

- *Human chorionic gonadotropin (hCG): Increased in cancer:* Gestational trophoblastic tumors, seminomatous and nonseminomatous testicular cancers, ovarian tumors, pancreatic islet cell cancer, liver, stomach, and less valuable in lung cancers and lymphoproliferative diseases. Useful to monitor testicular tumors. *Noncancer: Increased* in hydatidiform mole (gestational trophoblastic neoplasms), neoplasm of stomach, colon, pancreas, lung, and liver, or multiple pregnancy. Levels double every 48 hours during early pregnancy. *Decreased* in 48 hours in ectopic pregnancy and abortion. Not increased in endodermal sinus tumors.

Interfering Factors
- Produced in normal pregnancy.
- Some tumors produce predominantly hCG fragments or "nicked" hCG, which may cause falsely low results.

Normal Cell Products

Reference Values

Normal
- *Protein-Specific Antigen (PSA):* <2.5 ng/mL or <2.5 μg/L
- *B_2-Microglobulin (B_2M):* HLA system (B_2M): ≤2.7 μg/mL or ≤2.7 mg/L
- *5-Hydroxyindole Acetic Acid (Serotonin):* 1–9 mg/24-hour urine or 5–48 μmol/2-day urine
- *Immunoglobulins: Monoclonal proteins* (M proteins) (monoclonal gammopathy): Normally absent
- *Lactate dehydrogenase (LDH). Increased* isoenzymes I and II; total LDH: 166–280 U/L
- *Neuron-Specific Enolase (NSE):* Normal staining
- *Alkaline phosphatase (ALP):*
  Adults (20–60 years): 30–90 U/L or 0.50–1.50 μkat/L
  Elderly: Slightly higher
  Children (<2 years): 40–115 U/L or 0.67–1.92 μkat/L
  Young persons (2–21 years): 30–200 U/L or 0.50–3.33 μkat/L
- *Prostatic acid phosphatase (PAP):*
  Adults: <0.6 U/L or <0.6 U/L
  Children: 8.1–12.6 U/mL or 8.1–12.6 U/mL
  Newborns: 10.4–16.4 U/mL or 10.4–16.4 U/mL
- Levels increase with stage of cancer and age of the individual.
- *Other enzymes:* Gamma-glutamyl transpeptidase (GGT); muramidase, creatinine, phosphokinase isoenzyme BB, beta-glucuronidase, terminal deoxynucleotidyl transferase, ribonuclease, histaminase (medullary cancer of thyroid), amylase, cystine amino peptidase and CK BB isoenzyme (prostate and small-cell lung cancers). (See other areas of text for discussion of these enzymes.)
- *Calcitonin (CT):*
  Serum
      Adults: <40 pg/mL or <40 ng/L
  Plasma
      Men: <19 pg/mL or <5.5 pmol/L
      Women: <14 pg/mL or <4.1 pmol/L

- *Other hormones:* (See Oncofetal Antigen); ACTH (lung oat cell), PTH (lung-epidermoid), insulin (lung), glucagon (pancreas), gastrin (stomach and other carcinomas), prostaglandin and erythropoietin (kidney). (See other areas of text for discussion of these hormones.)
- *Tissue Polypeptide Antigen (TPA):* 80–100 U/L in serum.
- *Tumor-Antigen 4 (TA-4)* ≤2.6 ng/mL. Useful in the diagnosis and management of patients with squamous carcinoma of lung, cervix, or other sites. TA-4 is a protein specified from a cervical squamous carcinoma.
- *Other antigens:* Colon mucoprotein antigen (CMA), colon-specific antigen (CSA), Zino glycinate marker (ZGM-colon), pancreatic oncofetal antigen (POA), S-100 protein (malignant melanoma), sialoglycoprotein (wide variety of cancers), and "Tennessee" antigen (wide variety of cancers). (See other areas of text in alphabetical listing for discussion of these antigens.)

✐ Protein-Specific Antigen (PSA)

Clinical Implications

- *PSA increased in prostate cancer:* The higher the level, the greater the tumor burden. Successful surgery, chemotherapy, or radiation causes marked reduction in levels. Following radical prostatectomy, PSA should fall to undetectable levels by 3 months after surgery; PSA falls gradually, usually to within the reference range, by 6 months after radiation. A rising PSA after treatment almost always indicates recurrent cancer, with increase occurring an average of 1–2 years before clinical evidence of recurrence.
- *Noncancer: Increased* in benign prostatic hypertrophy, prostate massage, prostate surgery, and prostatitis. Acute inflammation or infarction of the prostate and acute renal failure produce transient increases in PSA, which may exceed 20 ng/mL (20 µg/L), whereas chronic prostatitis does not cause increased PSA. A transient (about 1 month) increase in PSA occurs after prostate biopsy but not by rectal examination if patient has normal PSA.

Interfering Factors

- PSA is approximately 25% lower during hospitalization; thus, PSA testing should ideally be done on outpatients.

Clinical Implications

- *B_2 Microglobulin: Increased in cancers*: Multiple myelomas, other B-cell neoplasms (B-cell lymphoma, lung cancer, chronic lymphocytic leukemia, hepatoma, and breast cancer). *Noncancer* *increases:* Sclerosing spondylitis, Reiter's syndrome, renal failure, and AIDS; *low* with renal tubular injury.

Interfering Factors

- False *low* levels occur because of increased urinary losses. Falsely elevated levels occur in renal failure. Nonspecific stimulation of the immune system in infection (particularly HIV infection) increases levels.

Clinical Implications

- *5-Hydroxyindole Acetic Acid (Serotonin): Increased 5-HIAA* in cancer is used to recognize and monitor patients with carcinoid tumors. *Noncancer increases:* Many foods, particularly nuts, and many fruits. Dietary intake must be controlled before specimen collection to avoid variation in test results not due to tumor.
- *Immunoglobulin: Monoclonal Protein: Increased in cancer:* Multiple myeloma, macroglobulinemia, amyloidosis, B-cell lymphoma, multiple solid tumors, chronic lymphocytic leukemia. *Noncancer increases: Cold agglutinin disease, Sjögren's syndrome, Gaucher's disease, lichen myxedematous, cirrhosis, renal failure, sarcoid, mycosis, and fungoides; cannot separate from other causes of monoclonal gammopathy by laboratory tests alone.*

Interfering Factors

- Drugs that may give false increases: Gamma globulins, hydralazines, isoniazid (INH), Dilantin, tetanus toxoid and antitoxin, and procainamide. Indicate on lab slip if the patient received vaccines or immunizations in the past 6 months.

Clinical Implications

- *Lactate Dehydrogenase (LDH): Increased in cancer:* Neuroblastomic carcinoma of testes. Elevated in 60% of those with stage 3 testicular cancer. Serial LDH may help detect recurrence of cancer. Ewing's sarcoma; acute lymphocytic leukemia; non-Hodgkin's lymphoma; LD-1 increased in germ cell tumors; LD-3 in leukemia; LD-5 in breast, lung, stomach, and colon cancers; elevated in metastatic carcinoma. *Noncancer increases include* cellular injury/hemolysis, myocardial infarction, hepatic diseases; see Cardiac Enzyme Tests.

Interfering Factors

- Hemolysis of blood can give false-positive results. Ascorbic acid decreases LDH levels; several drugs (aspirin, alcohol, narcotics, and anesthetics) increase LDH levels.

Clinical Implications

- *Neuron-Specific Enolase (NSE): Increased in cancer:* Neuroblastomas, small-cell lung carcinoma, medullary carcinoma of thyroid, pancreatic islet cell, Wilms' tumors, and pheochromocytoma.
- *Alkaline Phosphatase (ALP): Increased levels in cancer:* Osteosarcoma, hepatocellular, metastatic to liver, primary or secondary bone tumors, liver and bone leukemia, and lymphoma. *Noncancer increases:* Paget's disease, nonmalignant liver disease, normal pregnancy, healing fractures, hyperparathyroidism, osteomalacia and rickets, sprue, and malabsorption. Noncancer decreased levels in hypoparathyroidism, malnutrition, scurvy, and pernicious anemia.

Interfering Factors

- Drugs that elevate falsely include allopurinol, antibiotics, colchicine, fluoride, indomethacin, INH, oral contraceptives, probenecid. Drugs that falsely decrease LDH levels include arsenicals, cyanide, oxalates, zinc salts, and nitrofurantoin.

Clinical Implications

- *Prostatic Acid Phosphatase (PAP): In cancer:* High significant levels in metastatic prostate cancer. When used to monitor therapy with antineoplastic drugs, level drops in 3–4 days after successful surgery treatment and 3–4 weeks after estrogen administration. Moderate-level elevation in benign prostatic hypertrophy. Also, elevated in leukemia (hairy cell) and cancer metastasis to bone (osteoblastic lesions). *Noncancer elevated:* Noncancerous prostatic conditions, prostate palpation, hyperplasia, infection of prostate following cystostomy, prostate surgery, and chronic prostatitis. Other *conditions in which prostatic acid phosphatase is elevated:* Gaucher's disease (lipid storage disease), Nieman-Pick disease, Paget's disease, osteoporosis, renal osteopathy, hepatic cirrhosis, pulmonary embolism, and hyperparathyroidism.

Interfering Factors

- Drugs that elevate levels include androgens and clofibrate. Drugs that decrease levels include fluorides, phosphatase, oxalates, and alcohol.
- Falsely high levels after prostate, rectal exam, or instrumentation (ie, cystoscopy).

Clinical Implications

- *Calcitonin (CT): Increased in cancer:* Metastatic breast (greatly elevated). Limited in primary small tumor burden breast cancer because levels are lower; lung and pancreas hepatoma, renal cell carcinoma, carcinoid, medullary carcinoma of thyroid, and skeletal metastases. *Noncancer increases:* Zollinger-Ellison syndrome, pernicious anemia, chronic renal failure, pseudohypoparathy-roidism, apudomas, alcoholic cirrhosis, Paget's disease, pregnancy, benign breast, or ovary disease. *Decreased* with therapy and a rise after therapy suggests progressive disease.

- *Tissue Polypeptide Antigen (TPA): Increased in cancer:* Gastrointestinal, genitourinary tract, breast, lung, and thyroid cancer. *Noncancer increases:* Hepatitis, cholangitis, cirrhosis, diabetes, pneumonia, or urinary tract infections.

- *Tumor Antigen 4-(TA-4): Increased in cancer:* Squamous cancer of lung and cervix, especially in patients with advanced disease. Elevations correlate with stage of cancer and rising levels after surgery indicate recurrence.

Genetic Markers

Two types of genes are implicated in cancer: *oncogenes* (leukemia and some solid tumors) and *suppressor genes* (P_{53} is the major tumor suppressor gene). Oncogenes have not been widely used as tumor markers in clinical practice. Typically, tumor cells have mutations involving several oncogenes. The genes themselves can be detected only in tumor cells, which usually require tissue biopsy or examination of cells shed into body fluids. The p53 mutation is the most common genetic mutation in cancer. p53 antibodies are associated with the worst prognosis in breast, head, neck, and colon cancer. The mutation rate is 50% to 75% in small-cell lung cancer.

Markers of Host Response

Response to Tumor or Altered Cell Metabolism

These types of tumor markers are typically elevated only with advanced tumors and are commonly affected by benign disease. In some tumors, they may be the only marker that allows monitoring of treatment. These markers include nonspecific response to tumors (cytokinase)—increased production of acute phase reactant proteins; tumor lysis syndrome—tumor cells destroyed rapidly (therapy) and release of cell contents increase blood levels of LDH, K^+, and PO_4; abnormal amine accumulation (tumors have abnormal metabolism, causing accumulations of amines such as putrescine and spermidine with increased levels in CSF and urine and in brain and bladder tumors). **Interleukin** (also known as IL-2), a cytokine, T-cell growth factor I, is formed from T-helper cells and activated B cells; results are highly variable.

Cellular Markers Related to Prognosis

Cell markers predict prognosis or guide treatment—used most widely in breast cancer. Cellular tumor markers can be studied only when tumor cells can be sampled either through biopsy or, for tumors on mucosal surfaces, by exfoliative cytology. These markers include steroid receptors (exert their effects by binding to cytoplasmic or nuclear receptors, which alter DNA synthesis); DNA ploidy (tumor cells may have a different chromosome number than the normal cell, which has 46 chromosomes); cathepsin D, a protease (overproduction of cathepsin D in breast cancer has been associated with poor prognosis).

Interfering Factors
• Inadequate handling of biopsy specimen (requires rapid handling and freezing of tissue) will interfere with test outcomes.

Procedure
• A 10-mL venous blood sample is usually obtained for most tests; 24-hour urine testing may be done. Refer to Chapter 2 for specimen collection guidelines.
• Follow specific lab procedure for handling of each specimen.

Nursing Interventions
▸*Pretest*
• Assess patient's knowledge of test. Explain purpose and procedure of blood test and prepare the patient for possible test outcome indicative of cancer.

▸*Posttest*
• Evaluate outcomes; monitor and provide counseling.
• Provide support and educate regarding the need for follow-up tests, surgery, or further medical treatment.

Tumor Imaging

Nuclear Medicine, Tumor Imaging

Tumor imaging uses radiopharmaceuticals to identify tumors and stage cancers.

Indications

- Localize various tumors.
- Detect metastases.
- Monitor treatment regimen.

Reference Values

Normal

- Normal distribution of radiopharmaceutical; local distortion of primary and distant organs.
- No lymphatic spread; no lymph node enlargement.
- No vascular spread; no distortion of distant organs.

Clinical Implications

- Abnormal tumor uptake reveals cancer spread by the distortion of the primary tumors.
- Distortion of adjacent organs (local spread).
- Lymph node enlargement or lymphatic spread.
- Distortion of distant organs or vascular spread.

Procedure

Call the nuclear medicine department for specific protocols. Specifics of the protocol vary on the basis of instrumentation and radiopharmaceutical availability.

Specific Radiopharmaceuticals

- ^{99m}Tc sestamibi: Evaluate brain tumor viability; search for thyroid metastasis.
- TcV DMSA: Evaluate head and neck tumors.
- Pentetreotide (OctreoScan): Assess nonendocrine tumors (eg, carcinomas, gastronomas, and small-cell lung cancers).
- Capromab pendetide (ProstaScint): Assess those patients at high risk for prostate metastasis, for example, PSA >10 × upper limit or Gleason score of 3–7, Gleason stage > 8.

Nursing Interventions

▸*Pretest*

- Explain purpose and procedure for tumor scans.

▸*Intratest*

- Provide support during injection and assure the patient that delayed imaging is the usual procedure.

‣*Posttest*

- Assess for side effects of radiopharmaceuticals: rashes, nausea, or vomiting.
- Evaluate patient outcomes and, in collaboration with the physician, counsel appropriately regarding further tests and possible surgery.
- Monitor intravenous injection sites for extravasation, infection, or hematomas.
- Inform pregnant staff and visitors and family members to avoid prolonged exposure during the time from injection to delayed imaging.

URINALYSIS ROUTINE (UA): TESTS FOR BLADDER AND KIDNEY INFECTIONS OR METABOLIC (DIABETES) DISORDERS

Urine, Urinary Infection, Diabetes

Color, Appearance, Specific Gravity (SG), pH, Odor, Glucose, Ketones, Blood, Protein, Bilirubin, Urobilinogen Microscopic Examination of Sediment (Bacteria, Casts, Red Blood Cells, White Blood Cells, Crystals)

Urinalysis is the means of determining the various properties of urine, as well as any abnormal constituents, revealed by chemical determinations and microscopic examination of the sediment.

Indications

- Use as screening in routine physical examination, prehospital admission, and presurgical procedures.
- Diagnose and monitor treatment of kidney and urinary tract infections.
- Diagnose and monitor metabolic diseases (eg, diabetes, thyroid, liver) not related to urinary system.

Reference Values

Normal

ADULT VALUES

GENERAL CHARACTERISTICS AND MEASUREMENTS	CHEMICAL DETERMINATIONS	MICROSCOPIC EXAM OF SEDIMENT
Color: Pale yellow to amber straw: Normal with low specific gravity (SG) Amber: Normal with high SG	Glucose: Negative (diabetes main cause of glyco suria)	Bacteria: Negative; casts negative: rare hyaline casts (indicate damage to glomerular capillary membrane)
Appearance: Clear to slightly hazy. Series consists of mucus, pus, and epithelial (squamous) cells	Ketones: Negative (presence associated with diabetes or altered carbohydrate metabolism)	Red blood cells: Hemoglobin or myoglobin; negative or none (indicates trauma or damage to GU organs or systems)
SG: 1.015–1.025 with a normal fluid intake (ability of kidneys to concentrate urine)	Protein: Negative or trace (indicates renal disease)	Crystals: Negative (none) relative to pH of urine
Osmolality: 300–900 mOsm/kg of H_2O A precise measurement of SG per 24 hours	Bilirubin: Negative (monitor hepatitis and liver damage)	White blood cells: None or rare (0–4) Red blood cells: None
pH: 4.6–8.0 Average person has pH of about 6.0 (acid) Maintain constant body pH	Urobilinogen: 0.1–1.0 units/dL or <1 mg	Epithelial cells: Few, hyaline casts: 0–1/1 pF

GENERAL CHARACTERISTICS AND MEASUREMENTS	CHEMICAL DETERMINATIONS	MICROSCOPIC EXAM OF SEDIMENT
Odor: Aromatic (not offensive)	Nitrate for bacteria: Negative (presence indicates bacteria in urine)	
Volume: 600–2500 mL in 24 hours (fluid balance and kidney function)	Leukocyte esterase: Negative (indicates a urinary tract infection)	

Clinical Implications: Appearance

• Cloudy urine may indicate presence of pus (WBCs), red blood cells, or bacteria due to urinary tract infection, or shreds.

Interfering Factors: Appearance

• Foods, urates, phosphates, or vaginal contamination and degree of hydration or dehydration may affect appearance.

Clinical Implications: Color

• Abnormal-colored urine may be due to the presence of red blood cells (smoky), bilirubin (brownish yellow to yellow green), melanotic tumor or Addison's disease (black), alkaptonuria (black), and porphyria (port wine).

Interfering Factors: Color

• Color darkens on standing, certain foods (red/beets), medications (all colors), physiologic factors (stress/clear), excessive exercise (red), large fluid intake and alcohol (straw), fever (dark amber).

Clinical Implications: Odor

Abnormal odor may be due to foods (asparagus, garlic), medications (estrogen), bacteria (putrid), and ketones (sweet) and in PKU (musty, mousey), tyrosinemia (cabbage, fishy), maple syrup urine disease (burnt sugar), and oasthouse urine disease (brewery odor).

Clinical Implications: Specific Gravity (SG)

• *Low specific gravity* (1.000–1.010) may occur in patients with diabetes insipidus (decreased or absent ADH), glomerulonephritis with pyelonephritis, severe renal damage. (See TABLE 3.8.)
• *High specific gravity* (above 1.025) can occur in diabetes mellitus, increased secretion of ADH, nephrosis, congestive heart failure,

(text continues on page 589)

TABLE 3.8 CORRELATING CHEMICAL, PHYSICAL, AND MICROSCOPIC URINALYSIS (UA) FINDINGS WITH RENAL DISORDERS*

DISORDER AND CAUSE	SIGNS/SYMPTOMS	URINE APPEARANCE
Acute Glomerulonephritis Antibasement membrane smoky antibodies associated with strep infection, variety of infectious agents, toxins, allergens	Rapid appearance of hematuria, proteinuria, casts. Hypertension, renal insufficiency, and edema. More commonly seen in children and young adults	Gross hematuria, turbidity
Test Outcome: Protein <1.0 g/dL; positive for blood. Increased RBC, WBC, renal tubular epithelial casts; RBC, granular cast, occasional WBC and renal		
Chronic Glomerulonephritis Represents end-stage result of persistent glomerular damage with continuing and irreversible loss of renal function. Progresses to end-stage renal	Edema, hypertension, anemia, metabolic acidosis, oliguria progressing to anuria	Hematuria
Test Outcome: Protein >2.5 g/dL. Small amount of blood. SG low and fixed. Increased RBC, WBC, renal epithelial. Casts: Granular, waxy, broad		
Nephrotic Syndrome Glomeruli whose basement membranes have become highly permeable to plasma proteins of large molecular weight and lipids, allowing them to pass in the tubulars.	Massive proteinuria, edema, high levels of serum lipids and low levels of serum albumin	Cloudy
Test Outcome: Protein >3.5 g/dL. Small amount of blood. Increased RBC, oval fat bodies, free fat, renal epithelial. Casts: Fatty, waxy, renal		

Acute Tubular Necrosis

Destruction of renal tubular epithelial cells. Usually following a hypotensive (shock), toxic element, or drugs, and heavy metals

Oliguria and complete renal failure

Slightly cloudy

Test Outcome: Protein <1.0 g/dL. Positive for blood. SG low. Increased RBC, WBC, renal, epithelial. Casts: Renal, granular, waxy, broad

Cystitis (Lower Urinary)

Urethritis (urethra in males)

Infection of the bladder most commonly caused by *Escherichia coli* (85%)

Frequent and painful urination

Cloudy, foul smelling

Test Outcome: Protein <0.5 g/dL. Small amount of blood. Nitrite positive (usually); leukocyte esterase positive (usually). Increased WBCs, bacteria, RBCs. Transitional epithelial

Acute Pyelonephritis (Upper Urinary)

An infection of the kidney or renal pelvis. Caused by infectious organism that has traveled through the urinary tract and invaded the kidney tissue

More frequently in women with repeated urinary tract infections

Turbid, foul smelling

Test Outcome: Protein <1.0 g/dL. Positive for blood. Leukocyte esterase positive (usually). Increased WBC (clumps), bacteria, renal epithelial. Casts: WBC, granular, renal, occasionally waxy

(table continues on page 588)

TABLE 3.8 (continued)

DISORDER AND CAUSE	SIGNS/SYMPTOMS	URINE APPEARANCE
Chronic pyelonephritis Permanent scarring of the renal tissue.	Polyuria and nocturia develop as tubular function is lost. With disease progression there is hypertension and altered renal and glomerular flow	Cloudy
Test Outcome: Protein <2.5 g/dL. Nitrite positive (usually). Leukocyte esterase positive (usually). SG low. Increased WBCs. Casts: Granular, waxy, broad		
Acute Interstitial Nephritis Inflammation of the renal interstitium caused by drug toxicity or an allergic reaction.	Fever, eosinophilia, skin rash	Cloudy
Test Outcome: Protein <1 g/dL. Positive for blood. Leukocyte esterase positive (usually). Increased WBCs. Increased eosinophils. Increased RBCs. Increased epithelial. Increased casts: Granular, renal, hyaline		

Adapted from Finnegan, K. (1998). Routine urinalyses. In Lehman, C. A. (Ed.), *Saunders manual of clinical laboratory science.* Philadelphia: W. B. Saunders, pp. 773–805.

*See "Protein" in the alphabetical listing for more information.

toxemia of pregnancy, and excessive water loss (eg, in dehydration, fever, vomiting, diarrhea).

- *Fixed specific gravity* of 1.010 that does not vary from specimen to specimen indicates severe renal damage.

Interfering Factors: Specific Gravity (SG)

- Low specific gravity caused by diuretics, excessive fluid intake, coffee, or alcohol.
- High specific gravity can be caused by radiopaque x-ray contrast media, minerals, dextran, detergent residue, cold specimen temperature, and proteinuria.

Clinical Implications: pH

- *Acidic urine* (pH < 7.0) occurs in metabolic acidosis (diabetic ketosis), diarrhea, starvation, urinary tract infections caused by *E. coli*, and respiratory acidosis (carbon dioxide retention).
- *Alkaline urine* (pH > 7.0) occurs in urinary tract infections caused by urea-splitting bacteria, renal tubular acidosis, chronic renal failure, and respiratory alkalosis (due to hyperventilation).

Interfering Factors: pH

- Acidic urine: Mandelamine and ammonium chloride medications, ascorbic acid, high protein intake, and some fruits such as cranberries and pineapple.
- Alkaline urine: Prolonged standing of specimen (bacteria split urea and produce ammonia). Chemicals such as sodium bicarbonate, potassium citrate, and acetazolamide. Diet high in fruits, vegetables, and legumes; also, normal response after meal.

CLINICAL ALERT

- An accurate measurement of urinary pH can be made only on a freshly voided specimen. If the urine is to be kept for any length of time before analysis, it must be refrigerated.
- If pH of 9 is reported, obtain a blood specimen.

Clinical Implications: Glucose/Sugar

- *Increased amounts* (glycosuria) in patients with diabetes mellitus, brain tumors, brain injury, myocardial infarction, infections, lowered renal threshold (positive *urine* glucose, normal *blood* glucose), hyperthyroidism, asphyxia, gastrectomy, obesity, and glycogen storage disease.

Interfering Factors: Glucose

- Pregnancy, lactation, stress, excitement, ketonuria, testing after a heavy meal, IV glucose, some medications (ascorbic acid [vitamin C], Keflex [cephalosporin]); use of deteriorated reagent strips.

CLINICAL ALERT

- Urine glucose: >1000 mg/dL or >55 mmol/L (4+). Notify the physician and begin appropriate treatment.

Clinical Implications: Ketones

- *Increased amounts (ketonuria):* Diabetes mellitus, renal glycosuria, glycogen storage disease, starvation, fasting, high-fat or -protein diets; low-carbohydrate diet, prolonged vomiting, eclampsia, thyrotoxicosis, and severe prolonged exercise and stress.

Interfering Factors: Ketones

- Ketonuria can occur with dietary increase of fat and protein, along with the decrease of carbohydrates, stress, and pregnancy.
- Many drugs (insulin, Pyridium [phenazopyridine], phenothiazines, levodopa, and many others) may affect the test outcomes.

Clinical Implications: Bilirubin

- Bilirubin is always abnormal and warrants further investigation.
- *Increased levels* occur in hepatitis and liver disease (owing to infections or a toxic agent), obstructive biliary tract, and parenchymal injury.
- Urine bilirubin gives negative results in hemolytic disease.

Interfering Factors: Bilirubin

- Light exposure to specimen and many drugs affect test outcomes.

Clinical Implications: Urobilinogen

- See Liver Function Tests in alphabetical list for this item.

Clinical Implications: Proteins

- See Protein in alphabetical list for this item.

Clinical Implications: Blood/Hemoglobin

- *Presence of blood/hemoglobin* (hemoglobinuria) occurs in excessive burns and crushing injuries, transfusion reaction, febrile intoxication, chemical agents, snake venom, malaria, and other parasites, hemolytic disorders (sickle cell anemia), strenuous exercise (march hemoglobinuria), paroxysmal hemoglobinuria, kidney infarction, disseminated intravascular coagulation (DIC), and fava bean sensitivity.

- *Increased red blood cells* (hematuria) occur in acute urinary tract infections (cystitis), benign prostatic hypertrophy, glomerulonephritis, SLE, benign familial hematuria, and urologic cancer, trauma to kidneys, malignant hypertension, pyelonephritis, and polycystic kidney disease.

Interfering Factors: Blood

- Strenuous exercise, smoking, menstruation contamination, and many drugs (ascorbic acid, antibiotics toxic to kidney, anticoagulants, salicylates, bromides, copper, and iodine) may affect test outcomes.
- Myoglobulin gives a false-positive result for RBCs and hemoglobin.

 CLINICAL ALERT

- The appearance of blood in urine is one of the early indications of renal disease.
- Any instance of hematuria should be rechecked on a freshly collected specimen.

Clinical Implications: Bacteria/Nitrate or Leukocyte Esterase Dipstick Methods

- Positive nitrate is a reliable indicator of bacteriuria and is a cue for performing a urine culture.
- Positive leukocyte esterase indicates pyuria (WBCs present).

 CLINICAL ALERT

- The presence of bacteria and WBCs (pyuria) indicates the need for urine culture. Notify physician, record results in the patient's record, and begin treatment per orders/protocols.
- A negative nitrate test should never be interpreted as an indication of the absence of bacteria. Some bacteria do not produce nitrates.

Interfering Factors: Bacteria/Nitrate

- Vaginal discharge, trichomonas, parasites, and heavy mucus can cause false-positive results.
- Azo dye metabolites, high specific gravity, and ascorbic acid (vitamin C) may affect test outcomes.

DISPLAY 3.10 **Microscopic Examination of Urine Sediment**

Urine Sediment Component	Clinical Significance
Bacteria	Urinary tract infection
Casts	Tubular or glomerular disorders
Broad casts	Formation occurs in collecting tubules; serious kidney disorder
Epithelial (renal) casts	Tubular degeneration
Fatty casts	Nephrotic syndrome
Granular or waxy casts	Renal parenchymal disease
Hyaline casts	Acidic urine, high salt content
Red blood cell casts	Acute glomerulonephritis
White blood cell casts	Pyelonephritis
Epithelial cells	Damage to various parts of urinary tract
Renal cells	Tubular damage
Squamous cells	Normal or contamination
Erythrocytes	Most renal disorders; menstruation; strenuous exercise
Fat bodies (oval)	Nephrotic syndrome
Leukocytes	Most renal disorders; urinary tract infection; pyelonephritis

---

Clinical Implications: Microscopic Examination of Sediment

- Appearance of *bacteria* in urinary tract infections and renal *epithelial cells* in tubular disease. *Leukocytes* (WBCs) and *erythrocytes* (RBCs) in most renal disorders, urinary tract infections, and strenuous exercise. *Hyaline casts* occur in many types of renal diseases. *White cell casts* indicate the renal origin of leukocytes, are most frequently found in patients with acute pyelonephritis, but are also found in patients with glomerulonephritis. *Red cell casts* indicate renal origin of hematuria and suggest glomerulonephritis, including lupus nephritis, but are also found in malignant hypertension. *Epithelial casts* are most suggestive of glomerulonephritis but are also found in other disorders. *Granular casts* are found in a wide variety of renal diseases. *Waxy casts* are found especially in chronic renal diseases but occur in diabetic nephropathy, other forms of chronic renal disease, and glomerulonephritis. (See DISPLAY 3.10 and TABLE 3.9.)

(text continues on page 595)

TABLE 3.9 Urine Crystals

Type of Crystal	Color	Shape	Clinical Implications
Acidic Urine			
Amorphous urates	Pink to brick red	Granules	Normal
Uric acid	Yellow brown	Polymorphous—whetstones, rosettes or prisms, rhombohedral prisms, hexagonal plate	Normal or increased purine metabolism, gout
Sodium urate	Colorless to yellow	Fan of slender prisms	
Cystine (rare)	Colorless, highly refractive	Flat hexagonal plates with well-defined edges, single or in clusters	Cystinuria—cystine stones in kidney, crystals also in spleen and eyes
Cholesterol (rare)	Colorless	"Broken window panes," with notched corners	Elevated cholesterol, chyluria
Leucine (rare)	Yellow or brown, highly refractile	Spheroids with striations; pure from hexagonal	Protein breakdown, severe liver disease
Tyrosine (rare)	Colorless or yellow	Fine, silky needles in sheaves or rosettes	Protein breakdown, severe liver disease
Bilirubin	Reddish brown	Cubes, rhombi plates, amorphous needles	Elevated bilirubin
Acidic, Neutral, or Slightly Alkaline Urine			
Calcium oxalate	Colorless	Octahedral resemble envelopes, often small, colorless. Use high-power microscope for visualization	Normal; large amounts in fresh urine may indicate severe chronic renal disease

(table continues on page 594)

593

TABLE 3.9 (continued)

TYPE OF CRYSTAL	COLOR	SHAPE	CLINICAL IMPLICATIONS
Hippuric acid (rare)	Colorless	Rhombi plates, four-sided prisms	No significance
Alkaline, Neutral, or Slightly Acidic Urine			
Triple phosphate	Colorless	"Coffin lids" 3- to 6-sided prism; occasionally like fern leaf	Urine stasis and chronic infection
Alkaline Urine			
Calcium carbonate	Colorless	Needles, spheres, dumbbells	Normal
Ammonium biurate	Yellow opaque brown	"Thorn apple" spheres, dumbbells, sheaves of needles	Normal
Calcium phosphate	Colorless	Prisms, plates, needles	Normal; large amounts in chronic cystitis or prostatic hypertrophy
Amorphous phosphates	White	Granules	Normal

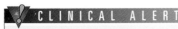

> CLINICAL ALERT
>
> • Specific drugs may cause increased levels of their own crystals. Unless toxicity is suspected, they are of little clinical significance.

Interfering Factors: Microscopic Examination
• Traumatic catheterization, alkaline urine, vaginal discharge, and improper specimen collection and storage.
• Volume less than 2 mL.

> CLINICAL ALERT
>
> • A urine culture should be done if elevated urine WBC counts are found.
> • Pyelonephritis may remain completely asymptomatic, even though renal tissue is being progressively destroyed. Therefore, careful examination (using low power) of urinary sediment for leukocyte casts is vital.

Procedure for Urinalysis
• Collect fresh random midstream or 24-hour urine specimen following collection guidelines in Chapter 2.
• First, the physical characteristics of the urine are noted and recorded. Second, a series of chemical tests are run. A chemically impregnated dipstick can be used for many of these tests. Standardized results can be obtained by processing the urine-touched dipstick through special automated instruments. Third, the urine sediment is examined under the microscope.
• Microscopic elements should be correlated with the physical and chemical findings. (See TABLE 3.10.)

Nursing Interventions
▶*Pretest*
• Explain the test purpose and procedure and the need to follow appropriate urine collection procedures.

▶*Intratest*
• Provide privacy during urine collection.

▶*Posttest*
• Evaluate patient compliance in specimen collection and outcomes and counsel the patient appropriately.

TABLE 3.10 COMMON CORRELATIONS IN URINALYSIS

MICROSCOPIC ELEMENTS	PHYSICAL EXAMINATION	DIPSTICK MEASUREMENT*
Red blood cells	Turbidity; red color	Blood
White blood cells	Turbidity	Protein Nitrate Leukocytes
Epithelial cast cells	Turbidity	Protein
Bacteria	Turbidity, odor	pH Nitrite Leukocytes
Crystals	Turbidity, color†	pH

*Positive result.
†See TABLE 3.9.

URINE CULTURE

Urine, Bladder, and Kidney Infection

Urine culture is done to identify the specific causative organisms in suspected infections of kidneys, ureter, bladder, and urethra.

Indications
- Isolate microorganisms that cause clinical infections of urinary tract.
- Evaluate effectiveness of medication therapy for existing urinary infection.
- Evaluate suspected urinary TB: Three consecutive early morning specimens.

Reference Values

Normal
- Adults: Negative (<10,000 organisms per milliliter of urine). Any bacteria found are either contaminants from the skin or invading pathogens.
- Pediatric: Same as adult.

Clinical Implications
- Bacterial count of 100,000 or more per milliliter of urine indicates infection. When the colony count is between 10,000 and 100,000

or when two or more organisms are recovered, the decision to identify and perform susceptibility tests is made on an individual basis. Colony counts of 30,000 are usually considered significant in catheter or suprapubic specimens.

- A significant titer of the following organisms in urine is considered pathogenic: *E. coli, Enterococcus, Enterobacter, Klebsiella* sp., *Mycobacterium tuberculosis, Proteus* sp., *Pseudomonas aeruginosa, Staphylococcus saprophyticus, Trichomonas vaginalis*, and *Candida albicans* and other yeasts.

Interfering Factors

- Dilute urine with a reduction in bacteria colony count when patients have been forcing fluids.
- Specimens not taken to laboratory immediately or refrigerated (approximately 24 hours). Urine at room temperature allows growth of many organisms.
- Not following collection procedure accurately.
- Urine contaminated during collection may lead to false test results. Sources of contamination include hair from perineum; bacteria from beneath prepuce in men; bacteria from vaginal secretion, vulva, or urethra in women; and bacteria from hands, skin, or clothing. Many women have small numbers of WBCs in urine.

Procedure

- Collect a clean-catch midstream specimen according to specimen collection guidelines in Chapter 2.
- Two successive clean-catch specimens should be collected to be 95% certain that true bacteria are present and results are not a result of urine contamination.
- The specimen that is collected should preferably be an early morning one, when the bacterial count is likely to be highest (urine concentrated), and before initiating antibiotic therapy.
- A sterile urine specimen may be collected by urethral catheterization, suprapubic catheter aspiration, or directly from an indwelling catheter (see Chapter 2 guidelines for collection of this type of specimen).

Nursing Interventions

▸*Pretest*

- Assess patient's knowledge of the test, signs and symptoms, and medication usage. Explain purpose and procedure for collection of clean-catch midstream urine specimen.
- Provide patient with necessary supplies, including sterile specimen container and antiseptic sponges.

⧫*Intratest*
- Usually, the patient collects this specimen if able to do so physically and comprehends directions. If not, the nurse collects specimen. Provide privacy during collection procedure. If patient assistance is needed, wear gloves.
- Send the specimen to the laboratory immediately. Place in a biohazard bag.

⧫*Posttest*
- Counsel the patient in relation to any lifestyle changes necessary to treat and prevent further urinary tract infections, such as proper perineal cleansing after bowel and urinary elimination, avoiding tight, restricting clothes (pants, hose), and drinking sufficient fluids.

 URODYNAMIC STUDIES

Special Study, Incontinence

Cystometrogram (CMG), Urethral Pressure Profile (UPP), Rectal Electromyogram (EMG), Cystourethrogram

These tests identify abnormal voiding patterns in persons with incontinence or inability to void normally.

Indications
- Evaluate incontinence, abnormal voiding patterns, dysuria, enuresis, and infections.
- Measure status of neuroanatomic connections between spinal cord, brain, and bladder.
- Evaluate neurogenic bladder dysfunction and assess neuropathies such as those associated with multiple sclerosis, diabetes, and tabes dorsalis.

Reference Values

Normal
- Normal bladder sensations of fullness, heat, and cold.
- Normal adult bladder capacity: 400–500 mL; residual urine less than 30 mL; desire to void: 175–250 mL; sensation of fullness: 350–450 mL; strong, uninterrupted stream.
- Normal voiding pressures and muscle coordination.

• Normal rectal EMG readings; urethral pressure profile readings normal.

Interfering Factors
• Inability of the patient to cooperate (eg, disorientation).
• Bladder capacity varies with age.

Clinical Implications
• Motor or sensory deficit of pelvic floor muscle or internal sphincter; disturbed muscle coordination.
• Detrusor muscle hyperreflexia (due to upper or lower motor neuron lesions such as cerebrovascular aneurysm, Parkinson's disease, multiple sclerosis, cervical spondylosis, spinal cord injury above the conus medullaris).
• Hyperreflexia—caused by benign prostatic hypertrophy or stress urge incontinence.
• Detrusor areflexia—difficulty emptying bladder without a residual volume because of inadequate detrusor muscle response to innervation. (*Causes:* trauma, spinal arachnoiditis, birth defects, diabetes, phenothiazines, reduced estrogen levels in menopause.)

Cystometrogram (CMG) Procedure

Residual urine is measured by inserting an indwelling catheter into the bladder after the patient voids. Flow rates, pressures, and urine amounts are recorded during voiding. After cystometric exam, cholinergics or anticholinergics may be administered to check bladder response to these drugs. The first cystometric is used as a control and a second cystometric is performed about 30 minutes after drug injection.

Rectal EMG Procedure

Electrodes are placed next to the anus and grounded on the thigh, or a needle electrode may be placed into the periurethral striated muscle. Measurements of EMG activity during voiding produce a recording of urine flow rate.

Urethral Pressure Profile (UPP) Procedure

A specially designed catheter coupled to a transducer records urethral pressures as it is slowly withdrawn.

Cystourethrogram Procedure

X-ray contrast material is instilled into the bladder via catheter until the bladder fills. X-ray films in several positions are taken. More x-ray films of contrast medium being voided through urethra are taken (voiding cystourethrogram) after the catheter is removed.

Nursing Interventions

▶*Pretest*
- Explain testing purpose, procedure, and collection of specimens. Be sensitive to cultural, social, sexual, and modesty issues.

▶*Intratest*
- Provide support and privacy.
- Observe patient for sensations or perceptions related to stages in the study.
- Assist as necessary with the actual procedure and collection of specimens.

▶*Posttest*
- Encourage increased oral fluid intake.
- Explain that minor burning or discomfort is a normal sensation immediately after the test and especially with the first voiding posttest.
- Instruct the patient to notify the physician STAT if fever, chills, tachycardia, or faintness occur—watch for hypotension as well.

CLINICAL ALERT

- Pre-existing urinary tract infections can precipitate a septic reaction.
- Some patients with cervical spine cord lesions may experience autonomic reflexia. This response produces hypertension, severe headache, bradycardia, flushing, and diaphoresis. Propantheline bromide (Pro-Banthine) can alleviate these symptoms.

VANILLYLMANDELIC ACID (VMA)—CATECHOLAMINES, FRACTIONATED (EPINEPHRINE, NOREPINEPHRINE, DOPAMINE)

Timed Urine, Adrenal Gland

These tests measure the excretion of urinary catecholamines, the substances formed by the adrenal medulla, over a 24-hour period. Vanillylmandelic acid (VMA) is the primary urinary metabolite of the catecholamines.

Indications
- Evaluate hypertensive patients; diagnose pheochromocytoma, a tumor of the chromaffin cells of the adrenal medulla.
- Diagnose and follow-up malignant neuroblastoma in children.

Reference Values

Normal

- Normal vanillylmandelic acid (VMA): <9 mg/24 hours or <45 μmol/day
- Normal catecholamines (total): <100 μg/24 hours or <591 nmol/day

FRACTIONS

- Epinephrine: 0–20 μg/24 hours or 0–118 nmol/day
- Norepinephrine: 15–80 μg/24 hours or 89–473 nmol/day
- Dopamine: 65–400 μg/24 hours or 420–2600 nmol/day
- Children's levels differ from adult levels. Check with your laboratory.

Clinical Implications

- *Increased VMA* is found in pheochromocytoma, neuroblastomas, and ganglioblastoma carcinoid tumor.
- *Increased catecholamines* are found in pheochromocytoma, neuroblastomas, ganglioneuromas, myocardial infarct, hypothyroidism, and long-term manic-depressive states.
- *Decreased urine catecholamines* are found in diabetic neuropathy and Parkinson's disease.

Interfering Factors

- *Increased levels of VMA* are caused by starvation (test should not be scheduled while patient is NPO) and many foods containing caffeine, such as carbonated drinks, coffee, cocoa, chocolate, vanilla, fruit (especially bananas, fruit juice), foods containing artificial flavoring or coloring, foods containing licorice; increased levels are also caused by stress and strenuous exercise.
- Many drugs give false-positive results, such as antihypertensives, antibiotics, vasopressors, epinephrine (Adrenalin), aminophylline, levodopa, isopropanol, MAO inhibitors, alpha- and beta-blockers, chlorpromazine (Thorazine), sinus and cough medicines, and appetite suppressants.
- Decreased levels of VMA are caused by alkaline urine, uremia, x-ray iodine contrast agents, and specific drugs.

Procedure

- Collect urine for 24 hours in a clean plastic container. See timed specimen collection guidelines in Chapter 2. A small urine collection is okay for pediatric patients.
- Keep specimen refrigerated with preservative in a container (hydrochloric acid or acetic acid).

• Ensure that the pH of the urine collection is below 3.0; if not, more hydrochloric acid may be required.
• Note drugs that the patient is taking.

Nursing Interventions

▶Pretest

• Assess patient compliance and knowledge base before explaining test purpose and procedure.
• Restrict diet from foods listed in *Interfering Factors* for 3 days (2 days before testing and on the day of the test).
• Discontinue all drugs for 3–7 days before testing with physician's permission.

▶Intratest

• Accurate test results depend on proper collection, preservation, and labeling. Be sure to include test startup and completion times. Record drugs patient is taking on a lab slip or computer screen.

▶Posttest

• Evaluate outcome and provide counseling and support as necessary.

VIRUS CULTURE

Tissue, Urine, Sputum, CSF and Mucous Membrane Fluids, Viral Infection

Virus cultures are obtained to isolate micro-organisms in patients with suspected viral infections.

Indications

• Identify the virus causing severe disease.
• Determine if there is a possibility of nosocomial transmission; also a public health concern.
• Document the presence or absence of viral etiology so as to eliminate the use of inappropriate therapy.

Reference Values

Normal

• Negative for viral organisms.
• Positive viral cultures from these sources are diagnostically accurate. Autopsy specimens, buffy coat blood WBC smears, biopsies, CSF, cervix, eye, and fine-needle aspirates.

Procedure

- Specimens for viral culture are best collected when symptoms first present themselves. If specimens are collected a week after symptoms first appear, the diagnosis of viral infection will be compromised.
- The type of viral illness and the symptoms influence the specimens of choice for viral culture; for example, if pneumonia is the symptom, the specimen of choice would be sputum, bronchial alveolar lavage, or bronchial brushing. If meningitis is the symptom during summer months (enterovirus infection), specimens of choice would be CSF and rectal stool or throat swab.
- Viral specimens can be collected from sterile as well as non-sterile sites. Sterile specimens tend to be collected by some invasive procedure, such as phlebotomy, lower respiratory tract specimens (collected by nursing or respiratory therapist), and tissue biopsies (collected by physician). Specimens from nonsterile sites, such as conjunctivae, skin, vesicles, nose, throat, urine, and genital and rectal sites, may be collected by nursing personnel.
- Observe standard precautions. If the specimen is collected on a swab, it must remain moist during transport to the laboratory. Modified Stuart transport medium in a self-contained transport system is recommended. Do not use cotton swabs and wooden-shafted cotton swabs. Dacron or rayon swabs are a better choice.
- Nonsterile specimens not of a liquid nature, fine-needle aspirates, or tissue biopsies should be moistened in a small amount of sterile saline, tryptic soy broth, or viral transport medium. Liquid specimens should be collected in a sterile container. Place specimens in biohazard bags.
- Viruses that can be recovered in urine include CMV, enteroviruses, and rubella-, measles-, and mumps-causing virus. In cases of viremia, blood specimens collected in tubes containing heparin or EDTA are recommended. Place specimen in a biohazard bag.

Nursing Interventions

▶ Pretest

- Label specimen with patient's name, date and time collected, specific source of specimen, and type. A contact person or clinic should be included for the notification of a positive result.

▶ Intratest

- Specimens should be promptly delivered to the lab. If there is a delay in transport, specimens should be refrigerated (0°C–4°C). If transport will exceed 5 days, the specimen should be frozen.

▶*Posttest*
• Counsel patient regarding positive results and possible need for further testing.

VISUAL FIELD TESTING

Eye

This procedure is used in conjunction with basic eye tests to evaluate the visual field.

Indications
• Assess for glaucoma.
• Evaluate eye and optic nerve.

Reference Values

Normal
• Negative for blind spots

Clinical Implications
• Abnormal findings show the blind spots that appear in glaucoma.
• Repeat testing for positive findings will show larger spots and progression of the disease.

Procedure
• The patient is seated in front of the visual-field analyzer.
• The visual-field test presents dimmer and dimmer targets of what the eyes can see until they reach the limit.
• One eye is checked at a time.
• Procedure time is about 45 minutes for each eye.

Nursing Interventions
▶*Pretest*
• Explain the purpose and procedure of the test.
• Although there may be some slight discomfort during the procedure, assure the patient that there is no pain involved.
• Explain that elevated intraocular pressure, family history, age, and ethnicity are among the risk factors for developing glaucoma.

◆ *Posttest*
• Interpret test outcomes and counsel appropriately, especially about the need for further testing and possible treatment.

Vitamin Testing

Blood, Urine, Hair, Nails

Vitamin, an organic compound necessary to sustain life, is a combination of the words "vital" and "amine" (compound with hydrogen as the key atom). Both fat-soluble and water-soluble vitamins play a variety of physiologic roles in the body. Vitamin concentrations in blood, urine, and certain body tissues can be measured and reflect the nutritional status of the patient. Vitamin deficiency can be either primary (due to a lack in dietary intake) or secondary (disorder that prevents or limits absorption). Most vitamins cannot be stored in any appreciable amounts by the body; therefore, daily ingestion of vitamins is necessary. Sources of *fat-soluble* vitamins include ingested (dietary) substances and biologic or intestinal micro-organisms. The sources of *water-soluble* vitamins are dietary (ingested) substances and intestinal micro-organisms. These tests are measurements of nutritional status. Low levels indicate recent inadequate oral intake, poor nutritional status, and/or malabsorption problems. They may not reflect tissue stores. High levels indicate excessive intake, intoxication, or absorption problems.

Reference Values

Dietary Reference Intakes (DRIs), the most recent approach adopted by the Food and Nutrition Board, Institute of Medicine, and National Academy of Sciences, provide estimates of vitamin intake. The DRIs look beyond deficiency disease and include the role of nutrients and food components in long-term health. The DRIs consist of four reference intakes: Recommended Dietary Allowances (RDAs), Tolerable Upper Intake Levels (ULs), Estimated Average Requirements (EARs), and Adequate Intake (AI). When an RDA cannot be set, an AI is given as a normal value; both are to be used as goals for the patient. Levels are given for each individual vitamin. The RDAs are the amounts of ingested vitamins needed by a healthy person to meet daily metabolic needs, allow for biologic variation, maintain normal blood serum values, prevent depletion of body stores, and preserve normal body functions.

(text continues on page 630)

Reference Values

SUBSTANCE TESTED (SPECIMEN NEEDED), REFERENCE RANGE (RR), AND CRITICAL TOXIC RANGE (CR), AND DRIs WHEN AVAILABLE	PATIENT PREPARATION, SUBSTANCE FUNCTION, AND INDICATIONS FOR TEST	CLINICAL SIGNIFICANCE OF VALUES	
		INCREASED	DECREASED
FAT-SOLUBLE VITAMINS *Vitamin A* (retinol, beta-carotene) Retinol (serum) RR: 360–1200 µg/L or 0.70–1.75 µmol/L CR: <10 µg/dL or <0.35 µmol/L indicates severe deficiency, >120 µg/dL indicates hypervitaminosis A Carotene (serum) RR: 50–250 µg/dL or 0.9–4.6 µmol/L	Fasting. No alcohol 24 hours before blood draw Prevents night blindness and other eye problems and skin disorders (acne) Enhances immunity, protects against pollution and cancer formation Needed for maintenance repair of epithelial tissues Aids fat storage Protects against colds, infections	Activation of phagocytes and/or cytotoxic T cells Alopecia Amenorrhea Arthralgia (gout) Birth defects Carotenodermia/aurantiasis Cheilosis Chronic nephritis Cortical hyperostoses Excessive dietary or supplement intake Hepatosplenomegaly	Acute infections Arthralgia (gout) Bile duct obstruction Bitot's spots Celiac disease Cirrhosis of the liver Congenital obstruction of the jejunum Cystic fibrosis Duodenal bypass Fat malabsorption syndrome Giardiasis

CR: >250 µg/dL or >4.6 µmol/L indicates carotenemia
RR: Retinyl esters <10 µg/L when selected
Relative dose response (%)
RR: >20
CR: >50 deficiency
Children show an age-related rise in serum retinol, and values lower before puberty.
Levels in adults increase slightly with age.
Premenopausal women have slightly lower values than do men. After menopause, values are similar.
DRIs:
Men: 900 µg/retinol equivalent (RE)/day

Acts as antioxidant (protects cells against cancer and other diseases)
Evaluate night blindness, malabsorption disorders, acute chronic nephritis, acute protein deficiency, Bitot's spots, intestinal parasites, acute infections, chronic intake of >10 mg retinol equivalent (RE)

Hypercholesterolemia
Hyperlipemia
Peeling of skin
Permanent learning disabilities
Pregnancy
Premature epiphyseal closure
Pseudotumor cerebri
Spontaneous abortions
Nyctalopia (night blindness)
Oral contraceptives (carotene)
Pancreatic surgery
Protein-energy malnutrition (marasmus or kwashiorkor)
Perifollicular hyperkeratosis (Darier's disease)
Sprue
Xerosis of the conjunctiva and cornea

Immunity compromised (cell-mediated response, antibody response)
Insufficient dietary intake
Keratinization of lung, gastrointestinal tract, and urinary epithelia
Keratomalacia
Measles
Xerophthalmia

(continued)

Substance Tested (Specimen Needed), Reference Range (RR), and Critical Toxic Range (CR), and DRIs When Available	Patient Preparation, Substance Function, and Indications for Test	Clinical Significance of Values	
		Increased	Decreased
Women: 700 µg/retinol equivalent (RE)/day Upper intake level: 3000 µg/day *Vitamin D* (calciferol, cholecalciferol) 1,25-dihydroxycholecalciferol, calciferol (serum) RR: 14–60 ng/mL or 35–150 nmol/L Toxic: >150 ng/mL (>374 nmol/L) Deficient: <10 ng/mL (<25 nmol/L) CR: Serum calcium levels of 12–16 mg/dL (vitamin D toxicity)	Fasting Synthesized by skin exposure to the sunlight Required for absorption of calcium and phosphorous by the intestinal tract Necessary for normal development of bones in children Protects against muscle weakness, involved in regulation of heartbeat	Gastrointestinal symptoms (anorexia, nausea, vomiting, constipation) Infants: "elfin facies," hypercalcemia with failure to thrive, mental retardation, stenosis of the aorta Metastatic extraosseous calcification Renal colic	Anticonvulsants Familial hypophosphatemic rickets (diabetes mellitus, Fanconi's syndrome, hypoparathyroidism, renal osteodystrophy, renal tubular growth acidosis) High phosphate or phytate intake Inadequate diet

DRI: Adults: Cholecalciferol 5–10 µg/day or 200–400 IU of vitamin D Aged 19–50 years: 5 µg/day or 200 IU Aged 51–70 years: 10 µg/day or 400 IU Aged >70 years: 15 µg/day or 600 IU	Important in treatment/ prevention of osteoporosis and hypocalcemia Evaluate rickets, osteomalacia, fat malabsorption; disorders of parathyroid, liver, or kidney; prolonged supplement intake of 2000 IU/day	Supplements Williams' syndrome	Inadequate exposure to sunlight (especially in the elderly) Liver disease Malabsorption syndromes Osteomalacia (adults) Osteoporosis (adults) Rachitic tetany Rickets (children) Menstrual problems
Vitamin E (tocopherols, tocotrienols) alpha-tocopherol, α-T (most active) RR (plasma): Adults: 5.5–17 mg/L or 12–39 µmol/L Significant deficiency: <3 mg/L (<7 µmol/L) Significant excess: >40 mg/L (>93 µmol/L)	Fasting No alcohol 24 hours before draw Antioxidant Important in prevention of cancer and cardiovascular diseases Promotes normal blood clotting, healing Reduces wound scarring	Low-birth-weight infants (sepsis, necrotizing enterocolitis) Vitamin E supplementation Increased bleeding tendency Impaired leukocyte formation	Infertility (men and women) Biliary atresia Carotid deposits in muscle Cholestasis Dermatitis (flaky) Edema Malabsorption syndromes with steatorrhea

(continued)

SUBSTANCE TESTED (SPECIMEN NEEDED), REFERENCE RANGE (RR), AND CRITICAL TOXIC RANGE (CR), AND DRIs WHEN AVAILABLE	PATIENT PREPARATION, SUBSTANCE FUNCTION, AND INDICATIONS FOR TEST	CLINICAL SIGNIFICANCE OF VALUES	
		INCREASED	DECREASED
Note: Concentration of vitamin E in newborns is less than half that of adults DRI: Adults: 15 mg Alpha tocopherol equivalent (α-TE) 1 α-TE = 1.49 IU	Improves circulation; necessary for tissue repair; maintains healthy nerves and muscles while strengthening capillary walls Prevents cell damage by inhibiting the oxidation of lipids and formation of free radicals (antioxidants) Aids utilization of vitamin A Retards aging and may prevent premature-birth-weight infants, abetalipoproteinemia, malabsorption	Reduced cataract formation (with high beta-carotene and ascorbic acid levels)	Neurologic syndromes affecting the spinal posterior columns and the retina (abeta- or hyperlipoproteinemia), blinding loop syndrome, chronic pancreatitis, cystic fibrosis, inborn errors of metabolism, obstructive liver disease, short bowel syndrome) Premature infants (bronchopulmonary dysplasia, intraventricular hemorrhage, platelet dysfunction, low retinopathy)

Vitamin K		
Vitamin K (phylloquinone, menaquinone) Phylloquinone (K_1) plants; menaquinone (K_2 series) bacterial; menadione (K_2) synthetic RR: 1.3–1.9 ng/mL or 0.29–2.64 nmol/L PIVKA 11 test (proteins induced in vitamin K absence). This test is superior. Plasma prothrombin concentration 10.5–12.5 seconds	Fasting Needed for the production of prothrombin (blood clotting) Essential for bone formation and repair Necessary for synthesis of osteocalcin (the protein in bone tissue on which calcium crystalizes). Therefore, prevents osteoporosis Plays role in converting glucose into glycogen for storage in liver	Glucose-6-phosphate dehydrogenase deficiency Increased dietary intake or administered vitamin K preparation Low-birth-weight infants (increased menadione) Anemia with Heinz bodies Hyperbilirubinemia Kernicterus (bilirubin encephalopathy) Loss of sucking reflex Postkernicterus syndrome	Protein-energy malnourished children Reperfusion injury Platelet hyperaggregation, decreased erythrocyte survival, and increased susceptibility to hemolysis Breast-fed infants (no vitamin K received) Conditions limiting for absorption or synthesis of vitamin K Coumadin (warfarin) Excessive oral mineral oil Hypoprothrombinemia Dietary lack Lack of bile salts (external biliary fistulas, obstructive jaundice) Liver disease

(continued)

611

SUBSTANCE TESTED (SPECIMEN NEEDED), REFERENCE RANGE (RR), AND CRITICAL TOXIC RANGE (CR), AND DRIs WHEN AVAILABLE	PATIENT PREPARATION, SUBSTANCE FUNCTION, AND INDICATIONS FOR TEST	CLINICAL SIGNIFICANCE OF VALUES	
		INCREASED	DECREASED
DRI: Men: 120 µg/day Women: 90 µg/day	Antibiotics interfere with absorption of vitamin K Evaluate renal insufficiency and chronic antibiotic treatment		Nonabsorbable sulfonamides Salicylate therapy Megadoses of fat-soluble vitamin A or E are known to antagonize vitamin K Chronic fat malabsorption, pancreatic disease, gastrointestinal disease
WATER-SOLUBLE VITAMINS *Vitamin C* (ascorbic acid) RR: 0.4–1.5 mg/dL or 28–84 µmol/L plasma; 0.6–2.0 mg/dL or 34–113 µmol/L plasma,	Antioxidant needed for tissue growth and repair, adrenal gland function, and healthy gums	Decreased anticoagulant effect of heparin and warfarin (Coumadin) Diarrhea Overabsorption of iron	Adult scurvy (acne, listlessness, deep muscle hemorrhages, swan-neck deformity, gingivitis, perifollicular hemorrhages,

Function	Supplementation/Considerations	Clinical Conditions	Laboratory Values
Aids in production of antistress hormones and interferon; needed for metabolism of folic acid, tyrosine, and phenylalanine Increases absorption of iron Essential in neurotransmitter synthesis and metabolism Essential in the formation of collagen; promotes wound healing; protects against infection Enhances immunity Evaluate scurvy, poor diet, and nephrolithiasis	Supplementation (alteration of tests for diabetes and occult blood) Nausea Some patients with history of kidney stones are at an increased risk of oxalate stones with too much vitamin C intake	hyperkeratosis, and hypochondriasis) Alcoholism and drug abuse Anemia (microcytic hypochromic) Burns Cold or heat stress Edema, lower extremities Gastric ulcers Impaired iron absorption Inadequate diet (especially elderly men) Infantile scurvy (Barlow's disease, "pithed frog" position) Inflammatory diseases, oxidative damage (proteins, DNA, human sperm DNA) Lactation Petechiae and total ecchymoses Pregnancy	114–301 nmol/10³ cells (mixed leukocytes) CR: <0.2 mg/dL or <11 µmol/L plasma ascorbate, plasma ascorbate, <57 nmol/10³ cells (mixed leukocytes), <10 mg/10³ cells (mixed leukocytes) Women consistently show higher vitamin C levels in tissues and fluids than do men. Plasma values are the best indicator of recent dietary intake. Leukocyte vitamin C levels are indicative of cellular stores and body pool. Note: Salivary vitamin C levels are not consistent; urinary vitamin C levels are not useful.

(continued)

Substance Tested (Specimen Needed), Reference Range (RR), and Critical Toxic Range (CR), and DRIs When Available	Patient Preparation, Substance Function, and Indications for Test	Clinical Significance of Values	
		Increased	Decreased
DRI: Men: 90 mg/day Women: 75 mg/day Upper intake level: 2000 mg/day			Risk of cancer (esophagus, oral cavity, uterine, cervix) Smokers (decreased ascorbic acid half-life) Thyrotoxicosis Toxicity from chemical carcinogens (anthracene, benzpyrene, organochloride pesticides, heavy metals, nitrosamines) Poor wound healing Bleeding gums, dyspnea, edema, and weakness
Vitamin B₇ (biotin) (plasma)	Biotin is produced by the gut flora		Alopecia Anorexia with nausea Antibiotics

RR: 0.82–2.87 nmol/L (200–700 pg/mL)
CR: <1.02 nmol/L deficiency (<249 pg/mL)
Prenatal diagnosis of multiple carboxylase deficiency (MCD) by direct analysis of amniotic fluid for methylcitric acid or 3-hydroxyisovaleric acid.
DRI:
Adults: 30 µg/day

Aids in cell growth, fatty acid production, metabolism of fats, carbohydrates, and proteins, and utilization of other complex vitamins
Promotes healthy sweat glands, nerve tissue, and bone marrow
Needed for healthy hair and skin
Assess for ingestion of raw eggs, inflammatory bowel disease, alcoholism, sulfonamide therapy, depression

Biotin responsive MCD syndromes
Changes in mental status (depression)
Glossitis (magenta hue)
High fetal resorption rate
Hyperesthesia (algesia)
Immunodeficiency
Increased serum, cholesterol and bile pigments
Ingestion of large amounts (>6/day) of *raw* egg white, ingestion of raw avidin
Localized paresthesia
Maculosquamous dermatitis of the extremities
Myalgia
Pallor
Long-term total parenteral nutrition after gut resection, if not supplemented
High blood sugar

(continued)

SUBSTANCE TESTED (SPECIMEN NEEDED), REFERENCE RANGE (RR), AND CRITICAL TOXIC RANGE (CR), AND DRIs WHEN AVAILABLE	PATIENT PREPARATION, SUBSTANCE FUNCTION, AND INDICATIONS FOR TEST	CLINICAL SIGNIFICANCE OF VALUES	
		INCREASED	DECREASED
Vitamin B$_{12}$ (cobalamin, cyanocobalamin, hydroxycobalamin) (serum) RR: 200–835 pg/mL (146–609 pmol/L) CR: <100 pg/mL (<73 pmol/L) deficiency DRI: Adults: 2.4 µg/day	Overnight fast. Avoid heparin, ascorbic acid, fluoride, and alcohol before testing Aids folic acid in formation of iron; prevents anemia Required for proper digestion, absorption of food, synthesis of protein, and metabolism of fats and carbohydrates Prevents nerve damage, maintains fertility, production of acetylcholine (neurotransmitter that assists memory and learning)	Improved mental function in elderly receiving B$_{12}$ supplements Toxicity to vitamin B$_{12}$ has not been reported	Deficiency caused by malabsorption—common in elderly and those with digestive disorders Alcoholism Addisonian pernicious anemia Thalassemia Diet lacking microorganisms and animal foods (sole vitamin B$_{12}$ sources) Distal sensory neuropathy ("glove and stockings") sensory loss Total gastrectomy

Found mostly in animal sources, so strict vegetarians may need supplements

Regional enteritis

Evaluate strict vegetarian diet spanning 20–30 years, alcoholism, after gastrectomy, and parasitic infections

Gastric atrophy (superficial gastritis, hereditary—degenerative congenital)

Liver disease

Pigmentation of skin creases and nail beds (brownish)

Polyendocrinopathy

Pregnancy

Renal disease

Small intestine disorders (cancer, gluten-induced enteropathy—celiac disease, granulomatous lesions, intestinal resections, "stagnant bowel" syndrome, tropical sprue)

Subacute combined degeneration of the cord

Tapeworms

Tinnitus and noise-induced hearing loss

(continued)

Substance Tested (Specimen Needed), Reference Range (RR), and Critical Toxic Range (CR), and DRIs When Available	Patient Preparation, Substance Function, and Indications for Test	Clinical Significance of Values	
		Increased	Decreased
			Tongue—red, smooth, shining, painful
			Vegans (and their breast-fed infants)
			Visual loss from optic atrophy
			Zollinger-Ellison syndrome
Folate (Folic Acid) (pteroylglutamate, pteroylglutamic acid, 5-methyltetrahydrofolate) Red blood cell folate (best indicator of status) RR: 150–800 ng/mL (0.34–182 µmol/L) whole blood, corrected to packed cell volume of 45%	Fasting Needed for energy production and formation of red blood cells Strengthens immunity by aiding white blood cell functioning Important for healthy cell division and replication (DNA and RNA synthesis)	Folacin is dominant form in serum and RBCs Loss of seizure control Acute renal failure Active liver disease Red blood cell hemolysis Supplemental folate 400 µg/24 hours or 4 mg/day	Alcohol, alcoholics Elderly Breast-fed infants of mothers taking estrogen-progesterone contraceptives Cervical dysplasia Cigarette smoking Drug therapy (phenytoin, primidone, barbiturates),

Tissue folate depletion (serum dietary fluctuations): <160 ng/mL (<360 nmol/L)

RR: 3–21 ng/mL (11–36 nmol/L)

CR: <1.5 ng/mL deficiency

Negative folate balance: <3 ng/mL (<7 nmol/L)

DRI:

Adults: 400 µg/day

Other methods (infrequently used):

Deoxyuridine suppression test (DU or dUST), a functional indicator of folate status; in vitro laboratory test that defines presence of megaloblastosis and

Protein metabolism

Prevention of folic acid anemia

In pregnancy, regulates embryonic and fetal nerve cell formation, prevents premature birth

Works best when combined with vitamins B_{12} and C

Cooking destroys folic acid

Evaluate megaloblastic anemia, cancer, inflammatory bowel disease, alcoholism, drug treatment with phenytoin, cholestyramine, sulfasalazine, oral contraceptives

Side effects will be seen at >1500 µg/24 hours or >15 mg/day

methotrexate, metformin, cholestyramine, cyclosporine, azathioprine, oral contraceptives, antacids)

Depression

Hematopoiesis (thalassemia major)

HPV-16 infection

Hyperhomocysteinemia

Inadequate dietary intake

Increased mean corpuscular volume

Increased requirements

Infancy

Lactating women

Liver disease

Malabsorption syndromes (celiac disease, sprue, blind loop syndrome)

Malignancy (lymphoproliferative)

Megaloblastosis

(continued)

Substance Tested (Specimen Needed), Reference Range (RR), and Critical Toxic Range (CR), and DRIs When Available	Patient Preparation, Substance Function, and Indications for Test	Clinical Significance of Values	
		Increased	Decreased
identifies which nutrient deficiency is responsible (folate or vitamin B$_{12}$) Formiminoglutamic acid (FIGLU)—after histidine loading			Methotrexate-treated patients Neural tube defects (spina bifida, anencephaly) Pancytopenia Pregnancy Protection from malaria Psoriasis Renal dialysis Rheumatoid arthritis Scurvy Tongue papillae atrophy (shiny, smooth) Vitamin B$_{12}$ deficiency Methotrexate-treated patients

Vitamin B₂ (riboflavin) (serum or plasma) RR: 4–24 µg/dL (106–638 nmol/L) Urine—much more sensitive to nutritional status RR: >80 µg/g creatinine (>24 µmol/mol creatinine); >15 µg/dL erythrocyte (>40 nmol/dL erythrocyte) Creatinine indicates deficiency <27 nmol/dL (erythrocyte) vitamin B₆-deficient status, <10 µg/dL (erythrocyte)-deficient status Erythrocyte glutathione reductase assay, expressed in activity coefficients (AC). Test	Fasting	Necessary for red blood cell formation, antibody production, cell respiration, and growth Alleviates eye fatigue and important in treatment and prevention of cataracts Aids metabolism of fat, carbohydrates, and protein With vitamin A, maintains mucous membranes in digestive tract Helps absorption of iron and vitamin B₆ Pure, uncomplicated riboflavin deficiency is rare—if seen, it is usually accompanied by multiple nutrient deficiencies	Alcoholism Angular stomatosis Ariboflavinosis Barbiturate use (long-term) Cheilosis Chronic diarrhea Dyssebacia (shark skin) Glossitis Inadequate consumption of milk and other animal products Irritable bowel syndrome Liver disease Normocytic anemia Nutritional amblyopia Oroaggulogenital syndrome Perleche (*Candida albicans* infection with cheilosis) Photophobia and lacrimation of eye Sore throat Tongue (magenta hue)
	None		

(continued)

Substance Tested (Specimen Needed), Reference Range (RR), and Critical Toxic Range (CR), and DRIs When Available	Patient Preparation, Substance Function, and Indications for Test	Clinical Significance of Values	
		Increased	Decreased
cannot be used in persons with glucose-6-phosphate dehydrogenase deficiency AC <1.2 acceptable; AC 1.2–1.4 low; AC <1.4 deficient. Flavin adenine dinucleotide (FAD) stimulation test RR: (stimulation): <20% DRI: Men: 1.3 mg/day Women: 1.1 mg/day *Vitamin B₂*	Needed for metabolism of amino acid tryptophan, which is converted to niacin in the body Easily destroyed by light, antibiotics, and alcohol Increased need for vitamin B₂ with the use of oral contraceptives or strenuous exercise Assess poor dietary intake, as in congenital heart disease and some cancers		Use of phenothiazine derivative
(niacin, niacinamide) Nicotinic acid, niacinamide (urinary *N*-methylnicoti-	24-hour urine collection Essential for proper circulation and healthy skin	Abnormal liver function Hypocholesterolemia Use as hypolipidemic drug	Alcoholics Carcinoid syndrome Casal's necklace

namide, NMN) 24-hour urine CR: <0.8 mg/24 hours Deficiency: <5.8 μmol/day DRI: Men: 16 mg/day Women: 14 mg/day Upper intake level: 35.0 mg/day	Aids functioning of nervous system and metabolism of carbohydrates, fats, and protein in the production of hydrochloric acid for digestion Involved in normal secretion of bile and stomach fluids and synthesis of sex hormones Lowers cholesterol Helpful in schizophrenia and other mental diseases Evaluate antituberculosis drug therapy (isoniazid), malabsorptive disorders, and alcoholism	Atrial fibrillation Cystoid maculopathy Epigastric discomfort Glucose intolerance Gout Hyperglycemia Hypotension Pruritus Smooth, swollen tongue Upper body flushing	Central nervous system dysfunction Cirrhosis of the liver Diarrheal disease Diet lacking in niacin and tryptophan Dyssebacia Encephalopathic syndrome Gastrointestinal dysfunction Hartnup's disease Isoniazid therapy Organic psychosis Pellagra dermatosa; glossitis (scarlet, raw beef)
Vitamin B_6 (pyridoxine, pyridoxamine, pyridoxal)	Fasting or urine collection Needed for production of hydrochloric acid and	Infants: neurologic symptoms and abdominal distress	Alcoholism Anemias Asthma Breast cancer

(continued)

Substance Tested (Specimen Needed), Reference Range (RR), and Critical Toxic Range (CR), and DRIs When Available	Patient Preparation, Substance Function, and Indications for Test	Clinical Significance of Values	
		Increased	Decreased
RR (direct): Plasma vitamin B_6: 5–24 ng/mL (30–143 nmol/L)	absorption of fats and protein, sodium and potassium balance, and red blood cell formation	Peripheral neuropathy; progressive sensory ataxia; lower limb impairment	Cheilosis Coronary heart disease Depression and confusion Diabetes
Plasma pyridoxal: 5-phosphate >7 ng/mL (>30 nmol/L)	Required by nervous system for normal brain function	Photosensitivity	Drugs (isoniazid, cycloserine, penicillamine, ethinyl, estradiol, mestranol)
Plasma total vitamin B_6: >10 ng/mL (>40 nmol/L)	Tryptophan metabolism Niacin formation Gluconeogenesis	Neurotoxicity	Glossitis Hodgkin's disease Impaired interleukin-2 production
Urinary 4-pyridoxic acid (4rPA): <3.0 μmol/day (useful short-term index)	Synthesis of nucleic acids, RNA and DNA; activates many enzymes and aids in absorption of vitamin B_{12} Cancer immunity, prevents arteriosclerosis		Increased metabolic activity Infants (abnormal electroencephalogram pattern, confusions)
Urinary total vitamin B_6 >0.5 μmol/day (isoniazid,	Mild diuretic—reduces premenstrual syndrome		Irritability

penicillamine, cycloserine)
RR (indirect):
Erythrocyte alanine transaminase index (EALT/EGPT): >1.25 (EALT is a better indicator than EAST; standardized approach needed to compare tests).
Erythrocyte aspartic transaminase index (EAST/EGOT): >1.80 (valid but somewhat outdated indicator of hepatic vitamin B_6 status)
2-g L-tryptophan load; urinary xanthurenic acid >65 μmol/day; 3-g L-methionine

Diuretics and cortisone drugs block absorption of vitamin B_6
Antidepressants, estrogen therapy, and oral contraceptives increase need for vitamin B_6
Evaluate groups at risk, including newborn infants with low vitamin B_6, some cancers, excess alcohol

Lymphopenia
Peripheral neuropathy
Premenstrual syndrome
Seborrheic dermatosis
Sickle cell anemia
Smokers
Stomatitis

(continued)

Substance Tested (Specimen Needed), Reference Range (RR), and Critical Toxic Range (CR), and DRIs When Available	Patient Preparation, Substance Function, and Indications for Test	Clinical Significance of Values	
		Increased	Decreased
load; urinary (24-hour urine samples, several collected over 1–3 weeks) <350 µmol/day DRI: Men: Aged 19–50 years: 1.3 mg/day Aged >50 years: 1.7 mg/day Women: Aged 19–50 years: 1.3 mg/day Aged >50 years: 1.5 mg/day			

Vitamin B$_1$ (thiamine)			
RR: 10–64 ng/mL; 0.7–1.3 IU/g Hgb; nmol (whole blood) Late changes: <50 µg/24 hours or <148 nmol/day urine with elevated blood pyruvate Red blood cell transketolase measurement (most reliable method) Enzyme assays—using thiamine pyrophosphate (TPP): 79–178 nmol/L RR (stimulation): 0%–25%; deficiency, >20% DRI: Men: 1.2 mg/day Women: 1.1 mg/day	Fasting Enhances circulation and blood formation, carbohydrate metabolism, and production of hydrochloric acid Optimizes cognitive activity and brain function Has a positive effect on energy, growth, normal appetite, and learning capacity Needed for muscle tone of intestines, stomach, and heart Acts as antioxidant, protecting body from degenerative effects of aging, alcohol consumption, and smoking	Parenteral dosages High-carbohydrate diet increases need for vitamin B$_1$ Thiamin is poorly absorbed in adults with folate or protein deficiency	Antibiotics, sulfa drugs, oral contraceptives Alcoholism Beriberi—dry beriberi (peripheral neurologic changes; ie, symmetric foot drop); infantile beriberi; wet beriberi Cardiovascular (high-output congestive heart failure, low-output Shoshin disease) Wernicke-Korsakoff syndrome (acute hemorrhagic polioencephalitis) Cerebral beriberi Dependency states (thiamine-responsive megaloblastic anemia, lactic acidosis, ketoaciduria, subacute

(continued)

Substance Tested (Specimen Needed), Reference Range (RR), and Critical Toxic Range (CR), and DRIs When Available	Patient Preparation, Substance Function, and Indications for Test	Clinical Significance of Values	
		Increased	Decreased
	Evaluate alcoholism, impaired absorption, excess intravenous glucose infusion, in diets primarily of refined, unenhanced grain products		necrotizing encephalopathy, Leigh's disease) Dextrose infusions (frequent, long-continued, or highly concentrated) Folate deficiency High-carbohydrate diet (mainly from milled [polished] rice) Hyperthyroidism Impaired absorption (ie, long-term diarrheas) Impaired utilization (ie, severe liver disease)

Inadequate calorie or protein intake
Increased requirements
(fever, lactation,
pregnancy, strenuous
physical exertion)
Poor memory
Renal dialysis
Long-term total parenteral
nutrition
Unsupplemented

Adapted from Otten, J. J., Hellwig, J. P., & Meyers, L. D. (2006). *Dietary reference intakes—The essential guide to nutrient requirements*. Washington, DC: The National Academies Press, Institute of Medicine of the National Academies.

Interfering Factors
- Factors that affect vitamin levels include age, season of the year, diarrhea or vomiting, certain drugs, various diseases, and long-term hyperalimentation.

Procedure
- Blood, urine, hair, or nail samples are examined for vitamin levels.
- The types of specimens needed are listed in the table.
- Vitamins are tested by both direct and indirect methods.

Nursing Interventions
▶*Pretest*
- Assess overall nutritional status and address potential deficiencies. Oftentimes, one deficiency is accompanied by several nutrient deficiencies.
- Evaluate signs and symptoms of disrupted vitamin-related metabolic reactions that indicate the need for testing.
- Explain the purpose of the test before collecting blood, urine, hair, or nail specimens.
- Inform the patient that vitamins are micronutrients that can be detected in the blood and urine as an indication of nutritional deficiency (hypovitaminosis) or excessive (hypervitaminosis) states. Excessive dietary intake of some vitamins can reach potentially toxic levels.

▶*Posttest*
- Counsel the patient about abnormal results, follow-up tests, dietary changes, and treatment.
- Notify patients and clinicians about abnormal outcomes when values are too high or too low.

WEST NILE VIRUS, WEST NILE FEVER, AND WEST NILE ENCEPHALITIS

Blood, CSF

This test is used to measure antibodies IgM to IgG, which are produced early in the course of West Nile virus (WNV) disease.

Reference Values

Normal
Negative for the WNV IgM antibody by ELISA.
Negative for the WNV IgG antibody by ELISA.

CLINICAL ALERT

The blood test may be negative for WNV early in the course of the infection; however, within about 8 days of the onset of symptoms, 90% of infected people will become positive for WNV. The Centers for Disease Control and Prevention may perform a plague reduction neutralization test (PRNT) on a specimen for confirmation.

Procedure
- Collect either a blood or CSF sample.
- Not all laboratories are equipped to measure the antibody, and the sample may have to be forwarded to a commercial or public health laboratory.

Interfering Factors
Exposure to the St. Louis encephalitis virus may result in a false-positive test result for WNV.

Nursing Interventions
Pretest
- Explain purpose and procedure of the test.
- Follow Chapter 1 guidelines for safe, effective, informed *pretest* care.

▶*Posttest*
- Interpret test results, and monitor and counsel patient appropriately.

 CLINICAL ALERT

Treatment is aimed at the prevention of secondary infections (e.g., pneumonia and urinary tract infection), airway management, and good nursing care.

WHITE BLOOD CELL (WBC) SCAN: INFLAMMATORY PROCESS IMAGING

Nuclear Medicine Infection Imaging

This procedure is used for the localization of acute abscess formation. The premise of the results is that any collection of labeled white blood cells found outside the liver, spleen, and functioning bone marrow indicates an abnormal white blood cell localization.

Indications

- Used in both adults and children with signs and symptoms of a septic process, fever of unknown origin, osteomyelitis, and suspected intraabdominal abscess.
- Determine cause of surgical complications, injury, and inflammation of GI tract and pelvis.

Reference Values

Normal

- Normal WBC image: Normal concentration of WBCs in radiopharmaceutical distribution outside of the reticuloendothelial system.
- Normal concentration of WBCs and radiopharmaceutical distribution in liver, spleen, and bone marrow.

Clinical Implications

- Abnormal WBCs concentrations may indicate acute abscess formation, acute osteomyelitis, infection of orthopedic prosthesis, active inflammatory bowel disease, postsurgical abscess sites, and wound infections.

Interfering Factors

- False-negative results have been reported when the chemotactic function (movement of WBCs to an area of inflammation in response to certain chemical stimuli, eg, injured tissue) of the white blood cell has been altered as in hemodialysis, hyperglycemia, hyperalimentation, steroid therapy, and long-term antibiotic therapy.
- False-positive results may occur in the presence of gastrointestinal bleeding and in upper respiratory tract infections and pneumonitis when patients swallow purulent sputum.

Procedure

- A venous blood sample of 60 mL is collected, and the white blood cells are isolated and labeled radiopharmaceutically. The labeling process takes about 2 hours to complete.
- The white blood cells are labeled with radioactive indium oxide (^{111}In) or ^{99m}Tc hexamethylphosphoramide (HMPAO) and injected intravenously.
- The patient returns for imaging at 24 or 48 hours postinjection.
- Imaging time is about 1 hour each session.

Nursing Interventions

▶Pretest

- Obtain careful history of steroid therapy and long-term antibiotic therapy and prior gallium scans.
- Explain purpose of inflammatory imaging and the procedure.

▶Intratest

- Provide support.

▶Posttest

- Evaluate patient outcome and counsel appropriately regarding further tests and possible treatment.
- Monitor intravenous sampling and intravenous injection sites for infection, hematoma, and extravasation or infiltration of the radiopharmaceutical agent.
- Observe and treat mild reactions (per orders): pruritus, rashes, and flushing 2–24 hours after injection; sometimes nausea and vomiting may occur.

> ### CLINICAL ALERT
>
> - If the patient does not have an adequate number of WBCs to label for this procedure, then donor WBCs may be used. Additional blood may need to be drawn. Gallium imaging may be indicated if unable to isolate enough WBCs.

WOUND, ABSCESS, AND TISSUE CULTURES

Special Study, Infection, Fluid, Tissue

Wound cultures are obtained to isolate pathogenic microorganisms (both aerobic and anaerobic) in patients with suspected wound infections.

Indications

- Understand that wound infection and abscess occur as complications of surgery, trauma, or disease that interrupts at skin surface.
- Identify specific microorganisms in a wound infection, especially when amount, consistency, or odor of drainage changes significantly.
- Determine appropriate antibiotic therapy for an infection or evaluate effectiveness of treatment.

- Document absence of transmissible microorganisms, especially when isolation procedures are considered.

Reference Values

Normal
Negative for pathogenic microorganisms.

Clinical Implications
- A wound infected with pathogenic microorganisms such as *Pseudomonas* spp., *Staphylococcus aureus*, *Proteus*, *Bacteroides* spp., *Klebsiella*, *Fusobacterium* spp., *Serratia*, *Enterococcus*, *Nocardia* spp., *Actinomyces* spp., *Mycobacterium*, *Escherichia coli*, *Clostridium perfringens*, *Candida*, and *Streptococci* (B hemolytic).

Interfering Factors
- Antibiotic medications (either systemically or topically) administered before taking of culture.
- Cleansing of wound or irrigation with an antiseptic solution before culture may kill the organism and produce a false-negative culture report.

Procedure
- Obtain specimens for wound culture by aspiration, tissue biopsy, and swab culture. Pus from deep wounds is associated with a foul odor, necrotic tissue, or lower extremity ulcers from diabetic patients.
- Use a culture kit containing a sterile cotton swab or a polyester-tipped swab and a tube with a culture medium.
- Prepare wound before culture:
  Use normal saline. Cleanse to risk introduction of extraneous microorganisms into specimen—if you culture only the *external exudate*, you may miss the real cause of the infection. If *moderate- to-heavy* drainage, irrigate with normal saline until all visible debris has been washed away—use a sterile gauze to absorb excess normal saline and expose culture site. Culture highly vascular areas of granulation tissue.
  In *chronic wounds* such as decubitus ulcers, debridement may be necessary—debride loose necrotic tissue and culture clean area of granulation tissue. *If a wound has been treated with a topical antibiotic or antiseptic*, clean thoroughly to remove the residual prior to culture.

Incision wounds may require removing of a few staples or sutures to gain access to wound infection (or use needed biopsy procedures). Immediately place the swab into the appropriate transport container.

- Tissue samples for culture should be promptly delivered to the laboratory in sterile gauze or in a sterile container. Aspirations of fluid or pus collected in a syringe should have the syringe needle removed and a sterile syringe cap replaced at the end of the syringe.

Nursing Interventions

▶*Pretest*
- Explain test purpose and procedure for obtaining the culture specimen.
- Hold antibiotics or sulfonamides until after specimen has been collected.

▶*Intratest*
- Use standard universal precautions and sterile aseptic techniques.
- Label specimen with patient's name, date and time collected, anatomic site or specific source of specimen (chest incision wound), type of specimen (abscess fluid, postsurgical wound tissue), exam requested, patient's diagnosis, any topical or systemic medication currently administered, and isolation status.
- Place specimen in a biohazard bag. Transport the specimen to the laboratory immediately after testing (within 30 minutes).

▶*Posttest*
- Reapply sterile dressing to wound if required before wound culture.
- Notify the clinician or physician of any positive results so that appropriate antibiotic therapy can be initiated.

Standard Precautions

The term "standard precautions" refers to a system designed to reduce the risk of transmission of micro-organisms from both recognized and unrecognized sources of infections. Standard precautions direct safe practice and are designed to protect health care workers, patients, and others from exposure to blood-borne pathogens or other potentially infectious materials from any body fluid or unfixed human tissue from any person, living or dead.

Revised guidelines based upon new information about infectious disease patterns and modes of transmission are designed to be more user-friendly and contain two tiers of precautions. Tier 1, standard precautions, is designed to control nosocomial infections and reduce the risk of transmission of both known and suspected infections. Tier 2, or transmission-based, is used in addition to standard precautions, includes airborne, droplet, and contact, precautions, and airborne/contact to prevent the spread of known virulent pathogens.

Safe Practice

When handling specimens and performing or assisting with diagnostic procedures, it is important for all health care workers to protect and always take care of themselves first. Presume that all patients have hepatitis B virus (HBV), human immunodeficiency virus (HIV), hepatitis C virus (HCV), or other potential pathogens and practice standard precautions consistently. Use special care when collecting, handling, packaging, transporting, storing, and receiving specimens. Initial laboratory observations and specimen handling are to be performed under a laminar flow hood while wearing protective clothing, which includes, but is not limited to, gloves, gowns, face masks or shields, and eye protection. These same precautions prevail in the performance of invasive diagnostic procedures.

COMMON CATEGORIES OF BODY SUBSTANCES AND FLUIDS[*] (REGARDLESS OF WHETHER THEY CONTAIN VISIBLE BLOOD)

Blood and blood products	Respiratory secretions[**]
Urine[**]	Semen
Vaginal secretions	Synovial fluid
Saliva	Vomitus[**]

Pericardial fluid

Peritoneal fluid

Pleural fluid

Cerebrospinal fluid

Gastric fluid

Wound or ulcer drainage

Ascites

Amniotic fluid

Sweat[**]

[*]Standard precautions should also be taken when handling amputated limbs and during removal of body parts (during surgery, autopsy, or donation).

[**]Unless they contain visible blood.

🖋 Standard Precaution Guidelines and Practices

Personal Protection Equipment

- Take appropriate barrier precautions when exposure to skin and mucous membranes, blood, blood droplets, or other body fluids is anticipated.
- Use protective equipment devices to protect eyes, face, head, extremities, air passages, and clothing. This equipment must always be used during invasive procedures. Ensure proper fit.

Gloves

- Wear gloves when collecting and handling specimens; touching blood, urine, other body fluids, mucous membranes, or nonintact skin; or performing vascular access procedures or other invasive procedures.
- Wear gloves when handling items or surfaces soiled with blood, urine, or body fluids.
- Mandate the wearing of gloves when the health care worker's skin is cut, abraded, or chapped; during examination of a patient's oropharynx, gastrointestinal, or genitourinary tract, nonintact or abraded skin, or active bleeding wounds; and when cleaning specimen containers or engaged in decontamination procedures.

Possible exceptions to use of gloves include the following:

- When gloves impede palpation of veins for venipuncture (eg, neonates, morbidly obese patients).
- In a life-threatening situation in which delay could be fatal (wash hands and wear gloves as soon as possible).

Disposable gloves must be changed in the following situations:

- When moving between patients.
- When moving from a contaminated site to a cleaner site on a patient or on an environmental surface.

- When gloves are torn or punctured or their barrier function is compromised (do so as soon as feasible).

CLINICAL ALERT

Gloves, barrier gowns, aprons, and masks are worn only at the site of use. They are then disposed of appropriately at the site of use.

Gowns, Masks, and Eye Protection

- It is necessary to wear gowns, aprons, and/or fluid-impervious lab coats to cover all exposed skin whenever there is a potential for splashing onto clothing.
- Do not hang and reuse gowns or aprons.
- Wear masks correctly situated over the nose and chin and tied at the crown of the head and the nape of the neck. Do not hang the mask around the neck. Change the mask when it becomes moist.
- Wear a mask, a face shield, and goggles (or prescription glasses with side shields) when contamination of eyes, nose, or mouth from fluid is most likely to occur.
- Wear shoe covers in areas where contamination might occur (eg, operating room, obstetrics, or emergency department). These are disposed of at the site of care.
- Provide masks, Ambu bags, or other ventilation devices as part of emergency resuscitation equipment kept in strategic locations.

Disposal of Medical Wastes

- Pour fluids "low and slow" to prevent splash, spray, or aerosol effect.
- Take precautions to prevent injuries caused by needles, lancets, scalpels, and other sharp instruments and devices during and after procedures and when disposing of used needles. Do not recap needles under normal circumstances.
- Dispose of all disposable sharp instruments in specially designed, puncture-resistant containers. Do not recap, bend, break by hand, or remove needles from disposable syringes. Use forceps or cut intravenous tubing if necessary. Use care when transferring "sharps" to another person. Use forceps or put the "sharp" in a receptacle.
- Place and transport specimens in leakproof receptacles with solid, tight-fitting covers. Cap ports of containers. Before transport, specimens must be placed in a tightly sealed bag marked with a "biohazard" tag. Biohazard symbols warn of biologic hazards and must be displayed in the presence of these hazardous biologic agents or locations.

- Soiled linens and similar items must be placed in leakproof bags before transport.

Placement of Warning Tags and Signs

- Properly place warning tags to prevent accidental injury or illness to clinicians who are exposed to equipment or procedures that are hazardous, unexpected, or unusual.
- Require warning tags to contain a signal word or symbol, such as "Biohazard" or "Biochemical Material," along with the major message, such as "Blood Banking Specimen Inside." All specimens must be placed in biohazard bags.

General Environmental Cautions

- Use approved antimicrobial soaps between care activities of individual patients.
- Wash hands immediately after removing gloves.
- Wash hands and other skin surfaces immediately and thoroughly if contaminated with blood or other body fluids.
- Consider saliva, when blood is visible, to be potentially infectious, even though it has not been implicated in HIV transmission.
- Transmission of HIV/acquired immunodeficiency syndrome (AIDS) is possible from stool specimens, especially if there is a possibility of blood existing in the stool.
- Health care workers with open skin lesions or skin conditions should not engage in direct care until the condition clears up or does not present a risk to the patient.
- Development of an HIV infection during pregnancy may put the fetus at risk for infection.

In Case of Exposure to Human Immunodeficiency Virus or Hepatitis B Virus

- Identify, obtain consent, and test the source of exposure immediately for evidence of HIV, HBV, and HCV. If the patient refuses consent, a nonconsenting form must be signed. If nonconsenting testing is done on the source, the exposed staff member must also have testing.
- Advise the HIV-negative worker to seek medical evaluation postexposure. The worker may be offered postexposure prophylaxis. The health care worker should be retested for HIV at 6 weeks and 6 months after exposure.
- Note that a vaccine is available at no cost to health care workers to prevent hepatitis B infection. There is no vaccine for HIV/AIDS or hepatitis C.

Hand-washing Protocols

Unless the situation is a true emergency, hands must always be washed during the following circumstances:

- Before and after care activities that involve direct contact.
- Before and after removal of gloves in surgical or obstetric procedures.
- Before and after endoscopy.
- Before and after invasive procedures.
- Before and after direct contact with a patient.
- After contact with body fluids or tissues or with soiled equipment, supplies, or surfaces.
- After direct contact with patients in isolation units.

Bibliography

Centers for Disease Control and Prevention. (2001). Updated U.S. Public Health Service guidelines for the management of occupational exposures to HBV, HCV, and HIV and recommendations for postexposure prophylaxis. *Morbidity and Mortality Weekly Report, 50*(RR-11), 1–42.

Centers for Disease Control and Prevention. (2002). Guideline for hand hygiene in healthcare settings: Recommendations of the Healthcare Infection Control Practices Advisory Committee. *Morbidity and Mortality Weekly Report, 51*(RR-16), 1–44.

Centers for Disease Control and Prevention. (2003). Guidelines for environmental infection control in health-care facilities: Recommendations of CDC and the Healthcare Infection Control Advisory Committee. *Morbidity and Mortality Weekly Report, 52*(RR-10), 1–42.

Centers for Disease Control and Prevention. (2005). Updated U.S. Public Health Service guidelines for the management of occupational exposures to HIV and recommendations for postexposure prophylaxis. *Morbidity and Mortality Weekly Report, 54*(RR-09), 1–17.

Centers for Disease Control and Prevention. (2007). *Guideline for isolation precautions: Preventing transmission of infectious agents in healthcare settings.* (Online.) Available: www.cdc.gov/ncidod/dhqp/pdf/isolation2007.pdf.

Code of Federal Regulations. (Effective date: January 18, 2001). Needlestick Safety and Prevention Act. *Federal Register.*

Code of Federal Regulations. (Revised January 1, 2007). Occupational exposure to bloodborne pathogens. *Federal Register.* 29CFR 1910.1030.

References

American Association of Tissue Banks, Association of Organ Procurement Organizations, and Eye Bank Association of America. (2000, Nov. 30). *Model elements of informed consent for organ and tissue donation* (Joint Statement).

American Society of Anesthesiologists. (2002). Practice guidelines for sedation and analgesia by nonanesthesiologists. *Anesthesiology, 96*, 1004–1017.

Bakerman, P., & Strausbalch, P. (2002). *Bakerman's ABCs of interpretive laboratory data*. Scottsdale, AZ: Interpretive Laboratory Data Inc.

Burtis, C. A., & Ashwood, E. R. (2000). *Tietz fundamentals of clinical chemistry* (5th ed.). Philadelphia: WB Saunders.

Carpenito-Moyet, L. J. (2005). *Nursing care plans and documentation: Nursing diagnosis and collaborative problems* (5th ed.). Philadelphia: Lippincott Williams & Wilkins.

Carpenito-Moyet, L. J. (2007). *Handbook of nursing diagnosis* (12th ed.). Philadelphia: Lippincott Williams & Wilkins.

Carpenito-Moyet, L. J. (2009). *Nursing diagnosis: Application to clinical practice* (13th ed.). Philadelphia: Lippincott Williams & Wilkins.

Centers for Disease Control and Prevention. (1991). Two-step tuberculin skin test. In *Core curriculum on tuberculosis*. Atlanta, GA: Author.

Connolly, M. A. (1999). Postdural puncture headache. *American Journal of Nursing, 99*(11), 48–49.

Dasgupta, A. (2009). *Critical issues in alcohol and drugs of abuse testing*. Washington, DC: AACC Press.

Drug Facts and Comparisons 2009 Edition (63rd ed.). (2008). St. Louis, MO: Facts and Comparisons, A Wolters Kluwer Co.

Dufour, D. R. (1998). *Clinical use of laboratory data: A practical guide*. Philadelphia: Lippincott Williams & Wilkins.

Dufour, D. R., Lott, J. A., Noethe, F. S., et al. (2000). National Academy of Clinical Biochemistry. Diagnosis and monitoring of hepatic injury. II. Recommendations for use of laboratory tests in screening, diagnosis, and monitoring. *Clinical Chemistry, 46*(12), 2050–2068.

Fauci, A. S., Braunwald, E., Kasper, D. L., et al. (2009). *Harrison's manual of medicine* (17th ed.). Washington, DC: AACC Press.

Fischbach, F. T., & Dunning III, M. B. (2009). *A manual of laboratory and diagnostic tests* (8th ed.). Philadelphia: Lippincott Williams & Wilkins.

Hammer, S. M., Eron, J. J., Jr, Reiss, P., et al. (2008). Antiretroviral treatment of adult HIV infection. 2008 Recommendations of the International AIDS Society—USA Panel. *JAMA, 300*(5), 555–570.

Hammett-Stabler, C. A., & Dasgupta, A. (2007). *Therapeutic drug monitoring data: A concise guide* (3rd ed.). Washington, DC: AACC Press.

Hennessey, I., & Japp, A. (2008). *Arterial blood gases made easy*. Philadelphia: Elsevier Mosby Saunders.

Horne, C. (1999). Mastering ABGs. *American Journal of Nursing, 99*(8), 26–32.

Jacobs, D. S. (Ed.). (2001). *Laboratory test handbook.* Cleveland, OH: Lexi-Comp Inc.

Johnson, M., Mass, M., & Moorehead, S. (2000). *Nursing outcomes classification (NOC)* (2nd ed.). St. Louis, MO: Mosby.

Jones, S. L. (2001). *Clinical laboratory pearls.* Philadelphia: Lippincott Williams & Wilkins.

Kahan, S., Miller, R., & Smith, E. G. (2008). *In a page signs & symptoms* (2nd ed.). Philadelphia: Lippincott Williams & Wilkins.

Kost, G. J. (2002). *Principles and practice of point-of-care testing.* Washington, DC: AACC Press.

Kost, M. (2004). Moderate sedation/analgesia (2nd ed.). Philadelphia: Elsevier Mosby Saunders.

Krisman-Scott, M. A. (2000). An historical analysis of disclosure of terminal status. *Journal of Nursing Scholarship, 32*(1), 47–52.

Leavelle, D. E. (2001). *Mayo Medical Laboratories interpretive handbook.* Rochester, MN: Mayo Medical Laboratories.

Marques, M. B., & Fritsma, G. A. (2009). *Quick guide to coagulation testing* (2nd ed.). Washington, DC: AACC Press.

Marriott, E. (2002). *Plague.* New York: Metropolitan Books.

McCall, R. E. (2008). *Phlebotomy essentials* (4th ed.). Washington, DC: AACC Press.

McCormick, M. E. (1999). Endoscopic retrograde cholangiopancreatography. *American Journal of Nursing, 99*(2), 24HH–26HH.

McPherson, R. A., & Pincus, M. R. (2006). *Henry's clinical diagnosis and management by laboratory methods* (21st ed.). Philadelphia: Elsevier Mosby Saunders.

Meyers, T. A., Eichhorn, D. J., Guzzetta, C. E., et al. (2000). Family presence during invasive procedures and resuscitation. *American Journal of Nursing, 100*(2), 32–39.

Murray, R., Zineh, I., Becker, R. L., Root, C., & Valdes, R. (2009). *Personalized medicine and the clinical laboratory—what the future holds.* Washington, DC: AACC Press.

Myers, G. L., Christenson, R. H. M., Cushman, M., et al. (2009). National Academy of Clinical Biochemistry Laboratory medicine practice guidelines: Emerging biomarkers for primary prevention of cardiovascular disease. *Clinical Chemistry, 55*(2), 378–384.

Narayanan, S., & Young, D. S. (2007). *Effects of herbs and natural products on clinical laboratory tests.* Washington, DC: AACC Press.

Nettina, S. M. (2009). *Lippincott manual of nursing practice* (9th ed.). Philadelphia: Lippincott Williams & Wilkins.

Nursing 2010 Drug Handbook (30th ed.). (2009). Philadelphia: Lippincott Williams & Wilkins.

O'Neil, M. J. (2006). *The Merck Index: An encyclopedia of chemicals, drugs, and biologicals* (14th ed.). Washington, DC: AACC Press.

Poon, E. G., & Gandhi, T. K. (2004). I wish I had seen this test result earlier! *Archives of Internal Medicine, 164*, 2223–2228.

Reddy, V., Marques, M. B., & Fristma, G. A. (2007). *Quick guide to hematology testing*. Washington, DC: AACC Press.

Ruppel, G. L. (2003). *Manual of pulmonary function testing* (8th ed.). St. Louis, MO: Mosby.

Sainato, D. (2000). A cavalcade of cytokines—Will these versatile immunoregulators become standard diagnostic tools? *Clinical Laboratory News, 26*(11), 1, 6–7.

Salimbeno, S. (2000). *What language does your patient hurt in? A practice guide to culturally competent care*. Amherst, MA: Diversity Resources.

Sandler, M. P., Coleman R. E., & Patton, J. A. (2003). *Diagnostic nuclear medicine* (4th ed.). Philadelphia: Lippincott Williams & Wilkins.

Sherman, R. A., & Shimoda, K. J. (2001). Tuberculosis tracking: Determining the frequency of the booster effect in patients and staff. *American Journal of Infection Control, 29*, 7–12.

Soldin, S. J., Brugnara, C., & Wong, E. C. (2007). *Pediatric reference values* (6th ed.). Washington, DC: AACC Press.

Sturgeon, C. M., Hoffman, B. R., Chan, D. W., et al. (2008). National Academy of Clinical Biochemistry Laboratory medicine practice guidelines for use of tumor markers in clinical practice: quality requirements. *Clinical Chemistry, 54*(8), e1–e10.

Toffaletti, J. G. (2009). *Blood gases and electrolytes* (2nd ed.). Washington, DC: AACC Press.

Torres, L. S., Dulton, A. G., & Watson, T. A. (2009). *Patient care imaging technology* (7th ed.). Philadelphia: Lippincott Williams & Wilkins.

Turgeon, M. L. (2004). *Clinical hematology therapy and procedures* (4th ed.). Philadelphia: Lippincott Williams & Wilkins.

U.S. Preventive Services Task Force. (2008). Screening for prostate cancer: Recommendation statement. *Annals of Internal Medicine, 149*, 185–191.

U.S. Public Health Service, Centers for Disease Control and Prevention. (2004). *Shipping instructions for specimens collected from people potentially exposed to chemical terrorism agents*. (Online.) Available: http://www.bt.cdc.gov.

Van Kuilenburg, A. B. P., van Lenthe, H., Loffler, M., et al. (2004). Analysis of pyrimidine synthesis "de novo" intermediates in urine and dried urine filter paper strips with HPLC-electrospray tandem mass spectrometry. *Clinical Chemistry, 50*(11), 2117–2124.

Wallach, J. (2006). *Interpretation of diagnostic tests*. (8th ed.). Philadelphia: Lippincott Williams & Wilkins.

Ward-Cook, K. M., Lehmann, C. A., Schoeff, L. E., & Williams, R. H. (2006). *Clinical diagnostic technology, the total testing process: Vol. 3. The post-analytical phase*. Washington, DC: AACC Press.

Weiner, Z., Goldstein, I., Bombard, A., Applewhite, L., & Itzkovits-Eldor, J. (2007). Screening for structural fetal anomalies during nuchal translucency ultrasound examination. *American Journal of Obstetrics & Gynecology, 197*, 181.e1–181.e5.

Westman, J. A. (2005). *Medical genetics for the modern clinician*. Philadelphia: Lippincott Williams & Wilkins.

Wilde, K. D. (2004). Foodborne diseases: An update, Part 1. *BD Lab•O: Microbiology News & Ideas, 15*(3). (Online.) Available: www.bd.com/Clinical/labo/LabOv15n3.pdf.

Willig, J. L. (2004). Care over contamination. Nurses can take precautions to be ready for radiological terrorism. *Advance for Nurses, 6*(4). (Online.) Available: http://nursing.advanceweb.com.

Winter, W. E., Sokoll, L. J., & Jialal, I. (2008). *Handbook of diagnostic endocrinology* (2nd ed.). Washington, DC: AACC Press.

Wong, S. H. Y., Linder, M. W., & Valdes, R. (2006). *Pharmacogenomics and proteomics: enabling the practice of personalized medicine*. Washington, DC: AACC Press.

Yamada T., Hasler, W. L., Inadomi, J. M., Anderson, M. A., & Brown, R. S., Jr. (2005). *Handbook of gastroenterology* (2nd ed.). Philadelphia: Lippincott Williams & Wilkins.

Young, D. S. (2001). *Effects of drugs and clinical laboratory tests* (5th ed.). Washington, DC: AACC Press.

Young, D. S. (2007). *Effects of preanalytical variables on clinical laboratory tests* (3rd ed.). Washington, DC: AACC Press.

Young, D. S., & Friedman, R. B. (2007). *Effects of disease on clinical laboratory tests* (4th ed.). Washington, DC: AACC Press.

Young, D. S., & Huth, E. J. (1998). *SI units for clinical measurement*. Philadelphia: American College of Physicians.

Web Sites

Breast Cancer:

www.komen.org

Centers for Disease Control and Prevention:

http://www.cdc.gov/page.do/id/0900f3ec80112422

Eye Diseases:

www.bausch.com

National Cancer Institute: Breast cancer risk assessment tool, a Web tool to project risk for invasive breast cancer to age 90.

www.cancer.gov

Telephone Numbers

Breast Cancer:
Susan G. Komen Breast Cancer Foundation: 1.800 I'M AWARE
Cancer:
Cancer Information Service (CIS): 1.800.4.CANCER
Medical Product Reporting Programs:
FDA Medical Product Reporting Programs: Mandatory medical device reporting: Required from user facilities regarding device-related deaths and serious injuries: 1-301-427-7500.
FDA Medical Product Reporting Programs: MedWatch Adverse Event and Product Reporting Line: Designed for health care professionals to voluntarily report adverse effects from drugs and medical devices. The MedWatch form and desk guide are provided by fax or mail. Health care professionals reporting adverse events or product problem by phone should call 1-800-332-1088.

Index

Note: Italicized *d*, *f* and *t* refer to displays, figures and tables